MOTIVATIONAL INTERVIEWING

Motivational Interviewing

SECOND EDITION

Preparing People for Change

WILLIAM R. MILLER
STEPHEN ROLLNICK

THE GUILFORD PRESS
New York   London

© 2002 The Guilford Press
A Division of Guilford Publications, Inc.
72 Spring Street, New York, NY 10012
www.guilford.com

Printed in the United States of America

This book is printed on acid-free paper.

Last digit is print number: 9 8 7 6 5 4

Library of Congress Cataloging-in-Publication Data

Miller, William R.
  Motivational interviewing : preparing people for change /
by William R. Miller, Stephen Rollnick.-2nd ed.
    p.   cm.
  Includes bibliographical references and index.
  ISBN 1-57230-563-0 (hardcover)
    1. Compulsive behavior-Treatment. 2. Substance abuse-
Treatment. 3. Substance abuse-Patients-Counseling of.
4. Compulsive behavior-Patients-Counseling of. 5. Motivation
(Psychology) 6. Interviewing in psychiatry I. Rollnick, Stephen, 1952– .

  RC533 .M56 2002
  618.85′84-dc21   2001051250

To our parents,
Hazel and Ralph Miller
and
Sonia and Julian Rollnick

May we succeed in passing on
such love to the next generation

About the Authors

William R. Miller, PhD, is Distinguished Professor of Psychology and Psychiatry at the University of New Mexico and Codirector of UNM's Center on Alcoholism, Substance Abuse, and Addictions. Dr. Miller's publications encompass more than 300 articles and chapters, as well as 27 books, including, most recently, *Quantum Change: When Epiphanies and Sudden Insights Transform Ordinary Lives* (with Janet C'de Baca; Guilford Press, 2001). He maintains an active interest in pastoral counseling and the integration of spirituality and psychology. Dr. Miller is supported by a 15-year senior career Research Scientist Award from the National Institute on Alcohol Abuse and Alcoholism, which allows him to focus full time on clinical research.

Stephen Rollnick, PhD, is on the faculty in the Department of General Practice at the University of Wales College of Medicine. He has also worked for many years as a clinical psychologist in the British National Health Service. With a background in the addiction field, his interest turned to consultations about behavior change in wider health care practice, where practitioners try to encourage patients to change their lifestyle and use of medication. Dr. Rollnick's research and teaching activity is now focused on the behavior of practitioners and other topics. He has trained practitioners in many countries and continents, and has published a wide range of research papers and articles. His most recent book is *Health Behaviour Change: A Guide for Practitioners* (with Pip Mason and Christopher C. Butler; Churchill Livingstone, 1999).

Contributing Authors

Jeff Allison, MA, CertEd, was a specialist social worker and service manager in the U.K. addictions field. He is a member of the Motivational Interviewing Network of Trainers. Mr. Allison now runs an international training consultancy providing short courses and practice supervision in motivational interviewing and health behavior change techniques for a wide range of organizations and professional groups. His special interests include applications within the criminal justice and smoking cessation fields.

Hal Arkowitz, PhD, received his doctorate from the University of Pennsylvania. After a predoctoral internship in clinical psychology at the University of California at San Francisco Medical Center, he was a postdoctoral fellow at the State University of New York at Stony Brook. Following this, Dr. Arkowitz was an Assistant Professor of Psychology at the University of Oregon, and is presently Associate Professor of Psychology at the University of Arizona.

John S. Baer, PhD, is Research Associate Professor in the Department of Psychology at the University of Washington in Seattle. He is also the Director of the Interdisciplinary Fellowship in Substance Abuse Treatment at the VA Puget Sound Health Care Center, also in Seattle. Dr. Baer's research interests and activities focus on the etiology, prevention, and treatment of addictive behaviors. He has studied smoking cessation and relapse, developed and tested brief interventions for heavy drinking in both adolescents and young adults, and participated in multisite trials of pharmacotherapy and behavioral treatments of alcohol dependence.

Stephanie Ballasiotes, MC, a Health Behavior Consultant for the Fred Hutchinson Cancer Research Center in Seattle, Washington, provides training and consultation on motivational strategies for the Women's Health Initiative, a nationally funded disease prevention study with 60,000 participants in the United States. Ms. Ballasiotes previously trained health care and addictions treatment personnel in motivational and educational methods in working with HIV/AIDS/HCV issues, as well as authored numerous publications for use in the Seattle community. She also helped establish one of the first harm reduction community treatment programs for methamphetamine users in the Seattle area and provides community-based motivational interviewing training.

Tom Barth, PhD, is a clinical psychologist in Norway. Since 1980, he has worked in the Bergen Clinics Foundation in outpatient and inpatient settings with a variety of addictive behaviors. Currently, he is head of an outpatient clinic for addictions. Dr. Barth's clinical work has been based on motivational interviewing since 1983, with individual patients, with groups, and as a consultant to community-based treatment and prevention projects. He is also coauthor of a textbook on the Norwegian version of motivational interviewing.

Belinda Borrelli, PhD, is an Assistant Professor of Psychiatry and Human Behavior in the Center for Behavioral and Preventive Medicine at Brown Medical School. She currently has two federally funded grants (National Cancer Institute and National Heart, Lung, and Blood Institute) involving training home health care nurses to deliver a motivational interviewing-based smoking cessation treatment versus standard care; one trial targets home-bound medically ill smokers; the other focuses on promoting smoking cessation in parents of children receiving home care for asthma. Dr. Borrelli has trained nurses, psychology students, medical students, and psychiatric residents in motivational interviewing.

Brian L. Burke, MA, is currently completing his doctoral studies in clinical psychology at the University of Arizona. His research interests include a meta-analysis of motivational interviewing studies as well as a pilot study adapting motivational interviewing for the treatment of clinical depression.

Christopher C. Butler, MD, graduated in medicine from the University of Cape Town, South Africa, and after various hospital posts in urban and rural South Africa, completed residency training in general practice in the United Kingdom. After nearly 10 years in the Department of General Practice at the University of Wales College of Medicine, he joined the faculty at McMaster University, Canada, in 2001. Dr. Butler was awarded a doctorate for work on health behavior change in 1999 and is the coauthor of a book on consulting around health behavior change (with Stephen Rollnick and Pip Mason). In 2001, he was a visiting professor in Japan to advise on research into health behavior change. He has also published 35 peer-reviewed papers, helped win 12 research grants, and is a family physician in private practice.

Kelly Conforti, PhD, received her doctorate in clinical psychology from the University of Missouri-Columbia. She is the Psychologist-Manager of Psychotherapy Services and the Intensive Outpatient and Partial Hospital Programs at the University of New Mexico Health Sciences Center Mental Health Center. Dr. Conforti's clinical interests include combining cognitive-behavioral coping skills therapies and motivational interviewing in the treatment of individuals with dual disorders, while her research interests lie in the use of psychophysiological outcome measures.

Carlo C. DiClemente, PhD, is Professor and Chair of the Department of Psychology at the University of Maryland, Baltimore County. He is the codeveloper of the transtheoretical model of behavior change with James Prochaska. Dr. DiClemente is the author of numerous scientific articles and book chapters on motivation and behavior change and the application of this model to a variety of problem behaviors. He is coauthor of a self-help book based on this model of change, *Changing for Good,* as well as several professional books. For the past 20 years he has conducted funded research in health and addictive behaviors and is a member of the Project MATCH and COMBINE research groups. He also serves as a consultant to private and public treatment programs.

Colleen DiIorio, PhD, RN, FAAN, is a Professor in the Department of Behavioral Sciences and Health Education of the Rollins School of Public Health at Emory

University. She holds a secondary faculty appointment at the Nell Hodgson Woodruff School of Nursing, also at Emory University. Dr. DiIorio is a nurse by training and has extensive experience in health promotion and disease prevention, including HIV/AIDS prevention research. She has served on national review panels and advisory boards, is a fellow of the American Academy of Nursing, and has received awards for her research, teaching, and service to the community. She has numerous publications describing her work and presents frequently at national and international conferences.

Christopher Dunn, PhD, is a psychologist on the Psychiatry and Behavioral Sciences faculty at the University of Washington in Seattle. He specializes in brief interventions for substance abuse and other lifestyle changes among patients with a chronic medical disease. Dr. Dunn's research focuses on brief intervention outcomes among substance abusers and the training of primary care residents to perform brief behavioral change counseling.

Denise Ernst, MA, is a Senior Research Associate at the Kaiser Permanente Center for Health Research in Portland, Oregon. Her research interests include the application of motivational interviewing to health behaviors in medical and community settings.

Joel I. D. Ginsburg, PhD, received his doctorate in experimental psychology from Carleton University in Ottawa, Ontario, Canada. He is a National Trainer and Quality Control Coordinator for the Correctional Service of Canada's Substance Abuse Programs, and a member of the Motivational Interviewing Network of Trainers. Dr. Ginsburg's interests include motivational interviewing practice, research, and training in the criminal justice system.

Nancy Handmaker, PhD, is a Research Assistant Professor in the Department of Psychology at the University of New Mexico. She is experienced in the training and practice of motivational interviewing applications for health care settings and in substance abuse treatment facilities. Currently, Dr. Handmaker is engaged in the study of the effects of motivational interviewing on drinking during pregnancy toward the prevention of fetal alcohol syndrome and other alcohol-related neurodevelopmental disorders.

Jacki Hecht, RN, MSN, is a Motivational Intervention Coordinator at the Centers for Behavioral and Preventive Medicine, Brown Medical School and The Miriam Hospital. She currently works on numerous federally funded studies where she provides training and supervision in delivering motivational interventions and consultation on intervention design. Ms. Hecht recently copresented at the Introduction to Motivational Interviewing workshop at the Society for Behavioral Medicine meeting in 2001.

Alexander Kantchelov, MD, is a Senior Trainer and Managing Founder of the South-east European Institute for Motivational Interventions and Behavior Change, Deputy Director of the National Centre for Addictions at the Ministry of Health in Bulgaria, and Chair of the Expert Council of the National Drugs Council, Bulgarian Council of Ministers. Dr. Kantchelov is a member of the Society for Psychotherapy Research-European Continental Chapter, the Motivational Interviewing Network of Trainers, the Bulgarian Psychiatric Association, the Bulgarian Association of Cognitive and Behavioral Psychotherapies, and the Bulgarian Physicians' Union. He has written more than 40 publications and presentations for Bulgarian and international congresses, conferences, and magazines focusing on drug- and alcohol-related issues and implications of psychotherapy and treatment modalities in the addictions field.

Ruth E. Mann, MSc, is Head of Sexual Offender and Domestic Violence Treatment Programs in Her Majesty's Prison Service, in England and Wales. She oversees five programs for sexual offenders, running in approximately 30 prisons and treating over 1,000 sexual offenders per annum. Ms. Mann is currently studying part time for a doctorate, investigating schemas related to sexual offending. She has published a number of clinical and research articles and book chapters on the topics of relapse prevention, motivational interviewing, and sexual offender treatment in general.

John E. Martin, PhD, is Professor of Psychology at San Diego State University and a faculty member of the SDSU/UCSD Joint Doctoral Program in Clinical Psychology since 1986. He has conducted motivational interviewing training since 1996 with his doctoral psychology students, as well as for therapists, social workers, nurses, community action workers, addictions counselors, and probation officers in both California and South Africa. Dr. Martin's research and publications have focused on the behavioral and health aspects of smoking treatment in recovering alcoholics, diet, exercise, medical compliance, high-risk drinking and drug use in college students, and spiritual and behavioral approaches to change.

Richard Ogle, PhD, received his doctorate in clinical psychology from the University of New Mexico. He is currently a postdoctoral psychology fellow at the Center for Excellence in Substance Abuse Treatment and Education at the VA Puget Sound Health Care Center, Seattle Division. Dr. Ogle is a motivational interviewing trainer and his research interests include the role of alcohol in aggression and substance abuse treatment outcome research.

Michele Packard, PhD, is the Executive Director of Sage Institute, in Boulder, Colorado, specializing in training of mental health and substance abuse professionals. In 1997 she was the recipient of the Best Practices Award from the Managed Care Behavioral Health Interest Group, and in 1993 she was voted best trainer by Colorado substance abuse program directors. Dr. Packard's current areas of interest include curriculum development that integrates the use of motivational interviewing in the treatment of serious and persistent mental illness and treatment of co-occurring Axis I and Axis II disorders as well as treatment of affective and anxiety disorders. She has also developed manualized protocols for criminal justice and substance abuse treatment programs.

Peggy L. Peterson, PhD, MPH, is a Research Scientist at the Alcohol and Drug Abuse Institute at the University of Washington in Seattle. She has published in the areas of drug prevention and HIV risk reduction. Dr. Peterson's current research concerns testing a brief motivational interviewing intervention to reduce alcohol and drug risk among homeless adolescents.

Ken Resnicow, PhD, is a Professor in the Department of Behavioral Science and Health Education at Emory University's Rollins School of Public Health. His research interests include the design and evaluation of health promotion programs for special populations, particularly cardiovascular and cancer prevention interventions for African Americans; understanding the relationship between ethnicity and health behaviors; substance use prevention and harm reduction; motivational interviewing for chronic disease prevention; and comprehensive school health programs. Dr. Resnicow also serves as a co-investigator on several studies and has also published over 100 peer-reviewed articles and book chapters.

Gary S. Rose, PhD, is Clinical Instructor in Psychiatry at Harvard Medical School. He is a member of the Motivational Interviewing Network of Trainers and lectures widely on topics of motivation, treatment compliance, and behavior change in clinical health psychology and the addictive disorders. Dr. Rose teaches at the Massachusetts School of Professional Psychology and is also a consulting psychologist with the University of Massachusetts Medical Center Division of Behavioral Medicine and the Joslin Clinic, Harvard Medical School. He also maintains a private practice in behavior therapy in Chelmsford, Massachusetts.

David B. Rosengren, PhD, a clinical psychologist in Seattle, Washington, divides his time between research at the University of Washington's Alcohol and Drug Abuse Institute and private practice and community-based motivational interviewing training. His research focus has been on the application of motivational interviewing across addiction and nonaddiction settings. Dr. Rosengren was the first coordinator of the international association of motivational interviewing trainers (MINT) and is former editor of the MINT newsletter. He also has authored several journal articles and book chapters, as well as served as a guest editor for *Addictive Behaviors and Addiction.*

Frederick Rotgers, PsyD, received his doctorate in clinical psychology from Rutgers University. He has had extensive experience in corrections, and was a faculty member of the Rutgers Center for Alcohol Studies and Assistant Chief Psychologist at the Smithers Alcoholism Treatment and Training Center. He is currently an independent practitioner and consultant. Dr. Rotgers has published widely and is senior editor of *Treating Substance Abuse: Theory and Technique.* He was a member of the consulting team that designed the Differential Substance Abuse Treatment (DSAT) system that is being implemented in the State of Maine Department of Corrections and Drug Courts. DSAT is an assessment-driven, research-based approach that makes extensive use of motivational approaches.

Francisco P. Sanchez, PhD, is a staff psychologist in the New Mexico VA Healthcare System, where he works with seriously mentally ill patients and those who abuse substances. His research interests include the effects of spirituality on mental health and incorporation of spirituality in psychotherapy.

Johanna E. Soet, MA, is a Senior Associate Faculty member at the Rollins School of Public Health at Emory University. She provides training and supervision to several projects evaluating the effectiveness of motivational interviewing in health care settings.

Angelica K. Thevos, PhD, MSW, is Associate Professor of Psychiatry and Behavioral Sciences at the Medical University of South Carolina. Her experience in clinical research and treatment spans almost two decades and is reflected in numerous publications and scientific presentations. Her interests and expertise lie in the transfer of recent advances in behavioral science research to practical clinical applications in the community. She is internationally recognized as a cross-culturally competent trainer. Dr. Thevos is also Director of the Sahred Scientific Resources Core of the National Institute on Alcohol Abuse and Alcoholism-funded Charleston Alcohol Research Center and is a co-investigator for the Southeastern

Node of the National Institute on Drug Abuse-sponsored Clinical Trials Network. She also serves as a consultant to several international research and aid organizations and is on research journal editorial and advisory boards.

Georgy Vassilev, MD, is Director of the National Centre for Addictions at the Ministry of Health in Bulgaria and a Founder of the South-east European Institute for Motivational Interventions and Behavior Change. He is principal author of National Program for Prevention, Treatment and Rehabilitation of Drug Addiction for Bulgaria, 2001-2005. He is a member of the Motivational Interviewing Network of Trainers, the Bulgarian Psychiatric Association, the Bulgarian Association of Cognitive and Behavioral Psychotherapies, and the Bulgarian Physicians' Union. Dr. Vassilev has written more than 30 publications and presentations for Bulgarian and international conferences, symposiums, and magazines. Along with his administrative work, he is deeply involved with the introduction of motivational interviewing in Bulgaria.

Mary Marden Velasquez, PhD, is Associate Professor in the Department of Family Practice and Community Medicine at the University of Texas-Houston Medical School. Her background and training are in the areas of clinical psychology, health psychology, and public health. Dr. Velasquez is a motivational interviewing trainer and has presented many workshops in the United States and abroad integrating motivational interviewing with the transtheoretical model of change.

Christopher C. Wagner, PhD, is a clinical psychologist and faculty member in the Department of Rehabilitation Counseling at Virginia Commonwealth University and a consultant with the CSAT-funded Mid-Atlantic Addiction Technology Transfer Center. He hosts the motivational interviewing website at *www.motivationalinterview.org*. Dr. Wagner's research interests focus on interpersonal aspects of psychotherapeutic and other treatment relationships as well as incorporating individual and group motivational interviewing approaches into community treatment settings.

Scott T. Walters, MA, is a predoctoral intern with the VA Boston Healthcare System and Boston University School of Medicine. His research has focused on brief interventions for heavy-drinking college students, aspects of group dynamics, and philosophical and spiritual issues in treatment. Mr. Walters has authored several empirical and theoretical articles on addictions treatment.

John R. Weekes, PhD, is Manager of Program Policy and Information Management for the Correctional Service of Canada and Adjunct Research Professor of Forensic Addictions in the Department of Psychology at Carleton University in Ottawa, Ontario, Canada. He has served as a consultant on forensic substance abuse, harm reduction, and drug strategy issues for a large number of international correctional jurisdictions. Dr. Weekes has also served as a member of the American Correctional Association's (ACA) "Best Practices" Coordinating Council and as a member and Chair of ACA's Substance Abuse Committee.

Allan Zuckoff, MA, is Research Instructor of Psychiatry, University of Pittsburgh School of Medicine, and Codirector of Training, Center for Psychiatric and Chemical Dependency Services, Western Psychiatric Institute and Clinic, in Pittsburgh, Pennsylvania. He is also a PhD candidate in clinical psychology at Duquesne University. His work has focused on development and testing of adaptations of motivational interviewing to enhance treatment adherence in the areas of dual disorders, HIV risk reduction, traumatic grief, bipolar disorder, and depression. Mr. Zuckoff has coauthored a book as well as several articles and treatment manuals related to this work.

Allen Zweben, DSW, is Director of the Center for Addiction and Behavioral Health Research and Professor of Social Work in the School of Social Welfare, University of Wisconsin-Milwaukee. He has expertise in a variety of areas related to substance abuse treatment, including early detection and screening, brief intervention, family treatment, adherence/retention techniques, and patient-treatment matching. His publications have been focused primarily on innovative approaches in the treatment of alcohol problems. Currently Dr. Zweben is one of the principal investigators in the COMBINE study, a National Institutes of Health/National Institute on Alcohol Abuse and Alcoholism-funded multisite collaborative project studying the efficacy of combining pharmacotherapy and psychotherapy interventions for alcohol problems.

Preface

A decade has passed since we sat together in Sydney, Australia, and envisioned the first edition of *Motivational Interviewing*. Before we met in 1989, we had been working separately in the United States and the United Kingdom on methods for practicing and learning this clinical approach. Little had been written about it, and we imagined a book for clinicians, bringing together what had been learned about motivational interviewing, not only by ourselves but by others. The result was an unusual volume: half authored, half edited. We had no idea what would come of it.

By the time The Guilford Press approached us about preparing this second edition, much had changed. In the addiction treatment field, on which we had focused the original book, practice had shifted substantially away from the confrontational methods of the 1970s and 1980s. Meanwhile, applications of motivational interviewing had spread into many other areas, including general medical care, health promotion, social work, and corrections. Responding to rapidly growing requests for clinical training, we had prepared more than 300 trainers who formed an international organization of motivational interviewing trainers. The first edition had been published in Italian, German, Spanish, Portuguese, and Chinese, with several other translations in progress. A website had been developed (*www.motivationalinterview.org*), and various briefer adaptations of the clinical method had appeared.

As a result of these and other developments, this is quite a different book from the first edition. Its focus has been broadened from addictions to behavior change in general. With 10 more years of experience in seeing what seems to help or confuse people as they learn the clinical method, we have sharpened up some presentations and left out other material that seemed to be distracting. Among the stylistic changes, we have departed from citing references within the text of the first 14 chapters and have used citations more sparingly in endnotes. This and other changes are meant to render the narrative even more accessible and relevant to a broad range of clinicians, while we retain documentation for those who wish to pursue background reading and research.

Part I is almost entirely rewritten. We have removed most of the material that contrasted motivational interviewing with other counseling approaches, and the prior counterpoint with confrontation is gone. Instead we have focused on a clear description of what the method *is* rather than what it is *not*. We have removed from the first 14 chapters nearly all the material on approaches with which motivational interviewing has sometimes been confused: FRAMES, assessment feedback, motivational enhancement therapy, the transtheoretical stages of change, brief negotiation, and other brief adaptations. These topics are now covered in special chapters in Part IV.

We have taken a further step away from the traditional concept of resistance as motivated client defensiveness. We now present (in Chapter 5) change talk (formerly self-motivational statements) and resistance behavior as opposite sides of the same coin, simply reflecting the poles of a client's ambivalence. After some deliberation, we did decide to retain the term "resistance" because of its familiarity, but to rehabilitate it a bit. Alternative terms that we had tried out (e.g., countermotivational statements, counterchange talk) seemed no more satisfactory or less pejorative. Change talk and resistance are now presented as complementary behaviors, and we have a chapter on how to respond to each: Chapter 7 is completely new and Chapter 8 is a reworking of our prior chapter on handling resistance. We have removed (but still discuss) the concept of therapeutic paradox, distinguishing it from the clinical method of motivational interviewing.

Other chapters contain new material as well. This time we included a definition of motivational interviewing (Chapter 4). Chapter 9 is entirely new, addressing an issue on which we had been mostly silent before: What do you do when importance is high but confidence is low? We have introduced an approach to enhancing confidence that, while incorporating some familiar strategies, places them in the collaborative change-talk context of motivational interviewing. It is accompanied by case material, and new clinical dialogue appears throughout the book, although the extended case example (Chapter 11) has been retained with relatively little change. There is a new chapter, Chapter 12, on ethical aspects of practice.

Part III is almost entirely new. Instead of presenting specific techniques for teaching, we focus on how people learn motivational interviewing. We reflect on processes of learning (including our own) in Chapter 13, and then on broad ways for facilitating learning in Chapter 14.

Finally, Part IV consists of all new contributed chapters focused on various applications of motivational interviewing. We intentionally avoided chapters dealing with applications to specific problems or disorders, both because there are so many and because there is an insufficient research base in most specific problem areas at present. Instead these chapters focus on applications of motivational interviewing in particular contexts (e.g., correctional settings, groups, public health) and populations (e.g., medical patients, adolescents, and couples). Other chapters in Part IV examine the relationships of motivational interviewing to values (Chapter 19) and the transtheoretical stages of change (Chapter 15), and provide a review of outcome research on this method to date (Chapter 16).

Acknowledgments

There is little that is truly original in motivational interviewing. We have built on the extraordinary contributions of Carl R. Rogers and his students, particularly Thomas Gordon, who developed the methods of client-centered psychotherapy over the past 50 years. Also influential in our thinking about motivational interviewing was the work of James Prochaska and Carlo DiClemente on the transtheoretical model of change, Milton Rokeach on human values, and Daryl Bem on self-perception theory.

We cannot thank enough our colleagues from the international Motivational Interviewing Network of Trainers (MINT) for the enthusiasm, collaborative spirit, and sheer talent that they bring to our annual meetings, steering committee, newsletter, videotapes, website, and training workshops. One of the great joys of our work over the years has been the opportunity to meet and work with such remarkable people as the MINTies, whose creativity and generosity manifest what they teach. Our own thinking and approaches have been greatly enriched by their collaboration and friendship.

We particularly thank Gian Paolo Guelfi, who opened to us his summer home in the northern Italian village of Fumeri for a concentrated sabbatical during which we drafted most of this second edition. It was a wonderfully peaceful time when we traded in our offices, faxes, and e-mail for green hillside walks, birdsongs, and a wood-fired pizza oven. We are also indebted to our families and colleagues who made this time away possible. This is a much better book for it.

William Miller acknowledges with gratitude the ongoing support of the U.S. National Institute on Alcohol Abuse and Alcoholism, from which a senior research scientist award (No. K05-AA00133) has permitted him for the past 11 years to devote full-time effort to developing and evaluating new methods for the treatment of addictive behaviors.

Having worked on a variety of book projects over the years, we have come to appreciate greatly the qualities and invaluable contributions of a highly skilled editor. We have been fortunate to work with some of the very best. Seymour Weingarten saw promise in our first edition and began our long relationship with The Guilford Press. Kitty Moore shepherded this second edition from start to finish, always providing patient support and expert guidance. We received expert help from dozens of capable staff throughout the process of producing and releasing this second edition, for which we are most grateful.

Contents

PART I

Context

CHAPTER 1

Why Do People Change?

> Until one is committed, there is hesitancy, the chance to draw
> back, always ineffectiveness, concerning all acts of initiative and
> creation. There is one elementary truth, the ignorance of which
> kills countless ideas and splendid plans: that the moment one
> definitely commits oneself, then Providence moves too. All sorts of
> things occur to help one that would never otherwise have
> occurred. A whole stream of events issues from the decision.
> —JOHANN WOLFGANG VON GOETHE

Interest in the topic of motivation often begins with wondering why people *don't* change. It is a common frustration for health professionals and teachers, counselors and parents, and those who work in social service and judicial systems. It seems apparent that what a person is doing either isn't working or is self-destructive; you can see a better way, yet the person persists in the same behavior. In a way, it is captured in the words, "You would think . . . "

> You would think that having had a heart attack would be enough to persuade a man to quit smoking, change his diet, exercise more, and take his medication.
> You would think that hangovers, damaged relationships, an auto crash, and memory blackouts would be enough to convince a woman to stop drinking.
> You would think that it would be apparent to any teenager that getting a

good education is important to how one spends and enjoys the rest of one's life.

You would think that time spent in the dehumanizing privations of prison would dissuade people from reoffending.

You would think so, and yet medication compliance problems are the norm, even with life-threatening conditions such as diabetes, heart disease, and HIV infection. It is the hallmark of addictive behaviors that they persist despite what seems overwhelming evidence of their destructiveness. Increasing the severity of punishment seems to offer little deterrence. We are not always sensible creatures.

A more productive and fascinating question, we believe, is why people *do* change, for change also is the norm. In time, people adjust to new lifestyles. Most people with alcohol, drug, or gambling problems ultimately escape them and go on to lead reasonably normal lives, often without formal treatment. In spite of themselves, teenagers usually grow up. What is it that awakens us and causes a gradual course correction—or even a dramatic turnabout?

Why *do* people change?

PIECES OF A PUZZLE

Those who work in the helping professions often are inclined to believe that what causes change is the service provided, be it counseling, treating, advising, or teaching. Our own journey that led to motivational interviewing began with treating alcohol and other drug problems, which is why some of the research and examples we draw on in this book come from the addiction field. Addictive behavior is a wonderful field in which to study the phenomena of change, and research in this area has caused us to question many of our early assumptions about how and why change occurs. Here are some pieces of a puzzle, some of which emerged from research on addictive behaviors.

Natural Change

It is now widely accepted that in many problem areas, positive change often occurs without formal treatment. Most people who quit smoking or recover from alcohol and other drug problems do so without assistance from health professionals, or even from the widely available mutual-help groups. Such treatment-free recovery was once referred to as "spontaneous remission" and was considered to be a relatively rare and anomalous event. Yet the stages and processes by which people change seem to be the same with or without treatment. In this sense, treatment can be thought of as facilitating what is a natural process of change.

Brief Intervention Effects

It is also clear that it is possible to speed or facilitate change. One rather consistent finding is that even relatively brief interventions under certain conditions can trigger change. One or two sessions of counseling often yield much greater change in behavior than no counseling at all. Dozens of studies from many different countries now document the effectiveness of brief interventions in reducing heavy or problematic drinking.[1] Similar findings have emerged with brief interventions for other problems as well.[2] A little counseling can lead to significant change.

Dose Effects

If a little counseling helps, then one might reason that the degree of change will be related to the amount (dose) of counseling a person receives. In the alcohol field, at least, the evidence is mixed. In general, the more treatment a person voluntarily completes (whether sessions of counseling or doses of medication), the more benefit is seen in behavior change. It is possible, however, that both treatment adherence and positive outcomes are related to some third factor—like motivation for change.

What happens if one randomly assigns people to receive more versus less treatment? Here again, the evidence is rather consistent. In controlled trials, people typically show about the same level of benefit, whether they are assigned at random to longer or shorter treatment or to inpatient versus outpatient care for alcohol use disorders, for example. On average, brief interventions yield outcomes that are similar to those with longer treatment. In studies of outpatient treatment, much of the reduction in drinking that occurs (and remains over years of follow-up) happens within the first week or two, again suggesting that change is occurring after relatively little treatment.

This is not an argument to restrict treatment to a few sessions, of course. While the average profile shows that change occurs early in treatment, the length of time to response varies. The fascinating point is that so much change occurs after so little counseling. Most theories of psychotherapy focus on processes that would require a longer period of time to accomplish (e.g., acquiring new cognitive-behavioral coping skills or working through transference in the therapeutic relationship). These findings suggest that we need different ways to think about the critical conditions for change to occur.

Faith/Hope Effects

Another piece of the puzzle is found in research on the effects of faith and hope in facilitating change. Ask a person how likely it is that he or she will succeed in making a particular change, and the answer is a reasonably good predictor of the likelihood that actual change will occur. These days this effect is often called "self-efficacy," but healers in all ages have been aware of the power of faith and hope. The effect of believing that one is receiving an effective treatment is so strong that placebo (rather than no medication) is the standard against which new medications must be tested.

This phenomenon is not restricted to patients' beliefs. The counselor, doctor, or teacher also holds beliefs about a person's ability to change, and these beliefs can become self-fulfilling prophecies. In one study conducted in three different alcohol treatment programs, patients identified to staff as having high potential for recovery (but who in fact had been chosen at random) were significantly more likely to be sober and working a year after discharge. Perceived prognosis influences real outcomes.

Counselor Effects

This in turn leads to another piece of the puzzle. When someone seeks help from a treatment program, what factors determine whether that person stays or drops out and how that person will fare after treatment? Findings are typically inconsistent about patient characteristics. For example, in some studies those with less severe alcohol problems are more likely to benefit from treatment, but in others greater alcohol severity is associated with better outcomes.

One factor that does frequently make a difference, however, is the professional to whom the person happens to be assigned. Research indicates that across a broad range of schools of psychotherapy, certain characteristics of therapists are associated with successful treatment. Counselors working in the same setting and offering the same treatment approaches show dramatic differences in their rates of client dropouts and successful outcomes. These variations in effectiveness among staff frequently exceed the magnitude of differences between treatment approaches. A majority of client dropouts at a particular clinic may occur within the caseloads of a few staff members, and characteristics predicting high patient dropout rates can be as subtle as the doctor's tone of voice. In sum, the way in which one interacts with people appears to be at least as important as the specific approach or school of thought from which he or she operates.

Carl Rogers articulated and tested a theory about critical counselor skills for facilitating change.[3] He asserted that a client-centered interpersonal relationship—in which the counselor manifests three critical conditions—provides the ideal atmosphere for change to occur. Within the context of such a safe and supportive atmosphere, clients are able to explore their experiences openly and to reach resolution of their own problems. The counselor's role, in Rogers's view, is not a directive one of providing solutions, suggestions, or analysis. Instead, the counselor need only offer these three critical conditions to prepare the way for natural change: accurate empathy, nonpossessive warmth, and genuineness.

Subsequent evidence has supported the importance of these conditions of change, particularly accurate empathy. This condition should not be confused with the meaning of "empathy" as identification with the person or as having had similar past experiences. In fact, a recent personal history of the same problem area (e.g., alcoholism) may compromise a counselor's ability to provide the critical conditions of change because of overidentification.[4] As defined by Rogers, accurate empathy involves skillful reflective listening that clarifies and amplifies the person's own experiencing and meaning, without imposing the counselor's own material

Research indicates that counselor empathy can be a significant determinant of clients' response to treatment.[5] In one study at the University of New Mexico, we found that about two-thirds of the variance in 6-month drinking outcomes could be predicted from the degree of empathy shown by counselors during treatment.[6] Counselor empathy still accounted for half of the variance in outcomes at 12 months, and a quarter of the variance at 24 months after treatment.[7] Similar effects of counselor empathy have been reported by other investigators.[8] Conversely, confrontational counseling has been associated with a high dropout rate and relatively poor outcomes. In another New Mexico study,[9] we were able to predict clients' alcohol consumption 1 year after treatment from a single counselor behavior: the more the counselor confronted during treatment, the more the person drank.

It appears that counseling style characteristics manifest themselves rather early in the treatment process and, indeed, can have a significant effect within a single session. The therapeutic relationship tends to stabilize relatively quickly, and the nature of the client–counselor relationship in early sessions predicts treatment retention and outcome. Whatever it is that happens during treatment begins very early.

This is not a new insight. For decades it has been recognized that "nonspecific" factors contribute to treatment. The original use of this term implied that such factors are not specific to particular treatment methods but cut across all styles of therapy. They are, in essence, those mysterious common healing elements that are presumed to be present in all forms of therapy.

Yet there is nothing inherently mysterious about nonspecifics. Viewed in another way, this term simply means that these determinants of outcome have not yet been adequately specified. "Nonspecifics" are *unspecified* principles of change. If these factors account for a large part of treatment success, then it is important that they be specified, researched, discussed, and taught. It is not a safe assumption that all practitioners somehow know and practice these principles. To say that these principles of change are important, regardless of specific orientation, does not imply that they are manifested equally in all clinicians or treatment approaches. In fact, counselors can vary dramatically in their effectiveness, and specific treatment approaches and philosophies differ in the extent to which they foster certain therapeutic (or countertherapeutic) styles.

Waiting-List Effects

Another piece of the puzzle emerged from research in which a waiting-list control group was used as the standard against which treatments were compared. This was understood to be an ethically preferable alternative to a no-treatment control condition, in that those who were assigned to this group were given delayed treatment rather than none at all. Indeed, waiting lists occur naturally in community treatment programs where demand exceeds resources.

Several studies have used waiting-list conditions as a control against which to evaluate the efficacy of brief or self-help interventions among help-seeking people. As a control group, the waiting list worked well. Often clients on the waiting list show little or no change during the waiting period. In contrast, those who are given self-help materials and are told to initiate change on their own typically do so. As a result, by the end of the waiting period there is a large difference between the brief intervention and the control groups.

What is a bit odd, however, is that people who seek help usually show a drift toward positive change no matter what treatment they are given. Even those in no-treatment control groups often show some improvement, albeit less than that for treated groups. People placed on a waiting list, however, showed no change at all in our studies.[10]

One way to think about what is happening here is that people in the waiting-list group are doing exactly what they were told to do: they are *waiting*. The implicit message is that they are not expected to improve until they are treated. When at last they can begin treatment, they should improve. This suggests that it is possible to intervene (in this case by placing people on a "waiting list") in a way that makes it *less* likely that people will change than if we had left them alone.

There is a parallel here to the study of counselor empathy described earlier. When we compared counselors' rates of improvement among their patients, we found wide variability (from 25% to 100%). In this study we also had a group that was given self-help materials and sent home to work on their own. On average, clients working with a counselor and those working on their own showed similar outcomes, but averages can be misleading. Those treated by high-empathy counselors had higher success rates than those in the self-help condition. Those treated by low-empathy counselors, in contrast, were less likely to improve than if they had been sent home with a good book.

It appears that the way in which one communicates can make it either more or less likely that a person will change.

Change-Talk Effects

Most clinicians might agree that resistant people are less likely to change. Indeed, the more a person argues against change during a counseling session, the less likely it is that change will occur.[11]

Generally, though, what people *say* during counseling about the possibility of change is related to whether it will actually occur. Ask people how confident they are that they can succeed in making a particular change, and their answer is a reasonably good predictor of what will happen. Give them a questionnaire at the outset of counseling, asking about their level of readiness for change, and their scores predict the amount of change at follow-up.[12]

What fewer people appreciate is the extent to which change talk and resistance are substantially influenced by counseling style. Counsel in a directive, confrontational manner, and client resistance goes up. Counsel in a reflective, supportive manner, and resistance goes down while change talk increases. In one study,[13] counselors intentionally switched back and forth between these two styles in blocks of about 12 minutes within sessions. Clients' resistance behaviors increased substantially during the confrontational periods and dropped when the counselors changed to a client-centered style. In another study using the same system for recording behaviors of counselors and clients,[14] problem drinkers randomly assigned to confrontational counseling showed much higher levels of resistance (arguing, changing the subject, interrupting, denying a problem) than did those given a more client-centered motivational interviewing approach.

Putting the Pieces Together: Toward a Motivational Understanding of Change

How can one put all these pieces together?

Change occurs naturally.
What happens after formal interventions (counseling, treatment, therapy, etc.) mirrors natural change, rather than being a unique form of change.
Nevertheless, the likelihood that change will occur is strongly influenced by interpersonal interactions. Even relatively brief counseling can initiate change—too brief for most people to be acquiring new coping skills or experiencing personality change.
When behavior change occurs within a course of treatment, much of it happens within the first few sessions, and, on average, the total dose of treatment does not make all that much difference.
The clinician by whom one is treated is a significant determinant of treatment dropout, retention, adherence, and outcome.
Specifically, an empathic counseling style seems to facilitate change, and its absence may deter change.
People who believe that they are likely to change do so. People whose counselors believe that they are likely to change do so. Those who are told that they are not expected to improve indeed do not.
What people say about change is important. Statements that reflect motivation for and commitment to change do predict subsequent behavior

change, whereas arguments against change (resistance) produce less change. Both kinds of speech can be influenced substantially by interpersonal (counseling) style.

One way to put this puzzle together is to think of *motivation* as fundamental to change. There is reason to think this, as clients' level of motivation for change is often a good predictor of outcome. Motivation can be influenced by many naturally occurring interpersonal and intrapersonal factors and by specific interventions, too. It seems particularly sensitive to interpersonal communication styles. Effective brief interventions don't seem long enough to teach new skills or alter personality, but it is plausible that they affect motivation for change. But what is motivation?

READY, WILLING, AND ABLE

Perhaps there is wisdom in natural language, which in English contains the phrase "ready, willing, and able" to communicate a high level of motivation for change. The implication is that there are at least these three critical components of motivation: readiness, willingness, and ability.

Willing: The Importance of Change

One factor is the extent to which the person wants, desires, or wills change. We tend to talk about this dimension as the perceived importance of a particular change.

One can also think of this as the degree of discrepancy between status and goal, between what is happening at present and what one values for the future. Discrepancy is a key concept within self-regulation theory,[15] which postulates an ongoing self-monitoring process much like that of a thermostat. As long as present reality is found to be within desired limits, no change is indicated. When an out-of-range value is detected, however, a change process kicks in. It is when things are sufficiently discrepant from the desired or expected ideal that motivation for change begins.

A low level of perceived importance is sometimes viewed as pathology, as being "resistant" or "in denial." We prefer to take it at face value. A lack of sufficient discrepancy to motivate action is a normal stage in the process of change (see Chapter 15). It suggests that what one must do in this case, in order to instigate change, is to *develop* discrepancy: to enhance the perceived importance of change.

People are not all that simple, of course. Each person has dozens of hierarchical core values,[16] and each value implies a desired state: some of these values may be mutually contradictory. The importance of any particular change is only one part of the puzzle.

Able: Confidence for Change

Sometimes a person feels willing but not able to change. Smokers and prostitutes often acknowledge the risks of their behavior and the importance of change, but many feel pessimistic about their chances. "I wish I could" captures this combination of high importance and low confidence.

Again, self-regulation theory is helpful. When discrepancy becomes large enough and change seems important, a search for possible methods for change is initiated. Given sufficient importance, if people find an avenue for change that they believe will work (general efficacy) and that they believe they can do (self-efficacy), they will often pursue it through behavior change. If a person becomes alarmed by a discrepancy but perceives no way to change, however, then something else happens. Instead of changing behavior, people reduce their discomfort by shifting their thought processes and perceptions in a way that is often called "defensive." The classic "defense mechanisms" described by Anna Freud echo these patterns: denial ("It's not really so bad"), rationalization ("I didn't want it anyway"), and projection ("It's not my problem, it's theirs").

Ready: A Matter of Priorities

One would think that the combination of high importance and high confidence would be enough to instigate change, but a moment's reflection shows that it is not necessarily so. One can be willing and able to change, but not ready to do so. "Quitting smoking is important to me," one person said, "but it's not the *most* important thing right now." Assuming the presence of adequate importance and confidence, this third dimension, readiness, has to do with relative priorities: "I want to, but not now."

Like low importance, low readiness is also sometimes viewed as pathological. "I'll quit tomorrow" has become a symbol of self-deception. Again, relative priorities are a part of normal human functioning, and low readiness can be viewed not as character armor but as information about what the next step is toward change.

All three of these elements—ready, willing, and able—can be sources of the "yes, but . . . " dilemma—the phenomenon of ambivalence—to which we turn our attention in Chapter 2.

WHAT TRIGGERS CHANGE?

A certain folk belief seems to be embedded in some cultures and subcultures: change is motivated primarily by the avoidance of discomfort. If you can just make people feel bad enough, they will change. Punish undesired behavior, and withdraw the pain when the unwanted behavior stops. People would be motivated to change, then, by causing them to feel enough discomfort, shame, guilt, loss, threat, anxiety, or humiliation. It is this view that made the excesses of confrontational "attack therapy," Synanon, Scared Straight, and "therapeutic" boot camps seem warranted. In this view, people don't change because they haven't yet suffered enough.

We are suggesting quite a different understanding of motivation. Many of the clients we see have had no dearth of suffering. Humiliation, shame, guilt, and angst are not the primary engines of change. Ironically, such experiences can even immobilize the person, rendering change more remote. Instead, constructive behavior change seems to arise when the person connects it with something of intrinsic value, something important, something cherished. Intrinsic motivation for change arises in an accepting, empowering atmosphere that makes it safe for the person to explore the possibly painful present in relation to what is wanted and valued. People often get stuck, not because they fail to appreciate the down side of their situation, but because they feel at least two ways about it. The way out of that forest has to do with exploring and following what the person is experiencing and what, from his or her perspective, truly matters.

NOTES

1. Bien, Miller, and Tonigan (1993); Miller (2000).
2. Glasgow and Rosen (1978); Gould and Clum (1993).
3. Rogers (1959).
4. Manohar (1973).
5. Luborsky, McLellan, Woody, O'Brien, and Auerbach (1985); Miller, Taylor, and West (1980); Truax and Carkhuff (1967); Truax and Mitchell (1971); Valle (1981).
6. Miller et al. (1980).
7. Miller and Baca (1983).
8. Valle (1981).
9. Miller, Benefield, and Tonigan (1993).
10. Harris and Miller (1990); Schmidt and Miller (1983).
11. Miller et al. (1993).
12. Project MATCH Research Group (1997a, 1997b).
13. Patterson and Forgatch (1985).
14. Miller et al. (1993).
15. Brown (1998); Kanfer (1986); Miller and Brown (1991).
16. Rokeach (1973).

CHAPTER 2

Ambivalence

The Dilemma of Change

Where did all the sages get the idea that a man's desires must
be normal and virtuous? Why did they imagine that he must
inevitably will what is reasonable and profitable?
—FYODOR DOSTOYEVSKY, *From the Underground*

I WANT TO, AND I DON'T WANT TO

Feeling two ways about something or someone is a common enough experience. Indeed, a person who feels no ambivalence about anything is hard to
imagine. Feeling 100% clear about something that is important is probably
more exceptional than normal.

This phenomenon of ambivalence is often prominent in psychological difficulties. A person suffering from agoraphobia, for example, may say, "I want
to go out, but I'm terrified that I will lose control." So, too, a person who is
socially isolated, unhappy, and depressed may express ambivalence: "I want
to be with people and make closer friendships, but I don't feel like an attractive or worthwhile person." With certain problems, the part played by ambivalence is even more central. A person who is having an extramarital affair vac-
illates between spouse and lover in an intensely emotional ambivalence. A
compulsive hand washer or checker may desperately want to avoid going
through this disabling ritual time and time again, yet may feel driven to it by
fear. Such approach–avoidance conflict is characteristic of addictive behaviors

13

as well. People who are struggling with problem drinking, drug addiction, bulimia, or pathological gambling often recognize the risks, costs, and harm involved in their behavior. Yet for a variety of reasons they are also quite attached and attracted to the addictive behavior. They want to drink (or smoke, or purge, or gamble), and they don't want to. They want to change, and at the same time they don't want to change.

It is easy to misinterpret such ambivalent conflict as pathological—to conclude that there is something wrong with the person's motivation, judgment, knowledge base, or mental state. A sensible conclusion from this line of reasoning is that the person needs to be educated about and persuaded to take the proper course of action. We will explore the practical limitations of this conclusion in Chapter 3. For now, suffice it to say that we regard ambivalence to be a normal aspect of human nature; indeed, passing through ambivalence is a natural phase in the process of change. It is when people get *stuck* in ambivalence that problems can persist and intensify. Ambivalence is a reasonable place to visit, but you wouldn't want to live there.

In this way, ambivalence can be a key issue that must be resolved for change to occur. One reason that brief interventions (see Chapter 1) may work is precisely that they help people get unstuck from their ambivalence—they enable a person to make a decision and move on toward change. In this way, the "lack of motivation" that so often frustrates the work of health professionals, counselors, and teachers can be thought of as unresolved ambivalence. To explore ambivalence is to work at the heart of the problem of being stuck. Until a person can resolve the "I want to, but I don't want to" dilemma, change is likely to be slow-going and short-lived.

Conflict and Ambivalence

Conflict has been an important concept in many psychological theories, and conflicts have been described as coming in three varieties. In the *approach–approach* conflict, the person must choose between two similarly attractive alternatives, and the important choice factors are all positive. It's the candy store problem. If one must have a conflict, this is the kind to choose. One example is deciding which of two exciting and rewarding job offers to accept.

An *avoidance–avoidance* conflict, in contrast, involves having to choose between two evils—two (or more) possibilities, each of which involves significant fear, pain, embarrassment, or other negative consequences. This is being caught "between a rock and a hard place" or "between the devil and the deep blue sea." The important choice factors are all negative, things to be avoided. In a congested city or on a large university campus, for example, one may have to choose between parking far away from one's destination and parking closer but risking an expensive parking ticket.

Still more vexing is the *approach–avoidance* type. This kind of conflict seems to have special potential for keeping people stuck and creating considerable stress. Here the person is both attracted to and repelled by the same object. The term "fatal attraction" has been used to describe this kind of love affair: "I can't live with it, and I can't live without it." In alternating cycles, the person indulges in and then resists the behavior (relationship, person, object). The resulting yo-yo effect is a classic characteristic of the approach–avoidance conflict. Ambivalent cognitions, emotions, and behaviors are a normal part of any approach–avoidance conflict situation. Many wry examples are found in American jazz and country and western song lyrics (e.g., "I'm so miserable without you, it's almost like you're here"). A 1930s Fletcher Henderson tune quipped, "My sweet tooth says I want to, but my wisdom tooth says no."

The grand champion of conflicts, however, is the *double approach–avoidance* type, wherein a person is torn between two alternatives (lovers, lifestyles, etc.), each of which has both enticing positive and powerful negative aspects. As the person moves closer to option A, the disadvantages of A become more salient and the advantages of B seem brighter. When the person then turns and starts moving toward B, the down sides of B become clearer and A starts looking more attractive.

Decisional Balance

One helpful way of illustrating ambivalence is the metaphor of a balance or seesaw.[1] The person experiences competing motivations because there are benefits and costs associated with both sides of the conflict (see Figure 2.1). There are two kinds of weights on each side of the balance: one has to do with the perceived benefits of a particular course of action; the other has to do with the perceived costs or disadvantages of the course of action (such as taking medication to lower blood pressure).

Another way of conceptualizing this is through a balance sheet, which

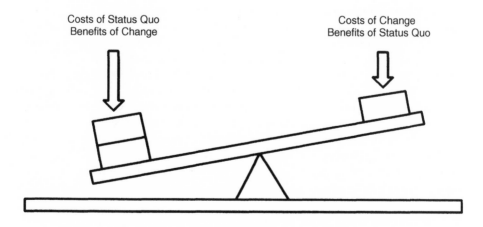

Costs of Status Quo
Benefits of Change

Costs of Change
Benefits of Status Quo

FIGURE 2.1. Decisional balance: Weighing the costs and benefits.

can be used to specify what a person perceives to be the benefits and costs associated with a behavior. An example regarding alcohol use is shown in Box 2.1. As shown here, the balance sheet (and hence the nature of a person's ambivalence) can be quite complex. It can comprise a set of pros and cons for each of the options open to the person. As is characteristic of a double approach–avoidance conflict, the person may experience ambivalence no matter which option is currently being exercised.

There is a danger of serious oversimplification here. We do not mean to imply that people are always (or even usually) consciously aware of this balancing process, or that when they are made aware, they will proceed like accountants toward rational decisions. The elements of this balance sheet, unlike the books or inventory of a business, do not add up in simple fashion. The value of each item may shift over time. Elements in the lists are interconnected, and a change in one may cause shifts in others. Almost by definition, a balance sheet will be full of contradictions: "I know it's bad for me, but I like it." "Sometimes I stop myself, and other times I want to but I just don't care." The experience of ambivalence can be confusing, perplexing, and frustrating.

SOCIAL CONTEXT

Social and cultural factors affect people's perceptions of their behavior, as well as their evaluation of its costs and benefits. Even across different neighborhoods and social groups within the same city, people may hold very differ-

---

BOX 2.1. A Decisional Balance Sheet

Continue to drink as before		Abstain from alcohol	
Benefits	Costs	Benefits	Costs
Helps me relax	Could lose my family	Less family conflict	I enjoy getting high
Enjoy drinking with friends	Bad example for my children	More time with my children	What to do about my friends
	Damaging my health	Feel better physically	How to deal with stress
	Spending too much money	Helps with money problems	
	Impairing my mental ability		
	Might lose my job		
	Wasting my time/life		

ent views about the pros and cons of the same behavior. In the United Kingdom, for example, the social meaning and value of drinking in rounds can vary dramatically among pubs in the same locality or even within the same pub. In certain U.S. communities and subgroups, drinking that results in a memory blackout, fighting, vomiting in the street, and passing out in one's car is regarded as just a normal part of a good time on a Friday night. Stealing, missing work, taking risks, and using drugs are much more acceptable within some subgroups than others. Asking a sexual partner to use a condom may communicate quite different messages, depending on the context. A person's motivational balance and ambivalence cannot be understood outside the social context of family, friends, and community.

Paradoxical Responses

It is also the case that ambivalent people may not respond in what would seem a logical manner. Unless one understands the dynamics of ambivalence, a person's responses can seem counterintuitive and puzzling.

A common example is found in the strategy of increasing negative consequences as a deterrent. It seems sensible that imposing harsher punishment for certain behavior should decrease the attractiveness of that behavior. In the context of a decisional balance model, adding more severe negative consequences to one side ought to favor a shift to the other. It does not always work this way, however; in fact, the opposite can occur. Nagging by family members, for example, may exacerbate rather than diminish a behavior. In *The Fatal Shore*, a historical account of Australia's first century as a British penal colony, Robert Hughes[2] recounted how convicts endured savage beatings and torture in order to continue smoking tobacco or drinking alcohol. He quoted the following chilling lyric of a song that was popular among Australian convicts in the 19th century:

> Cut yer name across me backbone,
> Stretch me skin across a drum,
> Iron me up to Pinchgut Island
> From today till Kingdom Come!
> I will eat your Norfolk Dumpling
> Like a juicy Spanish plum,
> Even dance the Newgate hornpipe,
> If you'll only give me rum!

The song defiantly expresses a willingness to risk torture (Pinchgut Island was a bare rock in the middle of Sydney Harbor, where convicts were chained without food—hence the name—and exposed to the elements for long periods), flogging (a "Norfolk Dumpling" was a whipping of 100 lashes with the steel-tipped cat-o'-nine-tails), and even execution (the "Newgate hornpipe" refers to the dancing of a hanged man's legs in midair) in order to get rum.

Clinicians know all too well that people with alcohol and drug problems can similarly persist in their habits, despite incredible personal suffering and losses. Obviously, a simple increase in painful consequences is not always successful in stopping such behaviors. Sometimes such consequences only seem to strengthen and entrench a behavior pattern.

How can such a seemingly paradoxical response occur? The theory of psychological reactance[3] predicts an *increase* in the rate and attractiveness of a "problem" behavior if a person perceives that his or her personal freedom is being infringed or challenged. Secondary effects of a change within the person's social environment may also account for detrimental shifts. For instance, the breakdown of a person's marriage—seemingly a terrible cost—may deprive him or her of the only social support that served to deter unhealthy behavior, resulting in ever greater excess. If all other sources of positive reinforcement are blocked, a person may persist in seeking the one remaining reward, albeit at great cost. Such seemingly paradoxical responses are neither mysterious nor uniquely pathological. Within the dynamics of ambivalence they are quite understandable and even predictable aspects of human nature.

Understanding the dynamics of ambivalence, then, provides an alternative to thinking of people as (and blaming them for being) "unmotivated." People are always motivated for something. Conflict arises when two people are motivated toward different goals. Those two people might be a doctor and patient, a parent and child, a wife and husband, or a counselor and client. When such conflict arises, one person may think of the other as "poorly motivated."

Readiness for What?

The proper question is not, "Why isn't this person motivated?" but rather, "For what *is* this person motivated?" It is unwise to assume that you already know the costs and benefits in another person's situation, or the relative importance that the person assigns to these factors. A stomach problem caused by work stress or drinking may be viewed with alarm by some, whereas others may regard it as something that they "just put up with." The threat of fines and imprisonment will deter many from engaging in illegal behavior, but for others it is just a risk that is part of the cost of doing business. What is highly valued by some (e.g., being healthy, employed, popular, slim, or pious) will be of little importance to others. Discovering and understanding an individual's motivations is an important first step toward change.

With specific regard to change, it is also important to understand what a person perceives and expects to be the outcome of different courses of action: What would happen if he or she continued on the present course, for example, or took a new road? People have particular expectancies about the likely results, both positive and negative, of certain courses of action. These expectations can have a powerful effect on behavior. Someone who desperately wants to stop smoking may still make no effort to do so, in the belief that all such efforts are futile. Gamblers may not want to consider quitting because they perceive (rightly or wrongly) that the thrill of gambling is the greatest source of excitement they have ever known and that life without it would be dull.

Instead of focusing, then, on why a person doesn't want to make a particular change, it is sensible to explore what the person *does* want. This is not to ignore the topic of change. Rather, it provides a context for change. Sometimes a behavioral course adjustment does not occur until people perceive that change is relevant to achieving or preserving something that *is* truly important or dear to them.

It is also the case that there are often multiple ways to approach a desirable goal. A person with marginally elevated blood pressure might consider dietary changes (such as reduction of salt and caffeine intake), weight loss, stress reduction, increased exercise, meditation, or medication. If one of these is prescribed, the person may be "unmotivated" to pursue it, even though desiring a reduction in blood pressure. Motivation can vary, depending on the specific course of action being considered. Given a choice of strategies to try, however, the person may find one that is acceptable as a starting point.

Motivation also varies across specific ends as well as means. A person who is using multiple licit and illicit drugs may be totally disinterested in changing one of them, willing to consider reducing another, and highly motivated to stop using yet another. Insisting that the person abstain from *all* drugs can be an obstacle to accomplishing positive changes (and associated harm reduction) that the person *is* willing to pursue.

To summarize, ambivalence is a common human experience and a stage in the normal process of change. Getting stuck in ambivalence is also common, and approach–avoidance conflicts can be particularly difficult to resolve on one's own. Resolving ambivalence can be a key to change, and, indeed, once ambivalence has been resolved, little else may be required for change to occur. However, attempts to force resolution in a particular direction (as by direct persuasion or by increasing punishment for one action) can lead to a paradoxical response, even strengthening the very behavior they were intended to diminish.

NOTES

1. Janis and Mann (1977).
2. Hughes (1987).
3. Brehm and Brehm (1981).

CHAPTER 3

Facilitating Change

Anyone who willingly enters into the pain of a stranger is truly a
remarkable person.
—HENRI J. M. NOUWEN, *In Memoriam*

THE RIGHTING REFLEX

Human beings seem to have a built-in desire to set things right. The strength
of this inclination varies from person to person and from one context to another. There are entire cultural and religious traditions, such as Buddhism, in
which detachment from this desire to meddle is encouraged. Yet it is common,
when we see something awry, to want to fix it. When people perceive a discrepancy between how things are and how they ought to be, they tend to be
motivated to reduce that discrepancy if it seems possible to do so.

Those of us who work in helping, healing, and teaching professions may
be particularly inclined to set things aright, for that broad desire is often what
draws people into such professions. See someone going astray, or even wandering aimlessly, and the reflex kicks in to set them back on the right path. It's
a noble desire, although people certainly differ in what they perceive the right
path to be.

Now consider what happens when someone with a righting reflex (R)
meets a person who is ambivalent (A). As A speaks to R about the dilemma of
ambivalence, R develops an opinion as to what the right course of action
would be for A to take. R then proceeds to advise, teach, persuade, counsel, or
argue for this particular resolution to A's ambivalence. One does not need a

doctorate in psychology to anticipate what A's response is likely to be in this situation. By virtue of ambivalence, A is apt to argue the opposite, or at least point out problems and shortcomings of the proposed solution. It is natural for A to do so, because A feels at least two ways about this or almost any pre-scribed solution. It is the very nature of ambivalence.

What happens next? R may respond to the challenge by turning up the volume and arguing more forcefully for the proposed resolution. The inclina-tion to do this may be particularly strong if R concludes that A is "in denial," "resisting," or otherwise impaired from seeing the truth. The natural response for A, of course, will be to intensify the counteraction, or perhaps begin to avoid or withdraw in discomfort—in either case confirming R's diagnosis of being in denial or resistant or recalcitrant.

Not every R takes the pugilistic route, however. Another natural response for R is to offer alternative solutions: "Well, all right, then how about *this* op-tion?" taking up another possible resolution to the person's problem. Again A's next line in the script is easy to anticipate. It is likely to have a "yes, but . . . " quality, expressing the other side of the ambivalence. Whichever of these two ways R goes—arguing more forcefully for R's preferred solution, or coming up with other possible resolutions—the conversation is likely to end with both being dissatisfied and frustrated. It can also have the paradoxical ef-fect of pushing A further toward the opposite of what R intended.

Why doesn't direct advocacy work in this situation? What R and A are doing, in essence, is acting out A's ambivalence. R takes one side, and naturallyA responds by defending the other. This might have some psycho-dramatic value, were it not for an important principle of social psychology: as a person argues on behalf of one position, he or she becomes more committed to it. In the language of self-perception theory,[1] "As I hear myself talk, I learn what I believe." In everyday language, we can literally *talk* ourselves into (or out of) things. If A is caused to take up the opposite side of the ambivalence dilemma, and to point out the down side of the course of action for which R is arguing, then that course of action (which R presumably favors) becomes *less* likely to occur. In effect, A is inadvertently talked out of it. Even if A respects the opinion and expertise of R, A is moved toward the other pole by the very act of defending it. This may explain our finding that the more "resistance" was evoked during a counseling session with a problem drinker, the more he or she was still drinking a year later. Conversely, the more a person's speech reflects increasing commitment to change over the course of a conversation, the more likely actual change is to occur.

What we have learned from this is that it can be important to inhibit the righting reflex. It is analogous to something that anyone must learn who is go-ing to drive a vehicle on snow and ice. When the tires begin to slide off the road to the right, there is a natural tendency to turn the steering wheel to the left, because that is where you want to go. Doing so, however, simply de-creases control and increases skidding toward the right. Wrong as it feels in the beginning, you must turn in the direction of the skid, turn the wheel to the right when the vehicle is skidding to the right. This provides traction that allows you to redirect momentum back onto the road.

MOTIVATION AS INTERPERSONAL PROCESS

What we are saying here is that motivation is in many ways an *interpersonal* process, the product of an interaction between people. This departs somewhat from the popular notion that motivation is internal, residing within the individual as a personal state or trait. Motivation for change can not only be influenced by but in a very real sense arises from an interpersonal context.

This clearly has implications for counseling. When someone comes for professional consultation, there may be an assumption that the person is already motivated for change. Indeed, many counseling approaches devote little attention to motivation and assume its presence. The person who does not follow through with advice that is given may then be faulted for being unmotivated, rather than considering that the difficulty (and the solution) may lie in the interpersonal context. Our perspective is that exploring and enhancing motivation for change is itself a proper task, at times even the most important and necessary task, within helping relationships such as counseling, health care, and education.

Developing Discrepancy

All of this points toward a fundamental dynamic in the resolution of ambivalence: *It is the client who should be voicing the arguments for change.* When you find yourself in the role of arguing for change while your client (patient, student, child) is voicing arguments against it, you're in precisely the wrong role. Counselor and client in this situation occupy complementary roles. Although the scripts are familiar and predictable, both parties often leave the interaction frustrated and dissatisfied, each perhaps blaming the other, and very little positive change occurs. Our colleague, Jeff Allison, suggested the useful analogy that such a relationship feels like wrestling, with each partner grappling to gain the advantage; wrestling leaves both participants tired and at least one of them feeling defeated. Motivational interviewing is more like dancing: rather than struggling against each other, the partners move together smoothly. The fact that one of them is leading is subtle and is not necessarily apparent to an observer. Good leading is gentle, responsive, and imaginative.

It is discrepancy that underlies the perceived importance of change: no discrepancy, no motivation. The discrepancy is generally between present status and a desired goal, between what is happening and how one would want things to be (one's goals). Note that this is the difference between two *perceptions*, and the degree of discrepancy (also a perception) is affected by a change in either. The larger the discrepancy, the greater the importance of change.

Because it involves perception, however, discrepancy is more complex than mere subtraction. For example, one's behavior can come into conflict with a deeply held value without there being a change in either. This happens particularly when there is a change not in the behavior but in the perceived *meaning* of the behavior. Consider this example:

> [A man] dates his quitting [smoking] from a day on which he had gone to pick up his children at the city library. A thunderstorm greeted him as he arrived there; and at the same time a search of his pockets disclosed a familiar problem: he was out of cigarettes. Glancing back at the library, he caught a glimpse of his children stepping out in the rain, but he continued around the corner, certain that he could find a parking space, rush in, buy the cigarettes, and be back before the children got seriously wet. The view of himself as a father who would "actually leave the kids in the rain while he ran after cigarettes" was . . . humiliating, and he quit smoking.[2]

Neither his smoking nor his value of being a good father had changed. It was the meaning of his smoking—the perception that it had become more important than his children—that suddenly became unacceptable to him. When a behavior comes into conflict with a deeply held value, it is usually the behavior that changes.[3]

There is an obvious overlap between ambivalence and discrepancy. Without some discrepancy, there is no ambivalence. For some people, then, the first step toward change is to *become* ambivalent. As discrepancy increases, ambivalence first intensifies; then, if the discrepancy continues to grow, ambivalence can be resolved in the direction of change. Conceptualized in this way, ambivalence is not really an obstacle to change. Rather, it is ambivalence that makes change possible.

Change Talk: Self-Motivating Speech

So the challenge is to first intensify and then resolve ambivalence by developing discrepancy between the actual present and the desired future. The righting reflex can lead one toward overtly directive and confrontational communications, intended to "make the person face up to reality," but, as we have discussed, this can have precisely the opposite effect to what was intended because it elicits counterchange arguments. Follow the instinct of the righting reflex, and you wind up asking exactly the wrong kinds of questions:

> "Why don't you want to change?"
> "How can you tell me that you don't have a problem?"
> "What makes you think that you're not at risk?"
> "Why don't you just . . . ?"
> "Why can't you . . . ?"

The literal answer to any of these questions is a defense of status quo, an explanation of why change isn't important or practical. In other words, such questions elicit just the opposite kind of speech to that which moves a person toward change.

Change is facilitated instead by communicating in a way that elicits the person's own reasons for and advantages of change. (We will discuss the practicalities of this approach in more detail in Part II.) Change talk generally falls into one of these four categories.

1. *Disadvantages of the status quo.* These statements acknowledge that there is reason for concern or discontent with how things are. This may or may not involve an admission of a "problem." The language generally reflects a recognition of undesirable aspects of one's present state or behavior.

2. *Advantages of change.* A second form of change talk implies recognition of the potential advantages of a change. Whereas the first type of change talk focuses on the not-so-good things about one's current status, this second type emphasizes the good things to be gained through change. Both kinds, of course, are reasons for change.

3. *Optimism for change.* A third kind of talk that favors change is that which expresses confidence and hope about one's ability to change. It may be stated in hypothetical (I *could*) or declarative form (I *can* do it). The common underlying theme is that change is possible.

4. *Intention to change.* As the balance tips, people begin to express an intention, desire, willingness, or commitment to change. The level of intention can vary from rather weak to very strong commitment language. Sometimes the intention is expressed indirectly by envisioning how things might be if change did happen.

In the discussion and chapters that follow, for convenience we have used the word "counselor" as a generic term for those in a helping or facilitating role and "client" for the person who is receiving such caring attention. The choice of these terms is arbitrary, however, and our underlying focus is on the process of communication that occurs between two people.

A Definition of Motivational Interviewing

Just as it is possible to counsel in a way that elicits resistance or counterchange talk, it is also possible to communicate in a way that elicits change talk and thereby nudges a person toward change. That is the starting point for understanding motivational interviewing.

First the choice of the term itself deserves comment. The "motivational" part is obvious enough, but why "interviewing"? The connotative meanings of "interview" in English are quite different from those of words like "therapy," "treatment," and "counseling." There is more of an egalitarian, sometimes even subordinate sense to the word "interview." Reporters interview famous people. Students interview experts to learn about a new topic. Of course, employers also interview potential employees. The word itself doesn't imply who has more power or is more important. It is an inter-view, a looking together at something. One image that we use is of two people sitting side by side, paging through a family album of pictures—one telling stories, the other listening with friendly and personal interest. The storyteller turns the pages. The listener wants to learn and understand and occasionally asks politely about a particular picture or a detail not mentioned. It is a rather different image from examination, treatment, therapy, or expert consultation. It is an inter-view, looking and seeing together.

We define motivational interviewing as *a client-centered, directive method for enhancing intrinsic motivation to change by exploring and resolving ambivalence*. The pieces of this definition merit some examination.

First, motivational interviewing is client-centered or person-centered in its focus on the concerns and perspectives of the individual, as well as in our heavy reliance on and indebtedness to the work of Carl Rogers and his colleagues. In this sense, motivational interviewing is an evolution of the client-centered counseling approach that Rogers developed. Motivational interviewing does not focus on teaching new coping skills, reshaping cognitions, or excavating the past. It is quite focused on the person's present interests and concerns. Whatever discrepancies are explored and developed have to do with incongruities among aspects of the person's own experiences and values.

Second, motivational interviewing differs from the method described by Rogers as it is consciously directive. The terms "client-centered" and "nondirective" are sometimes used interchangeably, but they refer to different aspects of counseling style. Motivational interviewing is intentionally addressed to the resolution of ambivalence, often in a particular direction of change. The interviewer elicits and selectively reinforces change talk and then responds to resistance in a way that is intended to diminish it. Motivational interviewing involves selective responding to speech in a way that resolves ambivalence and moves the person toward change.

Third, we emphasize that motivational interviewing is a method of communication rather than a set of techniques. It is not a bag of tricks for getting people to do what they don't want to do. It is not something that one does *to* people; rather, it is fundamentally a way of being with and for people—a facilitative approach to communication that evokes natural change.[4]

Fourth, the focus of motivational interviewing is on eliciting the person's intrinsic motivation for change. Motivational interviewing differs from motivational strategies that are intended to impose change through extrinsic means: by legal sanctions, punishment, social pressure, financial gain, and such. Behavioral approaches often seek to rearrange the person's social environment so that one kind of behavior is reinforced and another is discouraged. We mean to imply no judgment about such extrinsic approaches, which can be quite effective in modifying behavior. It is just that motivational interviewing focuses on intrinsic motivation for change, even with those who initially come for counseling as a direct result of extrinsic pressure (such as court mandate).

Fifth, the method focuses on exploring and resolving ambivalence as a key in eliciting change. It centers on the motivational processes within the individual that facilitate change. The motivational interviewing method is not (and, we believe, cannot be) used to impose change that is inconsistent with the person's own values and beliefs. In this way it differs from coercive methods for motivating change. Unless a change in some way is in the person's inherent interest, it will not happen. Within motivational interviewing, change arises through its relevance to the person's own values and concerns.

Limitations of Motivational Interviewing

Before we embark on an explanation of the style and practicalities of motivational interviewing, there are a few important points to be made. First, although we have had two decades of experience in developing and studying this approach, we believe we are only beginning to understand it. Clinical research evaluating the efficacy of motivational interviewing (reviewed in Chapter 16) has been encouraging, but it is still in a very early stage. There is reasonable evidence *that* motivational interviewing works in certain applications, but the data thus far are less clear in documenting *how* and *why* it works.

We also do not regard motivational interviewing to be a panacea, the answer to most or all counseling and behavior change problems. It is one method that can be used in concert with others. Neither do we believe that it is the best or only way to enhance motivation for change with everyone. In some contexts, it is entirely appropriate to educate, offer clear advice, teach skills, coerce, or make decisions for another. There are people who prefer, at least in some situations, simply to be told what to do and will then do it.

Neither is there clarity yet about the outer limits of motivational interviewing. We have no definitive answer yet to the question, "With whom should one *not* use this approach?" In search of its limits, there have been tests of motivational interviewing with ever more challenging populations: seriously alcohol-dependent or drug-dependent people, adolescents, court-mandated offenders, and those with chronic illnesses (see Part IV). There are already some indications from such studies that there may be certain subgroups who show more change when offered another approach—perhaps those who are less resistant and more ready for change at the outset of counseling. One very large study[5] of treatment for alcohol use disorders found that response to motivational enhancement therapy was not altered by sociopathy, severity of alcohol involvement, concomitant psychological problems, or cognitive impairment. In this same study, angry people fared particularly well with a motivational interviewing–based approach, whereas those less angry at the beginning of treatment did somewhat better in cognitive-behavioral or twelve-step counseling. Much remains to be learned about when motivational interviewing is most and least effective.

INTEGRATION WITH OTHER TREATMENT APPROACHES

Finally, we offer some reflections on ways in which motivational interviewing can be integrated with other methods for facilitating change. While motivational interviewing can be contrasted with different counseling approaches (as we did in our first edition), this in no way renders motivational interviewing incompatible with other methods. Fundamentally, motivational interviewing is intended to instigate change. For some people, this is all they need. Once they move from ambivalence to commitment, change proceeds apace without additional help. Others find that they need further assistance to carry out the change they desire after motivational interviewing. In that regard other change methods can follow naturally from motivational interviewing.

Our original conception of motivational interviewing, in fact, was that it would be a preparation for further treatment, enhancing motivation and adherence. In the beginning, it was not meant to be a stand-alone method. This realization came later, as research revealed change occurring soon after a session or two of motivational interviewing without further treatment, relative to control groups receiving no counseling at all. Several studies also show the effects originally intended: that clients who receive motivational interviewing at the beginning of treatment are likely to stay in treatment longer, work harder, adhere more closely to treatment recommendations, and experience substantially better outcomes than those who receive the same treatment program without motivational interviewing. In the treatment of substance use disorders, which is where the largest number of studies have been conducted to date, adding motivational interviewing has been found to facilitate treatments as diverse as cognitive-behavioral skill training, twelve-step and disease model counseling, and methadone maintenance.[6]

The most obvious integration, then, is to offer motivational interviewing as a first consultation, as a prelude to other services. This can be particularly useful in settings where duration of consultation is limited (e.g., employee assistance programs) and with populations where early dropout from treatment occurs at a high rate (e.g., drug dependence). In such cases, if motivational interviewing is the only intervention that one has the opportunity to offer, there is reason to believe that something helpful has been given. At the same time, motivational interviewing appears to increase the likelihood that people will return for additional treatment, increasing the opportunity to receive other services. For those who need or desire additional help in pursuing change, further treatment can be provided.

Surprisingly, it may also not matter if the subsequent treatment is in some way inconsistent with the principles of motivational interviewing. In one study,[7] for example, motivational interviewing was given (or not given) at intake to an inpatient treatment program with a confrontive and overtly directive approach. Yet program counselors (unaware of group assignment) perceived motivational interviewing recipients to be more motivated and compliant in treatment, and 12-month outcomes were substantially better in the motivational interviewing group than in people who were going through the same inpatient program without initial motivational interviewing.

Another way to think about integration is that motivational interviewing is a counseling and communication style that can be used throughout treatment, not simply as a prelude. There are already integrations of the motivational interviewing style with consultations as diverse as feedback of assessment results,[8] prenatal counseling,[9] and diabetes management.[10] The essential information and interventions are delivered in the style of motivational interviewing, which is both directive and client-centered. There is a dance back and forth between didactic material and asking for the person's reactions and perspectives.

Still another possibility is to keep motivational interviewing in the background, to be returned to as motivational issues emerge further down the line in treatment. Ambivalence does not usually disappear at the moment treatment begins. New motivational challenges may be encountered as homework assignments are given or as more difficult phases of treatment are reached. At such points it is possible to fall back to motivational interviewing in order to resolve new motivational issues as they arise.

As an illustration, all three of these applications of motivational interviewing—as a prelude, a permeating style, and a fall-back option—have been integrated into a comprehensive behavioral intervention for alcohol dependence in a multisite clinical trial.[11] The first session is strictly motivational interviewing—eliciting and listening to the person's concerns and reasons for change. Feedback of assessment results in a motivational interviewing style begins in the second session, followed by a thorough functional analysis of alcohol use in the person's life. All of this is then drawn together into a treatment plan, drawing on a menu of cognitive-behavioral skill-training modules to address specific goals for change. These modules are then delivered within a permeating motivational interviewing style, and the counselor can fall back to motivational interviewing whenever particular motivational issues or obstacles arise. Personal choice and autonomy are emphasized throughout treatment.

NOTES

1. Bem (1967, 1972).
2. Premack (1970), p. 115.
3. Rockeach (1973).
4. Rollnick and Miller (1995); Sobell and Sobell (1993).
5. Project MATCH Research Group (1997a, 1997b).

6. Aubrey (1998); Bien, Miller, and Boroughs (1993); Brown and Miller (1993); Saunders, Wilkinson, and Phillips (1995).
7. Brown and Miller (1993).
8. Miller, Zweben, DiClemente, and Rychtarik (1992).
9. Handmaker, Miller, and Manicke (1999).
10. Smith, Heckemeyer, Kratt, and Mason (1997); Trigwell, Grant, and House (1997).
11. Miller (in press).

PART II

Practice

CHAPTER 4

What Is Motivational Interviewing?

> If you treat an individual as he is, he will stay as he is, but if you treat him as if he were what he ought to be and could be, he will become what he ought to be and could be.
> —JOHANN WOLFGANG VON GOETHE

SPIRIT OF MOTIVATIONAL INTERVIEWING

In the 11 years since the first edition of this book, we have found ourselves placing less emphasis on techniques of motivational interviewing and ever greater emphasis on the fundamental spirit that underlies it. This happened in part because we encountered individuals who were mimicking some of the component techniques without understanding their overall context yet believing that they were doing (or teaching) the method itself. We also began to see descriptions and evaluations of interventions called "motivational interviewing" that bore little resemblance to our understanding of the method. The broader term "motivational interventions" (which might include anything from cash vouchers to cattle prods) has come into use and is further confused with motivational interviewing.

This is, of course, a common phenomenon in the diffusion of innovations.[1] One approach is to try to control use of the term, to certify practitioners, and to copyright procedures. In this way one can devote full-time effort to policing perceived misuse of a method. We decided instead to focus our limited time and efforts on doing what we could to promote quality practice, training, and research and to specify as clearly as possible what motivational interviewing is and is not.[2]

33

If motivational interviewing is a way of being with people, then its underlying spirit lies in understanding and experiencing the human nature that gives rise to that way of being. How one thinks about and understands the interviewing process is vitally important in shaping the interview.

Collaboration

Certainly one key component of the spirit of motivational interviewing is its collaborative nature. The counselor avoids an authoritarian one-up stance, instead communicating a partner-like relationship. The method of motivational interviewing involves exploration more than exhortation, and support rather than persuasion or argument. The interviewer seeks to create a positive interpersonal atmosphere that is conducive but not coercive to change. The collaborative nature of the method implies being attuned to and monitoring one's own aspirations. The interpersonal process of motivational interviewing is a meeting of aspirations, which frequently differ. Without awareness of one's own opinion and investment, one has only half the picture. (See Chapter 12 for further discussion of this ethical issue.)

Evocation

Consistent with a collaborative role, the interviewer's tone is not one of imparting things (such as wisdom, insight, reality) but rather of *eliciting*, of finding these things within and drawing them out from the person. To draw a parallel distinction from education, the Latin verb *docere* (a root of *doctor*, *doctrine*, and *indoctrinate*) implies an expert role, an imparting or inserting of knowledge in the student. In contrast, the verb *ducare* means "to draw," as one draws water from a well, so that *educare* is to draw out. It is the latter form of education, with Socratic roots, that is an apt analogy for the process of motivational interviewing. It is not an *instilling* or *installing* but, rather, an eliciting, a drawing out of motivation from the person. It requires finding intrinsic motivation for change within the person and evoking it, calling it forth.

Autonomy

In motivational interviewing, responsibility for change is left with the client—which, by the way, is where we believe it *must* lie, no matter how much professionals may debate what people can be "made" or "allowed" or "permitted" to do and choose. Another way to say this is that there is respect for the individual's autonomy. The client is always free to take counsel—or not. The overall goal is to increase intrinsic motivation, so that change arises from within rather than being imposed from without and so that change serves the person's own goals and values. As indicated earlier, when motivational interviewing is done properly, it is the client rather than the counselor who presents the arguments for change.

BOX 4.1. The Spirit of Motivational Interviewing

Fundamental approach of motivational interviewing	Mirror-image opposite approach to counseling
Collaboration. Counseling involves a partnership that honors the client's expertise and perspectives. The counselor provides an atmosphere that is conducive rather than coercive to change.	*Confrontation.* Counseling involves overriding the client's impaired perspectives by imposing awareness and acceptance of "reality" that the client cannot see or will not admit.
Evocation. The resources and motivation for change are presumed to reside within the client. Intrinsic motivation for change is enhanced by drawing on the client's own perceptions, goals, and values.	*Education.* The client is presumed to lack key knowledge, insight, and/or skills that are necessary for change to occur. The counselor seeks to address these deficits by providing the requisite enlightenment.
Autonomy. The counselor affirms the client's right and capacity for self-direction and facilitates informed choice.	*Authority.* The counselor tells the client what he or she must do.

HOW BROAD IS THE HORIZON?

A meta-issue to be dealt with here is the question of where motivational interviewing is applicable and where it is not. As the name implies, its intended focus is on motivational struggles, issues of change for which a person is not clearly ready and willing, or is ambivalent. Motivational interviewing itself is a skillful clinical method, a style of counseling and psychotherapy. It is not a set of techniques that one can learn quickly in order to deal with annoying motivational problems.

This has implications for both where and by whom motivational interviewing is practiced. There has been substantial interest, for example, in applications of motivational interviewing within medical settings, where motivational issues in patient behavior change are quite common but where practitioners may have only a few minutes to deal with them. The desire of practitioners in such settings is usually for something simple that can be done quickly to address patient reluctance to change health-relevant behavior. That desire is legitimate, and there are various simpler methods that can be useful in such contexts,[3] but we distinguish these from motivational interviewing as a clinical method (see Chapter 18 of this volume).

The difference is a bit like that between a fully trained physician and a paramedic or medical technician who is taught when and how to perform certain procedures skillfully. The physician, broadly trained in medicine, is able to draw flexibly from a wide array of clinical skills and knowledge in treating a range of health problems that patients bring. The paramedic learns more circumscribed skills that can be quite valuable, even life-saving, when applied in a timely manner within the context of relatively brief contact.

In the same way, a skillful motivational interviewer has learned and practiced the broad clinical method of motivational interviewing that can be applied flexibly to a wide range of motivational issues. There are practical subtleties and ethical complexities that are familiar to an experienced motivational interviewing clinician, who is prepared to adapt and apply the method with a broad range of people and problems.

This is not at all to say that busy health professionals cannot or should not learn the clinical method of motivational interviewing. There are many who are already superb listeners and have a long head start on developing clinical skillfulness in motivational interviewing. We have trained (among others) counselors, dieticians, exercise physiologists, forensic psychiatrists, nurses, physicians, pastors, probation officers, psychologists, remedial fitness instructors, caseworkers, and social workers.

As with the useful growth of paramedical practice, we have likewise been interested and involved in developing simpler techniques in the spirit of motivational interviewing, and these techniques can be applied in practice without learning and developing clinical skillfulness in the overall method of motivational interviewing. We have been careful not to call these adaptations "motivational interviewing," a term that we have reserved for the larger skillful clinical method. Some of these adaptations are discussed more fully in Chapter 18.

There are also motivational issues for which motivational interviewing is not an appropriate method, primarily for ethical reasons that are familiar to health care professionals. We would regard it as improper, for example, to apply the method of motivational interviewing in order to increase the likelihood of patients signing an informed consent to treatment or research. Ethical issues in the use of motivational interviewing are addressed in Chapter 12.

FOUR GENERAL PRINCIPLES

To help see the forest before we come to the trees, we next outline four broad guiding principles that underlie motivational interviewing. This is one step from the above-described general spirit, and toward greater specificity of practice. These represent a refinement of the principles originally outlined by Miller (1983) and of those described in our first edition. They are as follows:

1. Express empathy.
2. Develop discrepancy.
3. Roll with resistance.
4. Support self-efficacy.

We elaborate these four basic principles here, saving more specific "how-to" discussion for subsequent chapters.

1. Express Empathy

A client-centered and empathic counseling style is one fundamental and defining characteristic of motivational interviewing. We regard the therapeutic skill of reflective listening or accurate empathy, as described by Carl Rogers, to be the foundation on which clinical skillfulness in motivational interviewing is built. This style of empathic communication is employed from the very beginning and throughout the process of motivational interviewing.

The attitude underlying this principle of empathy is properly termed "acceptance." Through skillful reflective listening, the counselor seeks to understand the client's feelings and perspectives without judging, criticizing, or blaming. It is important to note here that acceptance is not the same thing as agreement or approval. It is possible to accept and understand a person's perspective while not agreeing with or endorsing it. Neither does an attitude of acceptance prohibit the counselor from differing with the client's views and expressing that divergence. The crucial attitude is a respectful listening to the person with a desire to understand his or her perspectives. Paradoxically, this kind of acceptance of people *as they are* seems to free them to change, whereas insistent nonacceptance ("You're not OK; you have to be different") tends to immobilize the change process. Family therapists call this sort of phenomenon "ironic process," because as in Greek tragedy, the action causes the very outcome that it was meant to avert. Happily, self-fulfilling prophecies work both ways. The attitude of acceptance and respect builds a working therapeutic alliance and supports the client's self-esteem, which further promotes change.

An empathic counselor seeks to respond to a person's perspectives as understandable, comprehensible, and (within the person's framework, at least) valid. Ambivalence is accepted as a normal part of human experience and change, rather than seen as pathology or pernicious defensiveness. Reluctance to change problematic behavior is to be expected in consultation and treatment settings; otherwise, the client would have changed before reaching this point. The client is not seen as uniquely pathological or incapable. Rather, the person's situation is understood as one of having become "stuck" through understandable psychological processes.

PRINCIPLE 1: EXPRESS EMPATHY.

Acceptance facilitates change.
Skillful reflective listening is fundamental.
Ambivalence is normal.

---

2. Develop Discrepancy

We certainly do *not* mean that the general goal of motivational interviewing should be to have people accept themselves as they are and stay that way. Neither do we advocate using reflective listening simply to follow people wherever they happen to wander. A person who presents with a health-threatening drug habit, for example, can be helped to change that behavior, and a person diagnosed with heart disease or diabetes is well advised to make significant changes in behavior. The question is how best to present an unpleasant reality so that the person can confront it and be changed by it.

Here motivational interviewing begins to depart from classic client-centered counseling. Motivational interviewing is intentionally directive—directed toward the resolution of ambivalence in the service of change. Totally exploratory client-centered counseling is legitimate for other purposes—for example, in helping people sort out their lives or make difficult choices. Motivational interviewing is specifically directed toward getting people unstuck, helping them move past ambivalence toward positive behavior change. (Of course, the definition of "positive" here has obvious ethical and value overtones, which are considered in Chapter 12.)

A second general principle of motivational interviewing is thus to create and amplify, from the client's perspective, a discrepancy between present behavior and his or her broader goals and values. In the original exposition of motivational interviewing,[4] this was described as creating "cognitive dissonance," borrowing a concept from Leon Festinger.[5] A more general and, we now believe, better way to understand this state is simply as a discrepancy between the present state of affairs and how one wants it to be. (This avoids invoking an inherent drive toward cognitive consistency.) Discrepancy may be triggered by an awareness of and discontent with the costs of one's present course of behavior and by perceived advantages of behavior change. When a behavior is seen as conflicting with important personal goals (such as one's health, success, family happiness, or positive self-image), change is more likely to occur.

We need to clarify here that discrepancy, as we use the term in motivational interviewing, has to do with the *importance* of change. This is different from the amount of behavior change to be accomplished, the distance that one's behavior would need to travel in order to reach the desired level (which for sake of discussion, we will term the "behavioral gap"). The two are easy to confuse, but importantly different. If the behavioral gap is very large, it can decrease motivation by diminishing confidence. The wider a chasm, the less the confidence in one's ability to jump it. A behavioral gap might be quite small, but the importance of jumping it very high. Whereas one can easily imagine a behavioral gap that is so large as to be demotivating, it is difficult to imagine a change that is too important to make. Just as importance and confidence are different aspects of motivation (see Chapter 6), so discrepancy and behavioral gap affect motivation in different ways.

Many people who seek consultation already perceive significant discrepancy between what is happening and what they want to happen. Yet they are also ambivalent, caught in an approach–avoidance conflict. A goal of motivational interviewing is to develop discrepancy—to make use of it, increase it, and amplify it until it overrides the inertia of the status quo. The methods of motivational interviewing seek to accomplish this within the person, rather than relying primarily on external and coercive motivators (e.g., pressure from the spouse, threat of unemployment, or court-imposed contingencies). This often involves identifying and clarifying the person's own goals and values with which the behavior may conflict. When skillfully done, motivational interviewing changes the person's perceptions (of discrepancy) without creating any sense of being pressured or coerced. This is because the discrepancy is between current behavior and goals or values that are important to the person. A sense of coercion arises when a person is pressured to change behavior because it is discrepant with *someone else's* goals or values.

The general approach is one that results in the client presenting the reasons for change, rather than the counselor doing so. People are often more persuaded by what they hear themselves say than by what other people tell them. When motivational interviewing is done well, it is not the counselor but the client who gives voice to concerns, reasons for change, self-efficacy, and intentions to change.

PRINCIPLE 2: DEVELOP DISCREPANCY.

The client rather than the counselor should present the arguments for change.

Change is motivated by a perceived discrepancy between present behavior and important personal goals or values.

---

3. Roll with Resistance

It follows from this that the least desirable situation, from the standpoint of evoking change, is for the counselor to advocate for change while the client argues against it. Such argumentation is counterproductive. Not only is the ambivalent person unlikely to be persuaded, but direct argument may actually press the person in the opposite direction that he or she is caused to defend.

If you don't argue for change, then what do you do? Jay Haley and other pioneers in the field of strategic family therapy made the analogy of psychological judo, referring to martial arts in which an attack is not met with direct opposition (as in boxing), but rather one goes with the attacker's momentum, using it to good advantage. It makes no difference what one throws at a master of this art. All blows fall on empty air, and the harder one attacks, the faster one falls into nothing.

This analogy can easily be taken too far. Motivational interviewing is not combat or even a chess match; it is not about winning and losing. The person is not an opponent to be outsmarted or defeated. Yet the illustration of rolling with resistance is useful. Resistance that a person offers can be turned or reframed slightly to create a new momentum toward change. The object that is in motion here is not a body but a perception. The problems and specifics of how this works will come later. For now, the point is that in motivational interviewing one does not directly oppose resistance but, rather, rolls or flows with it.

There is also an element here of great respect for the person. What to do about a problem, if anything, is ultimately an individual decision. Reluctance and ambivalence are not opposed but are acknowledged to be natural and understandable. The counselor does not impose new views or goals; rather, the person is invited to consider new information and is offered new perspectives. "Take what you want and leave the rest" is the permissive kind of advice that pervades this approach. It's an approach that is hard to fight against.

In motivational interviewing, the counselor also commonly turns a question or problem back to the person. It is not the counselor's job to provide all the answers and generate all the solutions. Doing so, in fact, invites the person to find the flaws in each idea ("Yes, but . . . "). It is assumed that the person is a capable and autonomous individual, with important insight and ideas for the solution of his or her own problems. Rolling with resistance, then, includes involving the person actively in the process of problem solving.

Finally, client behaviors that are labeled as "resistance" represent, in motivational interviewing, a signal for the counselor to shift approach. Resistance is an interpersonal phenomenon, and how the counselor responds will influence whether it increases or diminishes.

PRINCIPLE 3: ROLL WITH RESISTANCE.

Avoid arguing for change.
Resistance is not directly opposed.
New perspectives are invited but not imposed.
The client is a primary resource in finding answers and solutions.
Resistance is a signal to respond differently.

---

4. Support Self-Efficacy

A fourth important principle of motivational interviewing involves the concept of *self-efficacy*, which refers to a person's belief in his or her ability to carry out and succeed with a specific task. Self-efficacy is a key element in motivation for change and is a reasonably good predictor of treatment outcome. A counselor may follow the first three principles outlined here, and thereby develop a person's perception that he or she has an important problem. If the client perceives no hope or possibility for change, however, then no effort will be made, and the counselor's efforts have been in vain.

Although self-efficacy is a relatively recent term, healers have long recognized that hope and faith are important elements of change.[6] The counselor's own expectations about a person's likelihood of change can have a powerful effect on outcome, acting as a self-fulfilling prophecy.[7] A general goal of motivational interviewing is to enhance the client's confidence in his or her capability to cope with obstacles and to succeed in change.

Self-efficacy is the other side of personal responsibility for change. To assert that a person is responsible for deciding and directing his or her own change is to assume that the person is capable of doing so. The person not only can but must make the change, in the sense that no one else can do it for him or her. Motivational interviewing does not foster the view that the counselor will change the client. "I will change you" is not the intended message. A more appropriate message is, "If you wish, I can help you change." A person may also be encouraged by the success of others or by his or her own past successes in changing behavior.

PRINCIPLE 4: SUPPORT SELF-EFFICACY.

A person's belief in the possibility of change is an important motivator.

The client, not the counselor, is responsible for choosing and carrying out change.

The counselor's own belief in the person's ability to change becomes a self-fulfilling prophecy.

SUMMARY

Before learning and while practicing motivational interviewing, it is vital to understand the overall spirit and underlying assumptions of the method. Motivational interviewing honors and respects the individual's autonomy to choose. It is a collaborative, not a prescriptive, approach, in which the counselor evokes the person's own intrinsic motivation and resources for change. Implicit is the belief that such motivation and resourcefulness do lie within each individual and need to be evoked rather than imposed. We believe that each person possesses a powerful potential for change. The counselor's task is to release that potential and to facilitate the natural change processes that are already inherent in the individual. Motivational interviewing is about helping to free people from the ambivalence that entraps them in repetitive cycles of self-defeating or self-destructive behavior.

Motivational interviewing is a skillful clinical method, not a set of techniques that can be easily learned. It is more than a set of techniques for *doing* counseling. It is a way of *being* with people, which is likely to be quite different from how others may have treated them in the past. It is designed to resolve motivational issues that inhibit positive behavior change. Simpler techniques in the spirit of motivational interviewing have been adapted for use where training and consultation time is more limited, but these should not be understood to constitute the method of motivational interviewing.

Four broad principles underlie the specific methods that are described in the subsequent chapters of Part II. We have discussed them apart from practical how-to elements in order to provide a larger context regarding the "why" of practice. These principles bespeak the more general spirit and philosophy that underlie motivational interviewing. This way of being is not the whole story of change, of course. There are many specific treatment strategies that can be quite helpful as people pursue the course of change. Motivational interviewing is intended to get the person unstuck—to start the change process happening. Once begun, change may occur rapidly with relatively little additional assistance, or it may require a span of professional consultation and support.

We turn now to eight chapters addressing specific aspects of the practice of motivational interviewing. In Chapter 5 we discuss the polarity of change talk and resistance, which is the central dimension to which one attends in practicing motivational interviewing. In Chapter 6, we introduce methods that are important from the outset and which can help you avoid some common traps that await you. These methods are most appropriate for building motivation to change, the first of two major phases of motivational interviewing. In Chapters 7 to 9 we explain three key areas of skill that are fundamental to motivational interviewing: reflective listening, responding to change talk, and responding to resistance. Then in Chapter 10 we proceed to discuss methods appropriate for strengthening the commitment to change, the second phase of motivational interviewing. Chapter 11 offers a practical case from start to finish to illustrate how the methods of motivational interviewing are interwoven. Then in Chapter 12 we address issues of ethics, values, and priorities that arise when one practices motivational interviewing.

NOTES

1. Rogers (1995).
2. See Chapter 18, this volume; see also Rollnick and Miller (1995).
3. Rollnick, Mason, and Butler (1999).
4. Miller (1983).
5. Festinger (1957).
6. Frank and Frank (1991); Miller (1985); Shapiro (1971).
7. Jones (1977); Leake and King (1977); Parker, Winstead, and Willi (1979).

CHAPTER 5

Change and Resistance
Opposite Sides of a Coin

"Why are you drinking?" demanded the little prince.
"So that I may forget," replied the tippler.
"Forget what?" inquired the little prince, who already was sorry
  for him.
"Forget that I am ashamed," the tippler confessed, hanging his
  head.
"Ashamed of what?" insisted the little prince, who wanted to help.
"Ashamed of drinking!" The tippler brought his speech to an end,
  and shut himself up in an impregnable silence.
And the little prince went away puzzled.
"The grown-ups are certainly very, very odd," he said to himself.
                    —ANTOINE DE SAINT-EXUPÉRY, *The Little Prince*

CONSONANCE AND DISSONANCE

When things are going well in a motivational interview, there is a sense of moving together smoothly, like two dancers gliding across a ballroom floor. There may be some missteps, a small bump or loss of balance here and there, even occasional stepping on toes, but in general the two partners move together.

The feeling is quite different when instead of moving together, the counselor and client seem to be struggling against each other, grappling for control like two adversaries in a wrestling match. One opponent may be bigger or more powerful than the other, but each seeks to pin the other while warily avoiding being pinned. Consider this dialogue between probation officer and a man on probation, during a weekly check-in visit.

PROBATION OFFICER: What have you been doing this week?

CLIENT: Not much, really.

PROBATION OFFICER: What about finding a job?

CLIENT: Yeah, I've been looking.

PROBATION OFFICER: How seriously?

CLIENT: I've been looking, OK? I put in two applications this week.

PROBATION OFFICER: Good for you. Where?

CLIENT: At the gas station and the supermarket near my apartment. Listen, it would be a lot easier for me to find a job if I had my driver's license back, and if I didn't have to come here every week.

PROBATION OFFICER: So tell me why you don't have driving privileges.

CLIENT: I was driving with a suspended license . . . looking for a job!

PROBATION OFFICER: And your license was suspended because . . .

CLIENT: You know why. I didn't pay the fine for a couple of tickets. I could pay it if I could get to a job.

PROBATION OFFICER: And you're telling me that in a whole week you've only put in two job applications?

Although it sounds like these two are talking about the same topic, employment, in fact they have quite different agendas. Each wants something from the other. The probation officer wants this man to be employed and, more generally, to maintain a responsible lifestyle. The man wants greater freedom, and specifically he wants his driving license reinstated. Both evade the other's grasp and seek to shift the conversation to their own preferred topic.

We have chosen the terms "consonant" and "dissonant" as the two poles of a continuum for describing how a conversation (and counseling relationship) is going at any given time. Clearly, in the preceding example, the conversation was leaning toward the dissonant end of the scale. The ends of the scale might equally be anchored by the terms "dancing" and "wrestling." In either case, the terminology describes the present nature of an interaction. The counseling alliance or relationship fluctuates along this continuum of consonance versus dissonance.

The probation counselor might characterize the client's behavior in this example as defensive or resistant. From the counselor's perspective, "The client is not taking my lead." In preparing this second edition, we debated whether to retain or remove the term "resistance" in writing about motivational interviewing, for there are several aspects of the term that trouble us.

Chief among these is an implicit tone of blaming the person for being uncooperative, or at least attributing the problem to the client's pathology. What is happening in the preceding conversation is not the product of one person, but of two. It is a function of their interaction. Dissonance in a counseling relationship is not the product of resistance—of only one person's behavior.

As will be elaborated next, we decided to retain the concept of resistance and to rehabilitate it. Resistance is something that occurs only within the context of a relationship or a system. In the physics of electricity, it is an attribute related to current flow within a system. In human psychology, it is something that happens between people. A difficulty is that within the context of psychotherapy, resistance is usually used to describe the behavior of only one person, the client. Although transference has its countertransference in psychoanalysis, there is no corresponding concept of counterresistance to describe the counselor's role in evoking and maintaining this interaction. Later in this chapter, we propose such a term and offer a more specific behavioral definition for client resistance.

At a larger level, however, we wanted to describe the fluctuating nature of a relationship, and this is how we arrived at the continuum of consonance and dissonance. Drawing on the musical analogy, dissonance cannot be judged from a single note but involves the relationship between notes. There is a clear connotation of working together in a manner that is harmonious versus discordant, and unlike dancing and wrestling, these two terms are direct antonyms. Our only reluctance was the potential confusion of dissonance with cognitive dissonance, a concept that sometimes is used in conceptualizing motivational interviewing,[1] although not in this volume.

When a relationship is going dissonant, it is important to understand why. To use the term "resistance" as explanatory seems to suggest that things are not going smoothly because of something that one person (the client) is doing. We advocate a more relational view, in which client resistance behavior is, at most, a signal of dissonance in the relationship. In a way, it is oxymoronic to say that one person is not cooperating. It requires at least two people to not cooperate, to yield dissonance.

WHAT CAUSES DISSONANCE?

In the preceding dialogue, one important source of dissonance was that the two people clearly had different agendas, different aspirations. In part, the struggle was over whose agenda would be negotiated and whose aspirations fulfilled. As it went, there was not much negotiation happening at all. Each wanted something different and eluded the other's attempts to establish the topic of conversation.

There are many other possible sources of dissonant communication, besides the two parties having different goals. Some arise from a mismatch of counselor strategy to client readiness level, even when the two agree about the topic of conversation. If a person is ambivalent about a particular change, for example, and the counselor has jumped ahead to talk about how the person can take action to accomplish the change, there is dissonance. This happens not just in counseling relationships but in any interaction where one person communicates a level of request or demand for change that is higher than the other's level of readiness for change.[2] If either the client or the counselor brings into the room a high level of anger or frustration (as might occur if the client has been kept waiting for a long period of time), there can be dissonance at the outset. If a counselor, instead of listening, responds in the ways characterized in Chapter 6 as roadblocks, there is likely to be dissonance. A misunderstanding of the other's intent can yield dissonance.

Another important source of dissonance is particularly pertinent in understanding motivational interviewing, and that is a lack of agreement about roles in the relationship. This is common in parental interactions with teenagers. As adolescents mature, their relationship to their parents shifts, and dissonance emerges around issues of autonomy. The parent who rigidly maintains a stance of "I'm in charge here, and you will do whatever I tell you" may run headlong into an adolescent who asserts, "You can't tell me what to do." Their roles are defined, and the stage is set for a power struggle. Similar dynamics can emerge when counselor and client have different implicit assumptions about who is in charge and who determines what the client should do.

Remembering that consonance–dissonance is a fluctuating state, the next question is what happens when dissonance occurs. We believe it is the counselor's responsibility to perceive the dissonance, understand its source, and find ways to restore consonance in the working relationship. How to do this is a primary topic of Chapter 8.

CHANGE TALK AND RESISTANCE

This brings us back to the subject of resistance. We are using this term, as is customary, to describe certain kinds of client responses, albeit with the recognition that they occur in the context of and are influenced by interpersonal interaction. Whereas consonance–dissonance describes the current nature of a relationship and interaction, we use resistance (and change talk) to refer to client behavior. Putting these two constructs together, *client resistance behavior is a signal of dissonance in the counseling relationship.*

Client resistance is a meaningful signal. In counseling where the target behavior was problem drinking, we found that resistance, defined as we describe it here, predicted a lack of change in drinking. The more resistance responses occurred during a single session of counseling, the more the person was drinking 3 months, 6 months, and 12 months later.[3] This and other research further demonstrated that client resistance behavior is under the experimental control of the counselor; it can be increased or decreased, depending on how the counselor responds to it.[4]

Just as consonance and dissonance are opposite ends of a relationship continuum, resistance behavior has a conceptual opposite that we now call "change talk." (In the first edition we referred to this with the more unwieldy term "self-motivational statements," which we have found in training to be a confusing descriptor.) As a reminder from Chapter 3, we identify four categories of change talk: disadvantages of the status quo, advantages of change, optimism for change, and intention to change. Change talk reflects movement of the person *toward* change, while resistance represents and predicts movement *away* from change.

It is important, therefore, for the counselor to recognize both change talk and resistance responses. Within motivational interviewing, there are specific ways of responding to each of these client behaviors. In fact, ways of responding are the principal topic of Chapters 8 and 9. Motivational interviewing tends to evoke high levels of change talk and relatively low levels of resistance. In contrast, confrontational counseling tends to evoke high levels of resistance and relatively low levels of change talk, and this pattern predicts a lack of long-term behavior change.

There are many ways of defining client resistance responses. In our first edition, we focused on specific observable client behaviors (rather than inferring unconscious processes). The behavior categories shown in Box 5.1 are adapted from an observational system that was originally developed at the Oregon Research Institute to study client resistance during treatment sessions.[5] In this system, there are four major categories of client resistance responses. Each of these four of has been found to predict a *lack* of future behavior change.[6] To be sure, these categories can overlap. Except for certain research purposes, it is not necessary to be concerned about which category is the right classification for a particular client response. The point is that these responses signal dissonance in the counseling process and may indicate that the person is moving away from the direction of change.

As we explored further the dynamics of motivational interviewing, however, we began to encounter some shortcomings in defining resistance simply as behaviors such as disagreeing. For example, in both of the following examples, the client's response could be coded as arguing:

NURSE: Your diabetes is really unstable, and you've got to stop playing Russian roulette with sweets and insulin.

PATIENT: It's not that bad, really. I know what I'm doing.

NURSE: It may be that the freedom to eat whatever you want, whenever you want, is so important to you that you're willing to put up with the consequences, no matter how severe.

PATIENT: Well, I don't know if it's *that* important. I don't want to go blind or lose my feet or anything like that.

BOX 5.1. Four Process Categories of Client Resistance Behavior

1. *Arguing.* The client contests the accuracy, expertise, or integrity of the counselor.
   1a. *Challenging.* The client directly challenges the accuracy of what the counselor has said.
   1b. *Discounting.* The client questions the counselor's personal authority and expertise.
   1c. *Hostility.* The client expresses direct hostility toward the counselor.
2. *Interrupting.* The client breaks in and interrupts the counselor in a defensive manner.
   2a. *Talking over.* The client speaks while the counselor is still talking, without waiting for an appropriate pause or silence.
   2b. *Cutting off.* The client breaks in with words obviously intended to cut the counselor off (e.g., "Now wait a minute. I've heard about enough").
3. *Negating.* The client expresses an unwillingness to recognize problems, cooperate, accept responsibility, or take advice.
   3a. *Blaming.* The client blames other people for problems.
   3b. *Disagreeing.* The client disagrees with a suggestion that the counselor has made, offering no constructive alternative. This includes the familiar "Yes, but . . .," which explains what is wrong with suggestions that are made.
   3c. *Excusing.* The client makes excuses for his or her own behavior.
   3d. *Claiming impunity.* The client claims that he or she is not in any danger (e.g., from drinking).
   3e. *Minimizing.* The client suggests that the counselor is exaggerating risks or dangers, and that it "really isn't so bad."
   3f. *Pessimism.* The client makes general statements about self or others that are pessimistic, defeatist, or negativistic in tone.
   3g. *Reluctance.* The client expresses reservations and reluctance about information or advice given.
   3h. *Unwillingness to change.* The client expresses a lack of desire or an unwillingness to change, or an intention not to change.
4. *Ignoring.* The client shows evidence of ignoring or not following the counselor.
   4a. *Inattention.* The client's response indicates that he or she has not been following or attending to the counselor.
   4b. *Nonanswer.* In answering a counselor's query, the client gives a response that is not an answer to the question.
   4c. *No response.* The client gives no audible or nonverbal reply to a counselor's query.
   4d. *Sidetracking.* The client changes the direction of the conversation that the counselor has been pursuing.

Note. Adapted from a behavior coding system developed by Chamberlain, Patterson, Reid, Kavanagh, and Forgatch (1984).

Similarly, an interrupt may occur because a client vehemently disagrees with what the counselor is saying, or it could reflect a client's excitement about ideas and possibilities. That is, with the exception of negating responses, the verbal behaviors described here as resistance may, in some circumstances, represent movement *toward* change.

This led us to a new perspective: that resistance, like motivation and self-efficacy, is change-specific. A person may be quite motivated, for example, to stop using cocaine, but be unconcerned about alcohol and marijuana use. Change talk and resistance talk can be understood only in relation to a particular kind of change. Speech that reflects movement toward that particular change is what we originally referred to as self-motivational statements and now call change talk. Speech that reflects movement away from a particular change is what we mean by resistance. Viewed in this way, the same statement (such as, "I have decided not to break up with my boyfriend") could constitute change talk for one outcome (e.g., reconciling the relationship), but resistance for another (e.g., stopping drug use, if the boyfriend is a drug dealer).

We therefore define resistance as speech that signals movement away from a particular kind of change. In this way, it is the mirror image of change talk (see Box 5.2). Motivational interviewing involves recognizing and responding in particular ways to these two important forms of client speech.

COUNSELOR'S ROLE IN RESISTANCE

We have alluded in several chapters to counselor styles and behaviors that can elicit and intensify client resistance and thereby decrease the probability of behavior change. These are responses that, in essence, are complementary to client resistance, much as countertransference is complementary to and reinforces client transference. Here and elsewhere we have referred to such responses generically as "confrontational," and earlier in this chapter we suggested the idea of counterresistance.

What do these counselor behaviors look like? We have chosen the term "advocacy" to describe this set of counselor responses that tend to elicit and reinforce resistance behavior. The connotation of the term is to argue or plead for a particular cause. Thus—like motivation, self-efficacy, change talk, and resistance—advocacy is also change-specific, and the term itself is morally neutral. Many of Thomas Gordon's "roadblocks" (described in the next chapter) are examples of advocacy responses. (This usage should not be confused

---

BOX 5.2. Change Talk and Resistance

Change talk	Resistance talk
Disadvantages of status quo	Advantages of status quo
Advantages of change	Disadvantages of change
Intention to change	Intention not to change
Optimism about change	Pessimism about change

with "client advocacy," which denotes the clinician's role in promoting the rights and welfare of clients.)

We propose six broad types of advocacy responses, as shown in Box 5.3. They have in common an "I know best, listen to me" tone. Again, each of these responses is understood in relation to the particular change for which one is advocating. It is the case, however, that each of these advocacy responses can also have a more generic effect of damaging rapport and enhancing dissonance in the counseling relationship.

It can take relatively few such responses to sour an entire consultation, session, or counseling relationship. In one study[7] we found that counselors who were trained in motivational interviewing did show significant increases in the appropriate responses such as reflective listening, affirming, and asking open questions. These changes in counseling style endured 3 months later, and yet their clients were not responding any differently! It was then we noticed that while we had been successful in increasing the rate of some responses consistent with motivational interviewing, we had done nothing to decrease the rate of advocacy responses, and it seemed to take only a few of these to interfere with client motivation for change. The same is true in relationships more generally. It can take a long time to build trust and intimacy, but only a short time to destroy them.

BOX 5.3. Six Types of Counselor Advocacy Responses

1. *Arguing for change.* The counselor directly takes up the pro-change side of ambivalence on a particular issue and seeks to persuade the client to make the change.

2. *Assuming the expert role.* The counselor structures the conversation in a way that communicates that the counselor "has the answers." This includes the question–answer trap of asking many closed-ended questions, as well as lecturing the client.

3. *Criticizing, shaming, or blaming.* The counselor's underlying intent seems to be to shock or jar the client into changing by instilling negative emotions about the status quo.

4. *Labeling.* The counselor proposes acceptance of a specific label or diagnosis to characterize or explain the client's behavior. The focus is on what the client "is" or "has" rather than on what he or she does.

5. *Being in a hurry.* Sometimes a perceived shortness of time causes the counselor to believe that clear, forceful tactics are called for in order to get through. From his experience in working with horses, Monty Roberts[8] has observed the paradox that "if you act like you only have a few minutes" it can take all day to accomplish a change, whereas "if you act like you have all day," it may take only a few minutes. In counseling, this most often takes the form of getting ahead of your client's readiness.

6. *Claiming preeminence.* Finally, resistance is invoked when a counselor claims preeminence—that the counselor's goals and perspectives override those of the client. The quintessential form is a paternalistic, "I know what is best for you" approach.

As with the roadblocks in Chapter 6, we do not mean to say that it is always wrong to respond in advocacy terms. There are times when a client specifically requests the benefit of expertise, for example. A patient presenting with a distressing rash or infection usually wants the doctor's expert opinion and solution. Recognizing a valid diagnosis can be an important step in addressing bipolar disorder or tuberculosis. When it comes to consultations about behavior, however, advocacy responses are often counterproductive, and the focus needs to be on building the client's intrinsic motivation for change, the topic to which we turn in Chapter 6.

SUMMARY

Client responses must be understood within the context of the counseling relationship and are substantially influenced by how the counselor, in turn, responds to them. The counseling relationship fluctuates over time along a continuum from consonance to dissonance. Certain client responses, specifically change talk and resistance, are markers of consonance and dissonance, and they are also meaningful predictors of the probability of behavior change. Certain counseling responses evoke and exacerbate resistance, and it is important to remember to "First, do no harm," even and particularly when time is short. Within motivational interviewing, the counselor responds in particular ways to change talk in order to reinforce it, and to resistance in order to diminish it, both in the service of resolving ambivalence and promoting behavior change. Recognizing these two types of client behavior is therefore an important skill in motivational interviewing.

NOTES

1. Miller (1983).
2. Amrhein (1992).
3. Miller, Benefield, and Tonigan (1993).
4. Patterson and Forgatch (1985).
5. Chamberlain, Patterson, Reid, Kavanagh, and Forgatch (1984).
6. Miller et al. (1993).
7. Miller and Mount (2001).
8. Roberts (1997).

CHAPTER 6

Phase 1

Building Motivation for Change

What people really need is a good listening to.
—MARY LOU CASEY

A fool takes no pleasure in understanding, but only in expressing personal opinion.
—PROVERBS 18:2

We have conceptualized motivational interviewing as occurring in two phases, with somewhat different, albeit overlapping, goals. Phase 1 involves building intrinsic motivation for change. If the person is starting far down the mountain slope of motivation, this can feel like a long and gradual process, perhaps like snowshoeing upward one step at a time. At some point, importance peaks enough to begin talking about strategies rather than reasons for change. Phase 2 involves strengthening commitment to change and developing a plan to accomplish it. This is often the easier task, more like skiing down the other side of a summit, and the challenge is akin to avoiding moguls, trees, and cliffs on the way down.

Because the overall goal in Phase 1 is to resolve ambivalence and build motivation for change, the amount of work to be done will depend on the person's starting point. Some people come to counseling already quite convinced that there are ample reasons for them to make a change, and there is little left to do in Phase 1 except to gain a clear understanding of those reasons from the client's perspective. There is no point in prolonging Phase 1 if the person is ready to ski.

A dimension to which we gave insufficient attention in our first edition, however, is a person's confidence in his or her ability to change. Extending our mountaineering analogy, the person has reached a peak but has no skis.

IMPORTANCE AND CONFIDENCE

It is useful in understanding a person's ambivalence to know his or her perceptions of both importance and confidence. Both need to be addressed in Phase 1 because both are components of intrinsic motivation for change. One simple method that we have used is a ruler with gradations from 0 to 10 for each of these dimensions. Sometimes we directly ask the question using this scale.

"How important would you say it is for you to _____? On a scale from 0 to 10, where 0 is not at all important and 10 is extremely important, where would you say you are?"

0	1	2	3	4	5	6	7	8	9	10
Not at all important										Extremely important

And how confident would you say you are, that if you decided to _____, you could do it? On the same scale from 0 to 10, where 0 is not at all confident and 10 is extremely confident, where would you say you are?"

It is not necessary to show the client a ruler, though it can be helpful to do so. It works simply to describe the scale in language like that above. Some prefer not to use a formal scale at all, but just to talk about importance and confidence and get an informal sense of where the person is on each of these two dimensions. However you proceed, the idea is to end up knowing how important the client perceives change to be, and how confident the person is that he or she could do it. Notice that the second of these questions is phrased in the subjunctive: How confident are you that you *could* make this change? This allows confidence to be somewhat detached from importance. The client can give you an estimate of confidence without agreeing that the change is important to make.

Oversimplifying for the moment, assume that one can think of each of these two dimensions as being either high or low. This leaves four possible profiles (see Box 6.1).

For Groups A, B, and C, there is work to do in Phase 1. For A and B there is importance work, for unless the person comes to perceive change as suffi-

BOX 6.1. Four Client Profiles

Group A: Low importance, low confidence

These people neither see change as important nor believe that they could succeed in making such a change if they tried.

Group B: Low importance, high confidence

These people are confident that they could make the change if they thought it were important to do so but are not persuaded that they want to change.

Group C: High importance, low confidence

Here the problem is not in willingness to change, for these people express desire to do so. The problem is low confidence that they could succeed if they tried.

Group D: High importance, high confidence

These people see it is important to change and also believe that they could succeed.

---

ciently important, it is unlikely to happen. For Group C, perceived importance is already there. What they need is self-efficacy, an effective way of pursuing change in which they believe they can succeed. This is also a task for Group A, where both importance and confidence are low.

Reality is more complex than this. Instead of falling into two groups, high and low, people vary along a continuum on each dimension. Furthermore, these two scales address the willingness and ability aspects of motivation, but not the third dimension of readiness. Group D say they are willing (importance) and able (confidence) to change, but they still may not be ready to do so.

These three dimensions—ready, willing, and able—are related to each other in complex ways. Readiness implies at least some degree of both importance and confidence. A person who does not see change as important is unlikely to be ready to change. Similarly, people who see change as impossible are unlikely to say that they are ready to do it. If importance is high enough, those with low confidence still might say that they are ready to try. Importance and confidence can interact in other ways as well. A person with very low confidence may be reluctant to consider that change is important. High importance with low confidence (Group C) is a distressing place to be, because such people see the danger but no way to escape it, or they see a promise that is beyond their reach. Given low confidence, a person may be reluctant even to explore importance because "What's the point in thinking about it?" Why would anyone want to move from Group A to Group C? Low confidence can therefore be an obstacle, in Group A, to developing discrepancy (importance) during Phase 1.

Phase 1 therefore can involve either importance work or confidence work, or both. When both are needed, the order is flexible. It may be necessary to address confidence first, before the person will engage in discussing importance issues. Such might be the case with a demoralized smoker who has had many unsuccessful quit attempts. Others will grapple with importance first and then address confidence issues later. Often importance and confidence are discussed either simultaneously or by going back and forth between the two.

The focus of this chapter is on how to begin Phase 1. We describe here some opening methods for motivational interviewing that will allow you to put into practice the principles outlined in Chapter 5. We begin by explaining some traps that can be encountered early in motivational interviewing, with specific examples of counseling dialogue to illustrate how counselors may fall into or avoid these pitfalls. In essence, these traps are various forms of counselor advocacy, as described in Chapter 5.

SOME EARLY TRAPS TO AVOID

Question–Answer Trap

At the outset of a counseling process, it is easy to fall into a pattern whereby the counselor asks questions and the person gives short answers. This is similar to what may occur when a physician conducts a general health screening: The patient responds "Yes" or "No" to a long survey of potential problem areas. This can happen in part because the counselor feels a need for specific information. It may also be a response to anxiety—either in the counselor, who wants to keep control, or in the client, who is more comfortable with the safe predictability of this passive role. Indeed, counselor anxiousness has been associated with less empathic responding and may favor the structured format of question–answer.[1] In this trap, the "expert" counselor controls the session by asking questions, while the person merely responds with short answers. Here is an example. In this and subsequent interview segments, we designate the dialogue as occurring between a counselor-interviewer and a client.

INTERVIEWER: You're here to talk about your gambling, is that right?

CLIENT: Yes, I am.

INTERVIEWER: Do you think you gamble too much?

CLIENT: Probably.

INTERVIEWER: What is your favorite game?

CLIENT: Blackjack.

INTERVIEWER: Do you usually drink when you gamble?

CLIENT: Yes, I do usually.

INTERVIEWER: Have you ever gone seriously into debt because of gambling?

CLIENT: Once or twice, yes.

INTERVIEWER: How far into debt?

CLIENT: Once I had to borrow eight thousand to pay off a debt.

INTERVIEWER: Are you married?

CLIENT: No, I'm divorced.

INTERVIEWER: How long ago were you divorced?

CLIENT: Two years ago.

It can happen so easily. There are several negative aspects of this pattern. First, it teaches the client to give short, simple answers, rather than the kind of elaboration needed in motivational interviewing. Second, it subtly implies an interaction between an active expert and a passive patient: if you just ask enough questions, then you will have the answer. It affords little opportunity for a person to explore motivation and to offer change talk.

This trap is relatively easy to avoid. If you need concrete information at the outset, we recommend having clients complete a precounseling questionnaire and saving the other specifics for later. This saves you from going through an inventory of short-answer questions. The open-ended questions and reflective listening methods explained later in this chapter are also very helpful in getting around the question–answer trap.

There is a subtler form of this same trap, however, which involves open-ended questions. The optimal approach is usually to ask an open-ended question, then to respond to the client's response not with another question but with reflective listening. The use of a series of open-ended questions without sufficient reflective listening can have a very similar effect to that of a series of closed questions. The client is directed into a passive, question–answering role. As a general clinical guideline, avoid asking three questions in a row.

Trap of Taking Sides

From the perspective of motivational interviewing, taking sides is the most important trap to avoid, and a common trap it is. Counselors fall into it through their own good intentions and through a particular conception of motivational processes. If a counselor makes the wrong opening moves, most clients will readily play along with this pattern.

How does this trap happen? The familiar script is that the counselor detects some information indicating the presence of a problem (e.g., "alcoholism"), begins to tell the client that he or she has a serious problem, and prescribes a particular course of action. The client then expresses some reluctance about this, making statements along two general lines: "The problem isn't really *that* bad," and "I don't really need to change that much."

This response is quite natural and predictable. If people usually enter counseling in a state of ambivalence, they feel two ways about their current situation: They want it, and they don't want it. They think maybe they should change, and yet they are reluctant to give up their present pattern. They are in conflict. If the counselor argues for one side of the conflict, it is natural for the client to give voice to the other side. Here is a sample:

INTERVIEWER: Well, it seems clear to me that you have a serious drinking problem. You're showing a lot of the signs of alcoholism.

CLIENT: What do you mean?

INTERVIEWER: Well, you've had an alcoholic blackout, you're uncomfortable when you can't drink, and you're losing control of your drinking.

CLIENT: But a lot of people I know drink just like I do.

INTERVIEWER: Maybe so, maybe not. But we're not talking about other people here, we're talking about you.

CLIENT: But I don't think it's that serious.

INTERVIEWER: Not serious! It's just sheer luck that you haven't been arrested or killed somebody driving after drinking.

CLIENT: I told you, I can drive just fine. I've never had a problem.

INTERVIEWER: And what about your family? They think you're drinking too much, and they think you ought to quit.

CLIENT: Oh, Fran came from a family of teetotalers. There's nothing wrong with me. They think that anybody who has three drinks is an alcoholic.

By taking responsibility for the "problem-change" side of the conflict, the counselor elicits oppositional "no-problem" arguments from the client. As the counselor argues one side more adamantly, the client will defend the other with greater vigor. It is a familiar script, and probably one that the client has been through before with others. Clients in this situation can literally talk themselves out of changing. Hearing themselves vigorously arguing that they don't have a problem and don't need to change, they become convinced. Few people enjoy losing an argument or being proved wrong.

A counselor can fall into the taking-sides trap inadvertently, even if not consciously intending to defend or promote one particular side. Consider these two examples of counseling focused on choice in the midst of ambivalence—the decision whether or not to have children.

CLIENT: I guess the most pressing issue for me is a family. I'm over 30, and if I'm ever going to have children, it's time.

INTERVIEWER: Your biological clock is ticking.

CLIENT: Yes. I really have to decide about this.

INTERVIEWER: And so you're wondering now whether you want to have a family?

CLIENT: I guess I always thought I'd have kids at some point. It's just that both of us had to get school out of the way, and then we started working, and suddenly I'm 34.

INTERVIEWER: Of course, women are having babies at later ages now.

CLIENT: But isn't it risky?

INTERVIEWER: The risks do go up, yes, but they are still relatively low and there is good prenatal testing available.

CLIENT: If I got pregnant and then found out that there was something wrong, I don't know what I'd do.

INTERVIEWER: There are a number of options.

CLIENT: I know that, but I mean—I guess I'm just not sure if I really want to take the chance.

INTERVIEWER: Why not?

CLIENT: For one thing, it's such a long commitment. You give 20 years of your life—more, really, because being a parent never ends.

INTERVIEWER: Of course, there are certain rewards, too. It's a very special kind of relationship that you can never have with another human being in any other way.

CLIENT: I'm not sure, though, that I really want that kind of relationship with just one or two children. I'm a teacher, and in a way I can do a lot more good for children if I'm not tied up for 20 years in raising my own. And it's so *expensive* to raise children these days!

INTERVIEWER: And yet, there is that sense that you might be missing something.

CLIENT: I'd be missing something either way, really. If I have my own children, I miss out on all the opportunities that would have happened in the time I gave to them.

INTERVIEWER: What about just one child? How about that?

CLIENT: I don't think it's fair to make someone an only child. They need to have a brother or sister. It's a special relationship.

INTERVIEWER: Kind of like being a parent.

CLIENT: Well, yes and no. You usually don't spend the better part of your life raising a sibling.

INTERVIEWER: I guess what I'm saying here—what I'm worried about is that if you let your biological clock run out, you might regret it deeply later on.

CLIENT: But I think that's better than the opposite. I know parents who regret having had their kids. They usually don't say so, but deep down they wonder what their lives would have been like if they hadn't had children. I think kids can't help but sense that.

INTERVIEWER: I'm sure that does happen sometimes, but most parents find it very rewarding. It's true that being a mother demands a lot from you, and yet it also gives you something very special . . .

Now consider the same client and scenario, but this time the counselor happens for whatever reason to lean the other way at the outset.

CLIENT: I guess the most pressing issue for me is a family. I'm over 30, and if I'm ever going to have children, it's time.

INTERVIEWER: Your biological clock is ticking.

CLIENT: Yes. I really have to decide about this.

INTERVIEWER: And so you're wondering now whether you want to have a family.

CLIENT: I guess I always thought I'd have kids at some point. It's just that both of us had to get school out of the way, and then we started working, and suddenly I'm 34.

INTERVIEWER: So maybe it's getting a bit late to begin a family.

CLIENT: Oh, I don't know. Lots of people are having babies now who are older than we are. It's fairly common, really.

INTERVIEWER: I'm not saying that it's uncommon. I guess I was just hearing some reluctance in your voice.

CLIENT: Well, of course I'm somewhat reluctant. It's a major life change, but I've always felt like I would have children at some point, and now is the time.

INTERVIEWER: Why? What appeals to you about having a family?

CLIENT: It's hard to say, really—it's mostly a feeling I have. I guess it's good to have children when you get older—someone to look after you.

INTERVIEWER: Of course, that doesn't always happen.

CLIENT: I know. It's also an experience I don't want to miss out on. There's more to life than work. I just feel it would be nice to be a mother.

INTERVIEWER: What other advantages do you see?

CLIENT: Not *advantages*, really.

INTERVIEWER: It's not like you have children for what you can get out of them.

CLIENT: Right! There's something about being part of a new life, a part of the future.

INTERVIEWER: Sounds pretty romantic.

CLIENT: Well, I think it is! I know that it's not all roses, and it costs a fortune, and you open yourself up to pain. It takes a lot of time to raise children. You have to give a lot.

INTERVIEWER: It costs you a lot—not only in money but in time, too.

CLIENT: And yet I feel like it's worth it. . . .

The client might leave the first of these sessions feeling more committed to not have a family. In the second example, the same person's change talk, elicited by the counselor's taking one side, might steer the client in the other direction, toward choosing to have a child. The methods described in Chapter 8 can be particularly helpful in avoiding the trap of taking sides. In some cases, you will want to avoid taking sides at all. In situations where a more directive approach is appropriate, the art is to avoid this temptation to take the "good" side of the argument.

Expert Trap

An enthusiastic and competent counselor can unwittingly fall into the expert trap by conveying the impression of having all the answers. Like the question–answer trap, its most common effect is to edge people into a passive role, which is inconsistent with the basic goals of motivational interviewing— giving people the opportunity to explore and resolve ambivalence for themselves. A sincere desire to help can lead a counselor to try to "fix" the situation for a person, shift into problem-solving, and prescribe answers and solutions. There is an appropriate time for expert opinion (see Chapter 9), but the focus in Phase 1 is first on building the client's own motivation. This is unlikely to happen if the client is placed in the role of passive recipient of expert advice.

Within motivational interviewing, in a real sense it is the client who is the expert. No one knows more about his or her situation, values, goals, concerns, and skills. No one is in a better position to anticipate how change will fit into the person's life. It is worth remembering the image from Chapter 3, of two people seated side by side looking through a family album or scrapbook. It is quite different from the image of a pilgrim seeking enlightenment at the feet of a master. Motivational interviewing is about collaboration, not installation.

Labeling Trap

Counselors and clients can also easily be ensnared by the issue of diagnostic labeling. Some believe that it is terribly important for a client to accept (even "admit") the counselor's diagnosis ("You're an alcoholic," "You're in denial," etc.). Because such labels often carry a certain stigma in the public mind, it is not surprising that people with reasonable self-esteem resist them. Even in the field of alcohol problems, where emphasis on labeling has been high (at least in the United States), there is little evidence for any benefit from pressuring people to accept a label like "alcoholic," and the Alcoholics Anonymous (AA) philosophy specifically recommends against such labeling of others.

Often there is an underlying dynamic in a labeling debate. It may be a power struggle in which the counselor seeks to assert control and expertise. With family members, the label may be a judgmental communication. For some people, even a seemingly harmless reference to "your problem with . . . " can elicit uncomfortable feelings of being cornered. The danger, of course, is that the labeling struggle evokes dissonance, which descends into side-taking and, in turn, hinders progress.

We recommend, therefore, that you deemphasize labeling in the course of motivational interviewing. Problems can be fully explored without attaching labels that evoke unnecessary dissonance. If the issue of labeling never comes up, it is not necessary to raise it. Often, however, a client will raise the issue, and how you respond can be quite important. We recommend a combination of reflection and reframing, two techniques that will be discussed later in this chapter. Here is a brief example, again from the addiction field where this issue is often most intense. The counselor here quickly sides with the client's concern, and then offers a reframe.

CLIENT: So are you implying that I'm an addict?

INTERVIEWER: No, I'm really not concerned that much about labels. But it sounds like you are, that it's a worry for you.

CLIENT: Well, I don't like being called an addict.

INTERVIEWER: When that happens, you want to explain that your situation really isn't that bad.

CLIENT: Right! I'm not saying that I don't have any problems . . .

INTERVIEWER: But you don't like being labeled as "having a problem." It sounds too harsh to you.

CLIENT: Yes, it does.

INTERVIEWER: That's pretty common, as you might imagine. Lots of people I talk to don't like being labeled. There's nothing strange about that. I don't like people labeling me, either.

CLIENT: I feel like I'm being put in a box.

INTERVIEWER: Right. So let me tell you how I see this, and then we'll move on. To me, it doesn't matter what we *call* a problem. I don't care if we call it "addiction" or "problems" or "Rumpelstiltskin," for that matter. We don't have to call it anything. If a label is an important issue for you, we can discuss it, but it's not particularly important to me. What really matters is to understand how your use of cocaine is harming you, and what, if anything, you want to do about it. That's what I care about.

As a final note, we would add that we also see no strong reason to discourage people from embracing a label if they are so inclined. Members of AA, for example, often report that it was important for them to recognize and accept their identity as an alcoholic. There is little point in opposing such self-acceptance. The point here is to avoid getting into needless debates and struggles over labels.

Premature-Focus Trap

Even if the counselor avoids labeling and taking sides in the client's ambivalence, resistance may result if client and counselor wish to focus on different topics. Counselors often want to identify and hone in on what they perceive to be the client's problem. The client, in contrast, may have more pressing concerns and may not share the importance placed by the counselor on this "problem." In fact, the most common reason for clinical interest in motivational interviewing is the situation in which the client perceives less importance for a change than the counselor does.

The trap here is to persist in trying to draw the client back to talk about your own conception of "the problem." The probation counseling example in Chapter 5 is a clear example of such dissonance. The counselor wants to focus on one subject, and the client has different and perhaps broader concerns. A struggle may ensue regarding how much attention should be paid to what the counselor perceives to be the problem. Indeed, in the client's mind, the counselor's concern may be a relatively small part of the picture, and it may not be clear whether and how this is related to the client's larger life issues. If the counselor presses too quickly to focus the discussion, dissonance results and the client may be put off, becoming defensive. The point is to avoid becoming engaged in a struggle about the proper topic for early discussion. Starting with the client's concerns, rather than those of the counselor, will ensure that this does not happen. Very often, exploring those things that *are* of concern to the client will lead back to the topic of concern to the counselor, particularly when the areas of concern are related. In any event, spending time listening to the client's concerns is useful, both in understanding the person and in building the rapport that is a basis for later exploration of other topics.

A women's substance abuse treatment program in New Mexico illustrates this situation. The professional staff found that women who came to the program generally had many more pressing concerns than their use of alcohol and other drugs. They often had health care concerns, had parenting and child care problems, needed housing, and were traumatized by current or past physical and sexual abuse. These women had much to talk about, and if a counselor tried to focus on substance use early in treatment, the woman was likely to drop out. By contrast, if the counselor listened to and addressed the woman's immediate concerns, conversations invariably came around to the role of alcohol and other drugs in her life.

The point, then, is to avoid focusing prematurely on issues that are of concern to the counselor but of less concern to the client. When encountering dissonance around premature focus, start where clients' own concerns are, listen to their stories, and get a broader understanding of their life situation before coming back around to the topic.

Blaming Trap

Still another obstacle that can be encountered in the first session is a client's concern with and defensiveness about blaming. Whose *fault* is the problem? Who's to blame? If this issue is not dealt with properly, time and energy can be wasted on needless defensiveness. One obvious approach here is to render blame irrelevant within the counseling context. Usually this can be dealt with by reflecting and reframing the client's concerns. If this problem arises, for example, the client may be told:

> "It sounds like you're worried about who's to blame here. I should explain that counseling is not about deciding who is at fault. That's what judges do, but not good counselors. Counseling has a 'no-fault' policy. I'm not interested in looking for who's to blame, but rather what's troubling you, and what you might be able to do about it."

Concerns about blame may also be prevented by offering a brief structuring statement like this at the beginning of counseling. Once the client has a clear understanding of the purpose of counseling, worries about blaming may be allayed.

ABOUT THE FIRST SESSION

The very first session can be crucial as it sets both the tone and the expectations for counseling. The counselor's actions in even a single session can have a powerful influence on a person's change talk and long-term outcome. Rapport in the first session also influences whether the person will come back. It is important, then, to adopt the proper approach right from the beginning and to avoid falling into the traps (as just discussed) that can quickly undermine progress. This section discusses a few practical issues to keep in mind at the beginning. The next section then presents five clinical methods that are useful from the first session onward. As a reminder, we are focusing here on the overall clinical method of motivational interviewing, and we are not yet addressing adaptations to time-limited contexts such as general medical practice.

Opening Structure

People come to counseling with widely varying expectations. They may come expecting to be criticized, healed, advised, questioned, listened to, blamed, taught, medicated, or consoled. Prospective clients enter treatment with widely differing expectations, fears, hopes, and concerns. For this and other reasons, it can be useful at the outset to provide the client with a simple and brief structuring of the first session and of counseling in general. A good structuring statement can set the client's mind at rest and get counseling off to a good start. Some elements that may be included in a good structuring statement are the following:

- The amount of time you have available
- An explanation of your role and goals
- A description of the client's role
- A mention of details that must be attended to
- An open-ended question

Here is an example:

"We have about an hour together now, and in this time I want to get a beginning understanding of what brings you here. I'll probably spend most of this time listening, so that I can understand how you see things and what your concerns are. You must also have some hopes about what will and won't happen here, and I'll want to hear about those. Toward the end of this hour I'll need to ask you for some specific information that I need, but let's just get started now. What's on your mind?"

Agenda Setting

Agenda setting is an issue to keep in the back of your mind from the very beginning of the first interview. The basic question here is "What are we going to talk about?" Sometimes one topic is predefined by the context. If the client is referred by the court because of domestic violence or is meeting with the dietician in a diabetes management clinic, at least one topic of conversation is already identified. Even in these cases, however, the obvious subject is not necessarily *the* topic, the first and only matter to be discussed.

When there is doubt about the topics of conversation, it can be helpful to spend a few minutes exploring the client's view of what the agenda might be and also clarifying your own understanding. Here are two examples:

A *dietician to a patient seeking consultation in a diabetes management clinic*: "As you know, there are a number of things that we could discuss today—such as monitoring your blood sugar levels, healthy diet, exercise, and your medication—but what are you most concerned about? What would *you* like to talk about today? Perhaps there are other things that you feel are more important to discuss."

A counselor or probation officer to an offender referred after an arrest for domestic violence: "I see from the referral sheet that you are here to talk about what you've been through with an episode of violence last month, and we can do that. First, though, I'm interested in understanding how you feel about coming here and about what's happening in your life. What are *your* concerns that we should discuss?"

There can be an initial period of uncertainty as you discuss what the agenda will be. If so, then this period of listening is time well spent. It helps avoid the premature-focus trap of charging directly into what you assume to be the topic of conversation.

FIVE EARLY METHODS

There are five specific methods that can be useful from the first session on-ward and, indeed, throughout the process of motivational interviewing. We call them "early" methods not because they are used at the beginning and then abandoned but because it is important to be using them right from the start. Woven together, they begin to form the fabric of motivational interviewing. The first four are derived largely from client-centered counseling, although in motivational interviewing they are used for a particular purpose—that of helping people to explore their ambivalence and clarify reasons for change. These first four are summarized by the acronym OARS (Open questions, Af-firming, Reflecting, and Summarizing). The fifth method is more clearly direc-tive and is specific to motivational interviewing. It integrates and guides the use of the other four methods.

1. Ask Open Questions

During the early phase of motivational interviewing, it is important to estab-lish an atmosphere of acceptance and trust within which clients will explore their concerns. This means that the client should do most of the talking at this stage, with the counselor listening carefully and encouraging expression. When sessions with skillful motivational interviewing practitioners are ana-lyzed, the client is usually doing more than half of the talking that occurs. This is also important because part of the process of motivational interviewing in-volves eliciting and shaping certain kinds of client speech. The first four of these five early methods—the OARS—directly support this goal of encourag-ing client speech.

One key for encouraging clients to do most of the talking is to ask open questions: questions that do not invite brief answers. Some closed (short-answer) questions may be necessary, but they should be few and far between during the early phase of motivational interviewing. It is better to begin and continue with questions that open the door for the person to explore. Some people come in almost bursting to talk, and it takes only a simple invitation to elicit their story. Others are more reticent and require encouragement. How you respond to the person's initial answers will strongly influence what happens next, and that is addressed in the other methods. Our interest here is in how to ask good open questions.

If you know in advance or otherwise sense that the person has clear agenda to talk about, a simple opening of the door may suffice. Here are some examples:

> "I assume, from the fact that you are here, that you have some things you want to talk over. What would you like to discuss?"
>
> "I'd like to understand how you see things. What's brought you here?"
>
> "I understand that you have some concerns about _____. Tell me about them."
>
> "You said on the telephone that you have been having some trouble with _____, and you want to talk about it. Fill me in. How about starting from the beginning, and bringing me up to date?"

This may seem like a simple distinction between open and closed questions, but there are complexities. Box 6.2 contains a set of questions that a counselor might ask. How would you classify each of them: open or closed?

In discussing a focal problem with more ambivalent clients, it can be useful either to ask for both sides of the coin or to ask a connected cluster of relatively neutral open questions. Some counselors prefer to ask people first what they have liked about their current ("problem") behavior or situation, and then what the not-so-good side includes. Here are some sample openings:"

> "Tell me about your use of cocaine. What do you like about it? . . . [Then later:] And what's the other side? What are your worries about using it?"
>
> "Tell me what you've noticed about your marriage over the years. What changes have you seen, and how have these affected you?"
>
> "I understand that you're here to talk about your gambling. So help me see the big picture. What do you enjoy about gambling, and what's the not-so-good side?"

Remember that the guideline to avoid asking three questions in a row also applies to open questions. (Each of the clusters illustrated above is essentially a single open question, in that the client has not responded in between.) The process of motivational interviewing involves helping people openly explore their own experience, including ambivalence. Even open questions redirect a person's attention. The general pattern in motivational interviewing is

BOX 6.2. Is It an Open or a Closed Question?

	Open or Closed?
1. What do you like about drinking?	_____
2. Where did you grow up?	_____
3. Isn't it important for you to have meaning in your life?	_____
4. Are you willing to come back for a follow-up visit?	_____
5. What brings you here today?	_____
6. Do you want to stay in this relationship?	_____
7. Have you ever thought about walking as a simple form of exercise?	_____
8. What do you want to do about your smoking: quit, cut down, or stay the same?	_____
9. In the past, how have you overcome an important obstacle in your life?	_____
10. What would you like to set as your quit date?	_____
11. What possible long-term consequences of diabetes concern you most?	_____
12. Do you care about your health?	_____
13. What are the most important reasons why you want to stop injecting?	_____
14. Will you try this for 1 week?	_____
15. Is this an open or a closed question?	_____

Answers at the end of this chapter (p. 84).

to ask an open question, setting the topic of exploration, and then follow with reflective listening and the other responses described next.

These questions are just door-openers, providing opportunities for using other methods. Obviously, people will vary in how they react to open questions such as these. Some will respond eagerly to the opportunity to talk about their difficulties. In such cases, your job is a matter of guiding the client in this exploration, using the methods described in this and the following chapters. Others will volunteer relatively little and may change the subject or head off toward one of the traps described earlier. Skillful motivational interviewing involves particular ways of responding to what a person offers when open questions are asked.

2. Listen Reflectively

Reflective listening is one of the most important and most challenging skills required for motivational interviewing. In popular conceptions, listening just involves keeping quiet (at least for a little while) and hearing what someone has to say. The crucial element in reflective listening, however, is how the counselor responds to what the client says. Thomas Gordon[2] outlined 12 kinds of responses that are not listening:

1. Ordering, directing, or commanding
2. Warning, cautioning, or threatening
3. Giving advice, making suggestions, or providing solutions
4. Persuading with logic, arguing, or lecturing
5. Telling people what they should do; moralizing
6. Disagreeing, judging, criticizing, or blaming
7. Agreeing, approving, or praising
8. Shaming, ridiculing, or labeling
9. Interpreting or analyzing
10. Reassuring, sympathizing, or consoling
11. Questioning or probing
12. Withdrawing, distracting, humoring, or changing the subject

Gordon called these responses "roadblocks" because they tend to get in the way. They divert the person from pursuing the same path. In order to keep exploring in the same direction, the person has to deal with the roadblock, detour around it, and come back to the original train of thought. Roadblocks have the effect of blocking, stopping, diverting, or changing direction. As we will discuss later, there are times when such responses are used intentionally and directively, as in asking an open question to set a direction of discussion. Even then, once the question has been asked, it is time to listen.

Roadblocks also tend to imply an uneven or "one-up" relationship. The underlying message seems to be "Listen to me; I know best." Instead of continuing to explore the path, the person then has to deal with the roadblock. Consider this well-intentioned but unhelpful counselor talking with a client who feels two ways about an important decision. (The number of each corresponding roadblock from the preceding list is given in parentheses.)

CLIENT: I just don't know whether to leave him or not.

INTERVIEWER: You should do whatever you think is best. (#5)

CLIENT: But that's the point! I don't know what's best!

INTERVIEWER: Yes, you do, in your heart. (#6)

CLIENT: Well, I just feel trapped, stifled in our relationship.

INTERVIEWER: Have you thought about separating for a while to see how you feel? (#3)

CLIENT: But I love him, and it would hurt him so much if I left!

INTERVIEWER: Yet if you don't do it, you could be wasting your life. (#2)

CLIENT: But isn't that kind of selfish?

INTERVIEWER: It's just what you have to do to take care of yourself. (#4)

CLIENT: I just don't know how I could do it, how I'd manage.

INTERVIEWER: I'm sure you'll be fine. (#10)

This person has not been helped to explore ambivalence but instead is prematurely pressed toward one resolution. The counselor in this situation has never really listened—has never given the client a chance to keep on talking and exploring. The client's time has been spent dodging roadblocks.

What else is there? If one avoids all these roadblocks, what is there left to say? We don't mean to imply that it is wrong to use these 12 responses. There is a time and a place for each of them. We do mean to say that reflective listening is something different from any of these ways of responding.

The essence of a reflective listening response is that it makes a guess as to what the speaker means. Before a person speaks, he or she has a certain meaning to communicate. This is encoded into words, often imperfectly. People don't always say what they mean. The listener has to hear the words accurately and then decode their meaning. That means there are three steps along the way where communication can go wrong: encoding, hearing, and decoding. The reflective listener forms a reasonable guess as to what the original meaning was, and then gives voice to this guess in the form of a statement.

A statement? Why not a question? After all, the listener is not sure whether the guess is correct. The reason is very practical: a well-formed reflective statement is less likely to evoke resistance. In the dynamics of language, a question requires a response. Asking about meaning, through questioning, seems to distance people from experiencing it. They step back and begin to ask whether they really do or should feel what they have expressed. The difference is subtle, and not everyone notices it. Consider the difference in sound between these reflections:

"You're feeling uncomfortable?"
"You're feeling uncomfortable."

"You're angry with your mother?"
"You're angry with your mother."

The difference is an inflection. The voice tone goes up at the end of a question, but gently down at the end of a statement. Reflective listening statements should usually turn down at the end. They are statements of understanding.

To offer reflective listening, first train yourself to think reflectively. This includes the continual awareness that what you believe or assume people mean is not necessarily what they really mean. Most statements can have multiple meanings. Emotion words such as "depressed" or "anxious" can have very different meanings to different people. What could it mean for a person to say, "I wish I were more sociable"? Here are some possibilities:

"I feel lonely and I want to have more friends."
"I get very nervous when I have to talk to strangers."
"I should spend more time getting to know people."
"I would like to be popular."
"I can't think of anything to say when I'm with people."
"People don't invite me to their parties."

To think reflectively is to make this process more conscious. When hearing any utterance, one considers what it might mean and guesses about the most likely meaning. Many people then act as though this were the actual meaning, and react to it. Reflective listening is a way of checking, rather than assuming that you already know what is meant.

Reflective listening, then, involves making a statement that is not a roadblock but is, rather, a guess about what the speaker means. Often, but not always, the subject of the sentence is the pronoun "you." Here is an exemplary segment from a counseling session with an ambivalent problem drinker. For illustrative purposes, every counselor sentence in this segment is a reflective listening statement. Notice also that the counselor's reflections move forward rather than simply repeating what the client has said. In essence, the counselor is venturing the next sentence in the client's paragraph, instead of merely echoing the last one. This is a skillful form of reflection that we call "continuing the paragraph."

CLIENT: I worry sometimes that I may be drinking too much for my own good.

INTERVIEWER: You've been drinking quite a bit.

CLIENT: I don't really feel like it's that much. I can drink a lot and not feel it.

INTERVIEWER: More than most people.

CLIENT: Yes. I can drink most people under the table.

INTERVIEWER: And that's what worries you.

CLIENT: Well, that and how I feel. The next morning I'm usually in bad shape. I feel jittery, and I can't think straight through most of the morning.

INTERVIEWER: And that doesn't seem right to you.

CLIENT: No, I guess not. I haven't thought about it that much, but I don't think it's good to be hung over all the time. And sometimes I have trouble remembering things.

INTERVIEWER: Things that happen while you're drinking.

CLIENT: That, too. Sometimes I just have a blank for a few hours.

INTERVIEWER: But that isn't what you meant when you said you have trouble remembering things.

CLIENT: No. Even when I'm not drinking, it seems like I'm forgetting things more often, and I'm not thinking clearly.

INTERVIEWER: And you wonder if it has something to do with your drinking.

CLIENT: I don't know what else it would be.

INTERVIEWER: You haven't always been like that.

CLIENT: No! It's only the last few years. Maybe I'm just getting older.

INTERVIEWER: It might just be what happens to everybody when they reach 45.

CLIENT: No, it's probably my drinking. I don't sleep very well, either.

INTERVIEWER: So maybe you're damaging your health and your sleep and your brain by drinking as much as you do.

CLIENT: Mind you, I'm not a drunk. Never was.

INTERVIEWER: You're not that bad off. Still, you're worried.

CLIENT: I don't know about "worried," but I guess I'm thinking about it more.

INTERVIEWER: And wondering if you should do something, so that's why you came here.

CLIENT: I guess so.

INTERVIEWER: You're not sure.

CLIENT: I'm not sure what I want to do about it.

INTERVIEWER: So if I understand you so far, you think that you've been drinking too much and you've been damaging your health, but you're not sure yet if you want to change that.

CLIENT: Doesn't make much sense, does it?

INTERVIEWER: I can see how you might feel confused at this point.

Notice that the counselor does not insert any roadblocks throughout this process. It would have been easy enough to substitute some of the roadblocks for these reflections. This is avoided, however, because the purpose is to elicit talk, particularly change talk, from the client.

Reflective listening statements can be quite simple. Sometimes the mere repetition of a word or two will keep the client moving (in the preceding example, the first reflection could have been "Too much . . . "). A more sophisticated reflection substitutes new words for what the client has offered or makes a guess about the unspoken meaning. Sometimes it is helpful, too, to reflect how the person seems to be feeling as he or she speaks. Reflections that simply repeat what the person has said can yield slower progress; continuing the paragraph often adds momentum to the exploration process.

Depth of reflection increases with counselor skillfulness. Sometimes a counselor becomes frustrated with reflective listening because it seems to go around in circles, leading nowhere. We have found that the problem is usually insufficient depth of reflection; the counselor is staying too close to exactly what the client just said—like an echo—and the conversation literally is going nowhere. Skillful reflection moves past what the person has already said, though not jumping too far ahead. The skill is not unlike the timing of interpretations in psychodyamic psychotherapy. If the person balks, you know you jumped too far, too fast.

When using reflection to encourage continued personal exploration, which is the broad goal of reflective listening, it is often useful to understate slightly what the speaker has offered. This is particularly so when emotional content is involved. There is a rich array of language for describing emotion. Within any particular emotion, such as anger, there are descriptors that vary widely in intensity. There are low-intensity anger words like "annoyed" and "irritated," and high-intensity descriptors such as "outraged" and "incensed." Intensity can be diminished by adding words like "a little," "a bit," and "somewhat," or it can be increased by adding "quite," "very," or "extremely." As a general principle, if you overstate the intensity of an expressed emotion, the person will tend to deny and minimize it, backing off from the original statement. (This principle is applied intentionally in Chapter 8, in the method of amplified reflection for responding to resistance.) If you slightly understate the expressed intensity of emotion, however, the person is more likely to continue exploring and telling you about it. When reflecting emotion, err on the British side and understate:

Overstating

CLIENT: I just don't like the way she comments on how I raise my children.

INTERVIEWER: You're really angry with your mother.

CLIENT: Well, no, not angry really. She's my mother, after all.

Understating

CLIENT: I just don't like the way she comments on how I raise my children.

INTERVIEWER: You're a bit annoyed with your mother.

CLIENT: Yes, it just irritates me how she is always correcting and criticizing me.

Reflection is not a passive process. It can be quite directive. The counselor decides what to reflect and what to ignore, what to emphasize and deemphasize, what words to use in capturing meaning. Reflection can therefore be used to reinforce certain aspects of what a person has said or to alter its meaning slightly. In motivational interviewing, for example, change talk is preferentially reflected, so that people hear their own statements at least twice. These directive applications of reflection are discussed in Chapter 7.

We advise that reflective listening statements should constitute a substantial proportion of counselor responses during the early phase of motivational interviewing. Reflection is particularly important after open-ended questions. Once you have asked an open question, respond to the client's answers with reflective listening. Because questioning is a much less demanding skill (for the counselor) than empathic listening, it is easy to fall into the question–answer trap, asking a series of questions instead of reflecting the client's statements. This may evoke resistance more than change talk. Remember, therefore, to follow up a question with reflective listening rather than another question. Counselors skillful in motivational interviewing offer two to three reflections, on average, per question asked, and about half of all their responses (not counting the short "uh-huh" type of response) are reflections. In coding ordinary counseling sessions, in contrast, we find that questions often outnumber reflections by a ratio of 10 to 1, and reflections constitute a relatively small proportion of all responses.

3. Affirm

Directly affirming and supporting the client during the counseling process is another way of building rapport and reinforcing open exploration. This can be done in the form of compliments or statements of appreciation and understanding. The process of reflective listening can be quite affirming in itself, but direct affirmations have a place in counseling, too. Here are some examples:

> "Thanks for coming on time today."
> "I appreciate that you took a big step in coming here today."
> "You're clearly a resourceful person, to cope with such difficulties for so long."
> "That's a good suggestion."
> "I must say, if I were in your position, I might have a hard time dealing with that amount of stress."
> "It seems like you're a really spirited and strong-willed person in a way."
> "You enjoy being happy with other people, and making them laugh."
> "I've enjoyed talking with you today, and getting to know you a bit."

As with many aspects of conversation, norms vary from one culture or subculture to another. For instance, from a British perspective, American counselors can appear to be rather "over the top" with affirmations. One encounters similar issues in assertiveness training. The fundamental idea of assertiveness is sound—finding a middle ground between passive and aggressive responses—but there is wide variation in what constitutes an assertive versus aggressive response across societies, and so one adjusts content to social norms. Similarly, the appropriate level and frequency of affirmation within counseling will vary across social contexts. The point is to notice and appropriately affirm the client's strengths and efforts.

4. Summarize

The fourth OARS method to use early and throughout motivational interviewing is summarizing. Summary statements can be used to link together and reinforce material that has been discussed. When you are eliciting a person's change talk, for example, it is wise to summarize periodically:

> "So, this heart attack has left you feeling really vulnerable. It's not dying that scares you, really. What worries you is being only half alive—living disabled or being a burden to your family. In terms of things you want to live for, you've mentioned seeing your grandchildren grow up and continuing some of the work you've been doing that is especially meaningful to you, although maybe not with the intensity at which you'd been working before. What else?"

Such periodic summaries reinforce what has been said, show that you have been listening carefully, and prepare the client to elaborate further. They also allow a person to hear his or her own change talk for a third time.

At least three kinds of summaries are useful in motivational interviewing. The first of these, the *collecting* summary just illustrated, is offered during the process of exploration, particularly when you have heard several change talk themes. It's like collecting flowers one at a time and then giving them to the person in a little bouquet. Collecting summaries are usually short—just a few sentences—and should continue rather than interrupt the person's momentum. It is useful to end them with "What else?" or some other invitation to continue. (Notice, by the way, that "What else?" is an open question and invites continued exploration. "Is there anything else?" is a closed question [in that the literal answer is yes or no] and invites the answer "No.") Too-frequent collecting summaries can have an artificial feeling and can even be annoying, interrupting the natural exploration process. Use them judiciously when you have a number of new change-talk flowers to return (see Chapter 7).

Linking summaries tie together what a person has just been saying with material offered earlier, perhaps in a previous session. The border between collecting and linking summaries is grey, but their purpose is somewhat different. Collecting summaries draw together change talk and invite the person to keep going. Linking summaries are meant to encourage the client to reflect on the relationship between two or more previously discussed items. Linking summaries can be especially helpful in clarifying a person's ambivalence. The typical internal experience of ambivalence is to vacillate back and forth between thinking of reasons to change and reasons to stay the same. A linking summary is one way to allow a person to examine the positives and negatives simultaneously, acknowledging that both are present. When reflecting ambivalence, consider using "and" rather than "but" to link discrepant components, which has the effect of emphasizing the simultaneous presence of both.

use 'and' not 'but'

The conjunctions "yet" and "but" have a different function. They function like erasers, tending to soften and deemphasize what went before, and in this way they are more like the confusing back-and-forth thought process of ambivalence. Other linking phrases, such as "on the one hand . . . and on the other" and "at the same time," can also be useful:

> "It sounds like you're inclined in two different directions. On the one hand, you're somewhat worried about the possible long-term effects of your diabetes if you don't manage it well—blindness, amputations, things like that. Those are distressing to think about. The emergency room visit a while back also scared you, and you realize that if no one had found you, your children could be without a father. On the other hand, you're young and you feel fairly healthy most of the time. You enjoy eating what you like, and the long-term consequences seem far away. You're concerned, and at the same time you're not concerned."

Other sources of information can be incorporated into a linking summary as well. The results of objective assessment, or information from the courts or family members, can be combined with the person's own statements.

Finally there is the *transitional* summary, which marks and announces a shift from one focus to another. Such a summary can be used as a wrap-up toward the end of a session, and the transition from Phase 1 to Phase 2 is tested by such a summary (see Chapter 10). At the end of the first session in particular, it is useful to offer a substantial transitional summary, pulling together what has transpired thus far. Remember that in giving such summaries, you are deciding what to include and emphasize. When introducing a transitional summary, it can be helpful to use a prefacing statement that formally announces what is to follow. (We do not recommend doing this with collecting or linking summaries, which just fit into the flow of ongoing conversation.) Here is an example of a fairly complete transitional summary at the end of a first session, complete with prefacing statement:

> "Our time is running out, and I'd like to try to pull together what you've said so far, so we can see where we are and where we're going. Let me know if I miss anything important that we've covered. You came in because your husband is concerned about your drinking and your marijuana smoking. If he hadn't pushed you, you might not have come right now, but you've been very open in exploring this, and I appreciate that. I asked you about problems in your life that you think could be related to alcohol and marijuana, and you have mentioned several. You've been feeling quite depressed and tired, and, as we discussed, alcohol is a depressant. You said you're having a lot of trouble concentrating and that you're feeling as if you aren't motivated to do anything in your life. Again, rightly, you think this might be linked to your drinking and smoking, although you believe that's not the whole picture. You resent your

husband's sending you here alone, in a way, because you think he has a part in these problems, too. The tests that you completed indicate that you have developed a fairly significant dependence on alcohol and, to a lesser extent, on marijuana, and you realize that's something that can keep growing if you don't do something about it. When you were arrested that one time 2 years ago, your breath test showed that you were over 0.20, which is really quite intoxicated, even though you weren't feeling very drunk. We talked about how this kind of tolerance is in itself a risk factor. You're also concerned that you're not the kind of mother you want to be, in part because of drinking and smoking, and you don't want your kids to grow up with drug problems. Your doctor told you that your stomach problems are probably caused or at least made worse by your drinking. At the same time, you have liked alcohol and marijuana because you use them to relax and to get away from some heavy family stresses. You're not sure how you could handle life without drinking and smoking, and so you're not sure what to do at this point. Is that a fair summary so far? Anything I've missed?"

The transitional summary is a good way to draw the first session to a close. Notice the collaborative tone, allowing the client to add to or correct your summary. A somewhat shorter form of the same statement can be used at the beginning of the next session, building on progress made earlier.

5. Eliciting Change Talk

The preceding four skills, the OARS, are fundamental to motivational interviewing. If these were the only methods employed, however, it would be quite easy to remain stuck in ambivalence. It is important, therefore, to have a guiding strategy for resolving ambivalence. That is the underlying purpose of the fifth method, which is consciously directive. The other four skills can all be applied within this goal-directed approach.

In one sense, motivational interviewing is the opposite of a confrontational approach, in which the counselor advocates for the "problem-change" position and the client defends against it. We believe that such a confrontational dialogue is often detrimental, precisely because it causes the person to defend a no-change position. The idea in motivational interviewing is to have the client give voice to exactly the opposite kinds of statements, to present the arguments for change. It is the counselor's task to facilitate the client's expression of such change talk, referred to in our earlier writings as self-motivational statements.[3]

Because we are discussing an intentionally directive aspect, this seems a good place for a reminder of the consciously collaborative nature of motivational interviewing, as well. Some people misunderstand this method as a way of tweaking motivation, of manipulating or tricking people into doing what you want them to do. But both partners bring aspirations to the dance floor;

both have hopes for what will happen. The counselor's aspirations are not preeminent, not the model to which a client's will must be sculpted. Instead, motivational interviewing is a process of shared decision making, of exploration and negotiation. It is a process shaped and complicated by the opinions, investment, and relative power of the two partners. We explore some of these ethical aspects of motivational interviewing in Chapter 12.

As discussed in Chapter 3, change talk falls into four general categories. The first involves recognizing the disadvantages of the current situation, of the status quo:

Recognizing disadvantages of the status quo

"I guess there's more of a problem here than I realized."
"I never really thought that much before about how this affects my family."
"This is serious!"
"Maybe I have been taking foolish risks."
"I can see that in the long run, this is going to do me in if I don't make a change."

The other side of this coin is change talk that reflects potential advantages of change.

Recognizing advantages of change

"One thing is that I would have a lot more time, and it would help financially, too."
"My boys would like it. They're always after me to quit."
"Probably I'd feel a lot better."
"At least it would get the courts off my back."
"I'd probably be around to enjoy my grandchildren as they grow up."

Change talk can also express optimism about change. Such statements reflect self-efficacy to make a difference in the problem area:

Expressing optimism about change

"I think I could probably do it if I decided to."
"I'm a fairly stubborn person. If I put my mind to something, I don't let go until it's done."
"I did quit smoking a few years ago. That was tough, and it took a few tries, but I did it."

The fourth type of change talk is direct or implicit intention or determination to change:

Expressing intention to change

"I think it's time for me to think about quitting."
"I definitely don't want to keep going the way I have been."
"I've got to do something."
"This isn't what I want for my family. What can I do?"
"I don't know how I'm going to do it, but I'm going to get through this."

These four kinds of statements encompass cognitive, emotional, and behavioral dimensions of commitment to change. From our perspective, every statement of this kind tips the balance a little further in the direction of change.

Some people walk through the counselor's door already saying things like this and only need some help in confirming their commitment and planning a course of action. When this is not the case, how can a counselor evoke such statements from more ambivalent clients? Evoking change talk is one of the key motivational interviewing skills. It is also one of the most complex, precisely because there are so many ways in which to accomplish it.

METHODS FOR EVOKING CHANGE TALK

Asking Evocative Questions

The simplest and most direct approach is simply to ask the person for such statements. Open-ended questions can be used to explore the client's own perceptions and concerns. Don't ask whether the client has such concerns (e.g., "Do you think that you have a problem?"). Assume that he or she is feeling ambivalent and does have such concerns. Some questions for evoking each of the four categories of change talk are suggested in Box 6.3. Note that these are all open questions.

As discussed here and in the next chapter, the process requires more than just asking such questions. There are specific processes for reflecting and reinforcing change talk when the person offers it.

Using the Importance Ruler

The rulers described earlier in this chapter can be used to elicit change talk. Our usual method is to obtain the client's rating of importance and then ask two questions:

"Why are you at a _____ and not zero?"
"What would it take for you to go from _____ to [a higher number]?"

The answers to these questions will very likely be change talk. Note that one should not ask, "Why are you at a _____ and not 10?" because to answer that question is to argue *against* change.

BOX 6.3. Example Open Questions to Evoke Change Talk

1. Disadvantages of the status quo

   What worries you about your current situation?
   What makes you think that you need to do something about your blood pressure?
   What difficulties or hassles have you had in relation to your drug use?
   What is there about your drinking that you or other people might see as reasons for concern?
   In what ways does this concern you?
   How has this stopped you from doing what you want to do in life?
   What do you think will happen if you don't change anything?

2. Advantages of change

   How would you like for things to be different?
   What would be the good things about losing weight?
   What would you like your life to be like 5 years from now?
   If you could make this change immediately, by magic, how might things be better for you?
   The fact that you're here indicates that at least part of you thinks it's time to do something. What are the main reasons you see for making a change?
   What would be the advantages of making this change?

3. Optimism about change

   What makes you think that if you did decide to make a change, you could do it?
   What encourages you that you can change if you want to?
   What do you think would work for you, if you decided to change?
   When else in your life have you made a significant change like this? How did you do it?
   How confident are you that you can make this change?
   What personal strengths do you have that will help you succeed?
   Who could offer you helpful support in making this change?

4. Intention to change

   What are you thinking about your gambling at this point?
   I can see that you're feeling stuck at the moment. What's going to have to change?
   What do you think you might do?
   How important is this to you? How much do you want to do this?
   What would you be willing to try?
   Of the options I've mentioned, which one sounds like it fits you best?
   Never mind the "how" for right now—what do you want to have happen?
   So what do you intend to do?

Exploring the Decisional Balance

As mentioned earlier, it can be helpful to have people discuss both the positive and the negative aspects of their present behavior, of the status quo. They may be asked, for example, to say or list what they like about their present pattern, as a preface to inquiring about the down side. This has the advantage of getting people talking and feeling comfortable and also of clarifying both sides of their ambivalence. Often, simply asking about one side will elicit the other. It may be useful to fill in a decisional balance sheet, like the one illustrated in Chapter 2, to allow a person to see the pros and cons simultaneously—a direct picture of the ambivalence.

Elaborating

Once a reason for change has been named, it is often the counselor's tendency to move on and find others. It can be quite useful, however, to have the client elaborate on a topic before moving on. For one thing, it is a way of eliciting further change talk, and it helps reinforce the motivational theme.

There are several ways of eliciting elaboration once a reason for change has been raised. They include:

- Asking for clarification: In what ways? How much? When?
- Asking for a specific example:
- Asking for a description of the last time this occurred.
- Asking "What else?" within the change topic.

Here is an illustration:

CLIENT: One obvious place where this is a problem for me is money.

INTERVIEWER: In what ways is that a concern for you?

CLIENT: Well, I just spend a lot of money on gambling, and I'm not always paying my bills.

INTERVIEWER: Tell me about the last time that happened.

CLIENT: Just last week I went through about $600. I start out setting a limit, but then I lose that amount and decide to try to win it back.

INTERVIEWER: Over time it really adds up.

CLIENT: I'll say. I've lost about $30,000 over the last 6 months.

INTERVIEWER: And that's a lot for you.

CLIENT: We don't have that kind of money. At least we don't now.

INTERVIEWER: How much does this money issue concern you?

CLIENT: It's getting to be a big problem, and I worry about it all the time. I've got people coming to the door, calling on the telephone, sending nasty letters. I've got to do something.

INTERVIEWER: And in what specific ways does it affect you, to lose so much?

CLIENT: Nobody will give me credit any more, except the casinos. My husband finally noticed all the cash withdrawals, and he's hardly talking to me.

INTERVIEWER: What else?

CLIENT: He's worried about our retirement security, of course. And I can't buy things I want.

INTERVIEWER: Such as . . .

CLIENT: The other day I saw this nice dress in just my size, and I couldn't afford it. My credit cards have all been canceled. Then I get mad and do stupid things.

INTERVIEWER: Like what?

Early in motivational interviewing, if there is little change talk to elaborate, it may be useful to ask the person to walk you through a typical day in his or her life. This offers opportunities for asking in more detail about behavior patterns and mood changes, for example, and areas of concern often emerge quite naturally from such discussion.

Querying Extremes

When there seems to be little desire for change at present, another way to elicit change talk is to ask people to describe the extremes of their (or others') concerns, to imagine the extreme of consequences that might ensue:

> "What concerns you the most about your high blood pressure in the long run?"
> "Suppose you continue on as you have been, without changing. What do you imagine are the worst things that might happen to you?"
> "How much do you know about what can happen if you drink during pregnancy, even if you don't see this happening to you?"

At the other extreme, it can be useful to imagine the best consequences that could follow from pursuing a change:

> "What might be the best results you could imagine if you make a change?"
> "If you were completely successful in making the changes you want, how would things be different?"

Looking Back

Sometimes it is useful, in eliciting change talk, to have the client remember times before the problem emerged and to compare these times with the present situation:

> "Do you remember a time when things were going well for you? What has changed?"
>
> "What were things like before you started using drugs? What were you like back then?"
>
> "Tell me about how you two met, and what attracted you to each other back then. What was it like?"
>
> "What are the differences between the Pat of 10 years ago and the Pat of today?"
>
> "How has your pain changed you as a person, or stopped you from growing, from moving forward?"

Looking back at the past sometimes recalls a time before problems emerged and can highlight both the discrepancy with how things are at present and the possibility of life being better. If looking back yields a description of a period when problems were worse, you can explore what has happened to yield some improvement to date.

Looking Forward

Helping people envision a changed future is another approach for eliciting change talk. Here you ask the client to tell you how it might be after a change:

> "If you do decide to make a change, what do you hope might be different in the future?"
>
> "How would you like things to turn out for you 10 years from now?"
>
> "I can see that you're feeling really frustrated right now. How would you like things to be different?"

Similarly, you can invite the client to look ahead in time and anticipate how things might be if no changes are made:

> "Suppose you don't make any changes, but just continue as you have been. What do you think your life would be like 10 years from now?"
>
> "Given what has happened so far, what do you expect might be happening 5 years from now if you don't make any changes?"

There is some overlap here with querying extremes. In the looking-ahead method, however, you are asking for either the person's realistic appraisal of a future unchanged or his or her realistic hopes for a future changed.

Exploring Goals and Values

Still another approach is to ask the client to tell you what things are most important in his or her life. After all, no one is truly "unmotivated." Their priorities may be quite different from the counselor's, but every person does have goals and values. Exploring what those are provides some reference points against which to compare the status quo.

This method can overlap nicely with the looking-forward process. What values or goals does this person hold most dear? From the perspective of motivational interviewing, the purpose of this exploration is to discover ways in which current behavior is inconsistent with or undermines important values and goals for the person. When the client's highest or most central values and goals are defined, you can ask how the problem you are discussing (e.g., drinking) fits into this picture. The central point here is to explore and develop themes of discrepancy between these important goals or values and the client's current behavior. Chapter 19 describes some more specific methods for incorporating values in motivational interviewing.

SUMMARY

In motivational interviewing, eliciting change talk is a primary method for developing discrepancy. Hearing oneself state the reasons for change tends to increase awareness of the discrepancy between one's goals and present actions. The greater this discrepancy, the greater the perceived importance of change. The first four early methods for motivational interviewing (OARS) can be integrated with the fifth, eliciting change talk, by (1) asking open questions that pull for change talk; (2) affirming and reinforcing the client for change talk; (3) reflecting back, sometimes selectively, change talk that the client has voiced, which allows him or her to hear it a second time; and (4) offering collecting, linking, and transitional summaries of change talk, allowing the client to hear once again the statements that he or she has made. Other methods, such as objective feedback and values exploration, can also serve to increase perceived discrepancy. Phase 1 of motivational interviewing focuses primarily on this process of building intrinsic motivation through the amplification and clarification of discrepancy.

Eliciting change talk can be important, however, not only in early sessions, but throughout counseling. Ambivalence does not usually disappear but only diminishes in the transition to Phase 2 and the initiation of action toward change. Evoking change talk can serve as a continuing reminder of the reasons for commitment to change.

ANSWERS TO BOX 6.2

1. Open question.
2. Closed question, in that it asks for a specific piece of information. An open question (in imperative form) would be "Tell me about your growing-up years."
3. Closed question, in its rhetorical structure that implies a "Yes" or "No" answer. An open form would be "What gives meaning to your life?"
4. Closed question, answered by "Yes" or "No." An open form would be "What do you think about coming back for a follow-up visit?"
5. Open question.
6. Closed question, answered by "Yes" or "No." An open form would be "What would be the good things and not-so-good things about staying in this relationship?"
7. Advice veiled as a closed question, for which the literal answer is "Yes" or "No." An open version would be "If you decided to exercise more, what kinds of exercise might be most appealing or acceptable to you?"
8. Closed question. Drop the multiple-choice options at the end, and it becomes an open question.
9. Open question.
10. Closed question, asking for a specific piece of information—a date.
11. Open question.
12. Rhetorical closed question. An open form would be "In what ways is it important to you to be in good health?"
13. Open question.
14. Closed question answered by "Yes" or "No."
15. Closed question, two choices.

NOTES

1. Rubino, Barker, Roth, and Fearon (2000).
2. Gordon (1970).
3. Miller (1983).

CHAPTER 7

Responding to Change Talk

> It is the truth we ourselves speak rather than the treatment we receive that heals us.
> —O. HOBART MOWRER (1966)

WHEN IS MOTIVATIONAL INTERVIEWING DIRECTIVE?

In the preceding chapters we have defined motivational interviewing as a directive yet client-centered counseling style. In one sense, motivational interviewing is always directive, in that it is consciously directed toward the resolution of ambivalence in order to facilitate change. In another sense, however, the directiveness of motivational interviewing varies, depending on the extent to which its goal is to resolve ambivalence in the direction of a particular kind of change. Consider what might be the differences in doing motivational interviewing with these particular clients:

A couple trying to decide whether or not to adopt a child
An overweight person who has lost a significant amount of weight several
    times but has always gained it back
A person with diabetes, seen in emergency room because of poor
    glycemic control
A sex offender entering treatment as an alternative to incarceration

An obvious dimension along which these four examples vary is the extent to which the counselor is likely to have a clear sense of the desirable outcome of change. In the first case, the counselor may have no opinion or investment at all in which way the couple decides. With regard to being overweight, knowledgeable counselors vary in their opinions about the desirability of continued weight loss efforts. The life-threatening nature of out-of-control diabetes is likely to inspire clearer conviction about the desirable change—namely, improved glycemic control. Finally, in the case of an offender, there are potential victims to consider as well, along with society's general consensus as to the desirability of changed behavior.

There are clearly cases, then, in which motivational interviewing is directed toward a particular change goal that the counselor judges to be desirable, even though the person at the moment may or may not feel ready, willing, or able to pursue such change. That was, in fact, the context within which motivational interviewing was originally developed: to enhance intrinsic motivation for change in people with persistent addictive behaviors that are harmful to themselves and others. Such discrepancy between client and counselor goals raises complex and fascinating ethical issues that are explored in Chapter 12.

We realize, however, that a motivational interviewing style can also be used in helping people who are stuck to resolve ambivalence and move on with change, even when the counselor is truly indifferent to the direction of the change. Choice counseling is a legitimate and helpful process even (and perhaps especially) when the counselor has no particular opinion or investment about the choice that results.

How one responds to change talk within motivational interviewing will vary, then, depending on the extent to which the goal of counseling is to elicit intrinsic motivation for a particular kind or direction of change. We begin with the more familiar situation in which there is a particular change toward which counseling is directed.

WHEN MOTIVATIONAL INTERVIEWING IS DIRECTIVE

Just eliciting change talk is not enough when the intent of motivational interviewing is to enhance intrinsic motivation toward a particular change outcome. It is here that one responds differentially to client statements, depending on whether they move toward (change talk) or away from (resistance) the change goal. As noted earlier, counselors do this even without being aware of it, encouraging clients in a particular direction. The skillful motivational interviewer is consciously aware of and intentional in this process of differential responding.

It is worth an aside here to note that in this motivational interviewing context, the terms "change talk" and "resistance" are usually defined in relation to a particular type of change. One need only analyze a few counseling sessions to realize that people talk about making many different kinds of changes. In fact, talk directed toward one kind of change might be judged to be resistance if it favors change in the direction opposite to a counseling goal. Consider this example:

> "I know I really ought to get out of this relationship. It's tough to quit when the person you live with is constantly using. I'd like to have a life of my own and a real job, and to raise my kids in a better environment. But I do love him, and it's hard to think about leaving him."

What would be considered change talk or resistance in this example? It depends on how one thinks about the change goal(s). What counts as change talk would vary, depending on whether the person had come seeking career counseling, marital counseling, or treatment for drug dependence; had been referred because of concerns about possible child abuse; or was being sheltered as a victim of domestic violence. It depends on the identified goal(s) of change. In this context, then, change talk refers to speech that is directed toward the desired kind of change, and resistance refers to speech that moves away from the desired kind of change.

When there is a clear goal for change, motivational interviewing involves not only eliciting but also responding in particular ways to change talk. The methods for eliciting change talk have been described in Chapter 6. This section focuses on clinical aspects of how to respond when it does occur, with the general technical goal of reinforcing and increasing change talk. The four general strategies described are by now familiar: elaborating, reflecting, summarizing, and affirming change talk. Chapter 8 takes up the topic of how to respond to resistance (that is, to talk that moves away from the desired direction of change).

Elaborating Change Talk

Whether a person will continue to explore change talk or veer away from it depends on how you respond. When a client voices a change statement, even tentatively, respond with particular interest, both nonverbally (for example, with attention and a simple head nod) and by asking for elaboration.

Once the process has begun, straightforward encouragement to continue is often effective. The general form here is "What else?":

> "In what ways?"
> "Give me an example. When was the last time this happened?"
> "What else have you noticed or wondered about?"
> "What other concerns have you had about _____?"
> "What are some other reasons why you might want to make a change?"
> "What other things have people told you?"
> "Why else do you think you could succeed?"
> "How else could you do it?"

Reflecting Change Talk

Reflective listening both clarifies the person's meaning and encourages continued exploration of the content that is reflected. Simple reflection of change talk, then, is likely to elicit further elaboration and exploration.

Consciously or not, reflective listening is selective. One does not and cannot reflect all shades of meaning, explore all possible avenues, or capture all of the content offered or implied in the person's speech. For one thing, you can reflect only those aspects that you perceive. Within the range of perceived content, however, you select what to reflect and what to leave unsaid. In motivational interviewing, this selection process is conscious and purposeful. The person's change talk is reflected selectively.

Consider this example of how a counselor might respond to the ambivalent distress of the woman in the preceding example, if counseling her toward distancing from an abusive relationship:

CLIENT: . . . Maybe it's easier just to stay together and work on our relationship, at least until my daughter starts school.

INTERVIEWER: So one of the most important considerations for you is how staying together or separating would affect your daughter.

CLIENT: Right. I don't want to mess up her life, just because mine has been a mess. It might be better for her to have two parents around, I guess, but then in some other ways he's not the best influence on her.

INTERVIEWER: What are some of those ways?

CLIENT: Well, like I told you, he has a bad temper. He's never hit her so far, but she's seen him beat me up, and that really upsets her.

INTERVIEWER: It's not good, you think, for her to see him hurting you, and you also worry that eventually he might hurt her physically as well.

CLIENT: That's got to be bad. It was awful last time. She was screaming and crying, but it didn't stop him.

INTERVIEWER: She was really scared, but that didn't seem to matter; it didn't keep him from hurting you more.

CLIENT: Once he gets going like that, he doesn't care about anyone or anything. It's like he's in a blind rage.

INTERVIEWER: And that's terrifying for a 4-year-old girl, and for you as well. So even if you didn't mind particularly what happens to you, it's important to you to protect that little girl of yours.

CLIENT: She's so sweet. I just love her so much.

INTERVIEWER: Enough, perhaps, to make this really hard choice . . .

The righting reflex gets very strong in a situation like this. It is quite easy to imagine the counselor taking over with forceful advice, telling the mother her duty, warning, even ordering. Sometimes this may be necessary, but it is worth considering the assumptions that underlie and are communicated by the use of such roadblocks. They implicitly assume that the mother does not see and cannot appreciate the danger, is not capable of making the right decision on her own, and needs an outsider to take control and tell her what to do. There are situations in which this is exactly the appropriate thing to do, as in the case of an acutely depressed and intoxicated person with the means at hand to commit suicide and a plan to do so. In many other situations, however, we believe it is more effective to elicit the intrinsic motivation and plan for change from the person rather than trying to install them.

There is a danger in selective reflection of change talk that is worth noting. Remember that an ambivalent person may respond with the opposite when you seem to be taking up one side of the argument. Reflecting change talk, then, can sometimes have the paradoxical effect of evoking the other side of the ambivalence (resistance). If this occurs, it is easy enough to recover with a double-sided reflection. The point is not to fall into defending the change side while the client argues the other.

CLIENT: My parents really are too strict, and
I hate that, but I guess it's because they
worry about me.

INTERVIEWER: They care enough about you   *Reflecting one side . . .*
to set limits.

CLIENT: But their rules are just   *. . . elicits the other.*
unreasonable!

INTERVIEWER: You wish, sometimes, that   *A double-sided reflection*
they didn't care about you so much,   *recaptures both sides . . .*
because they go way overboard
in trying to protect you.

CLIENT: Right! I mean, I know they care   *. . . and restores a balanced*
about me. I'd just like them to give   *perspective.*
me more freedom and to trust me
more.

Always keep in mind that the overall purpose here is for the client to voice the change side of the conflict and, ultimately, to move in that direction.

Summarizing Change Talk

A third useful way to respond to change talk, besides reflecting and asking for elaboration, is to offer summaries that gather together bouquets of change statements that the person has offered. In the previous chapter we distinguished collecting, linking, and transitional summaries, but all three kinds serve a similar function: they allow the person to hear once again their own change talk.

Like reflections, summaries are consciously selective. Certain flowers are placed in the bouquet, while others are not. Some flowers are put up front in a prominent position, and others are put behind. In general, summaries are collections of change statements the person has made: disadvantages of the status quo, reasons for change, optimism about change, and desire to change (Chapter 6). Particularly in transitional summaries, that tend to be somewhat longer, it can be important to include in the background an acknowledgment of the other side of ambivalence, as well. Including both sides can head off the person responding to your summary with a "Yes, but . . . " Here is an example of a transitional summary that includes resistance themes sandwiched within prominently placed change talk:

> "What you seem to be thinking, then, is that you want to make a fairly significant change in your lifestyle. In fact, it sounds like the change needs to be large in order to work: moving to a different neighborhood, finding a whole new set of friends, getting a job to have more structure in your life, and maybe getting reconnected with a church. There's a part of you that has wanted to hold onto your old life, because you would be losing so much that is familiar to you now, but mostly you believe that it's time to move on with your life. One possibility that you're considering is enlisting in one of the armed forces, which could help you do all of this at once. You see a number of important reasons for taking this leap now, difficult though it will be. One of them is freedom. You see yourself headed for jail, maybe even a life in prison if you don't turn your life around very soon. You also have this feeling that it's time to grow up, that adolescence was fun but now it's time to be an adult. You had some sense of loss in that, too—giving up childhood and taking on responsibility—but you seem to be ready to move on. It's also really important to you to be there for your son and not have him grow up without you. All of that is why you want to make such a major change now."

Note some artful nuances of language here. Resistance themes are stated in past tense, change talk in present tense. In discussing summarizing in Chapter 6, we suggested using the conjunction "and" to capture ambivalence rather than "but," because the former acknowledges the simultaneous presence of both sides. Later in the process, however, as ambivalence begins to move toward change, it can be useful to alter the structure of language for describing the resistance side. This is illustrated in the preceding example. Points of reluctance (resistance) are stated first within a sentence, then joined by "but" to counteract points of change talk. The conjunction "but" has a partial eraser effect, directing attention toward what follows it and away from what goes before. It has a subtle effect of partially detracting from or invalidating whatever precedes it. Consider an example from a performance evaluation:

> "In general, Jones, you're doing a fine job here. You are reliable, and the quality of your work is good, but ... "

Suddenly, all that went before is forgotten, and the employee's attention is fixed on whatever comes next. The conjunction "but" (and its functional equivalents such as "however, "yet," and "although") can therefore be useful syntax when you wish to acknowledge the other side of ambivalence but direct momentum toward change.

Affirming Change Talk

Finally, one can reinforce change talk simply by commenting positively on it. A few examples will suffice:

> "That sounds like a good idea."
> "I can see how that would concern you."
> "I think that could work."
> "You're very considerate of how your actions affect other people."
> "That's a good point."
> "It's important to you to be a good parent."
> "I think you're right about that."

In closing this rather technical section, we are inclined to reiterate the overall spirit within which these methods are applied. Motivational interviewing is not a set of quick-trick techniques for making people change. The person's autonomy is always respected, and the reasons for change arise from the person's own values and goals. It is a collaborative process of shared decision making.

WHEN MOTIVATIONAL INTERVIEWING IS NONDIRECTIVE

There are other times when counseling is not directed toward any particular change outcome. There are still goals for the counseling, of course. A common one is to help the person get unstuck, resolve ambivalence, and move on with life. What we mean here is that the counselor is not interested in directing the resolution of ambivalence toward any particular kind of change.

The goal is to help people explore the options and their possible consequences in relation to their own values and goals. The counselor may provide requested information but has no directional advice to give, being truly indifferent to the direction chosen. Medical ethicists term this "equipoise," when the physician has no clear attachment to or recommendation for one resolution more than another.

In a way, this situation requires a still higher level of clinical skillfulness than the directive variety of counseling, because one must avoid inadvertently tipping the scales in one direction or the other (for examples, see Chapter 6). There is also the opposite risk, of negating each change statement by eliciting its opposite and thereby exacerbating and entrenching ambivalence:

CLIENT: I suppose it would be fun to go. I've never visited a place like Greneda, but I also hate to use up my holiday time.

INTERVIEWER: There are other things you'd like to do with your time off.

CLIENT: I have work to do in the house, and I would enjoy planting a garden in the back. It's nice sometimes just to stay home.

INTERVIEWER: Yet the adventure of visiting an exotic place is appealing, too.

CLIENT: It is! I like the idea of just taking off for some place I've never seen, and leaving everything else behind. I might not want to come back!

INTERVIEWER: And still, it's nice to relax at home, too, and accomplish a few things there.

Clarifying Ambivalence

One key task is to clarify the ambivalence, to explore each side in some depth. The back-and-forth process just illustrated can be quite frustrating. In fact, it resembles how people ordinarily remain stuck in ambivalence, going back and forth in thinking about pros and cons, until in exasperation they stop turning it over.

One approach is to thoroughly explore each side of the ambivalent conflict. This is best done by making it clear that you are exploring together one option at a time. (Note that there may well be more than two options under consideration: not ambivalence as much as mutivalence.) For the time being, the attractiveness of other alternatives is suspended, and together you go down one road at a time, exploring its good things and not-so-good things. Then the process is repeated for another option. It may be useful to keep decisional balance notes about the pros and cons of each option, making the arguments for each side visible simultaneously (see Chapters 2 and 6).

Summary reflections should contain the important elements of each side of the conflict. Double-sided reflections with "and" (not "but") conjunctions are a normal part of this process.

Clarifying Values

Once the ambivalence is clear, then what? The way out of ambivalence is like the way out of a deep forest. Pick a direction and keep moving in as straight a line as possible. The question is how to pick the direction.

A primary basis for resolving ambivalence is in relation to the person's values. What does the client hold most dear? What goals and values are central to his or her life? Which values particularly pertain to this choice point?

How would each possible resolution move the client toward or away from important values and goals? Looking ahead, where does the client want to be in 5 or 10 years? How would each possible resolution move the client toward or away from that envisioned horizon?

Here is an example of nondirective motivational interviewing with a person who is choosing between staying in her present community or moving to take a new job in another area. It illustrates briefly the methods described: double-sided reflection, clarifying ambivalence by exploring one avenue at a time, summary reflections, and incorporating values.

INTERVIEWER: Let me suggest that we try something here. It's easy to get stuck in a decision like this because as soon as you think of an advantage of one possibility, you then think of its down side or an advantage of the other possibility. Let's take the possibilities one at a time: stay here, or move. Let's begin with staying here. What are the advantages?

CLIENT: It's familiar—the devil you know, as they say. I'm not that happy at work, but I get along OK, and I know how to do my job well.

INTERVIEWER: So your job here is OK. What else?

CLIENT: I have plenty of friends here, including some really close friends. I'd miss them a lot. I say I'd write or telephone, but the truth is that I get busy and don't do it, and those friendships would drift away. Of course, I'm sure I could make new friends if I moved.

INTERVIEWER: But that's about option number two. Let's stick with option one for now: staying here. So far you've said that your work situation is satisfactory, not great but familiar, and that you have good close friends here who are important to you. What else?

CLIENT: It's kind of related, but the synagogue I attend is one that I really like, and it might be hard to find a community like that in a new city. It means a lot to me to go every sabbath, and I'm close to the rabbi and the people there. It builds me up spiritually.

INTERVIEWER: OK. You have a strong faith community here. What else?

CLIENT: It might be better for Alison to finish school here. She has three more years to go, and she doesn't want to move to a new school. And I like the weather here.

INTERVIEWER: Work, friends, synagogue, school, weather. What else would be good about staying here?

CLIENT: I guess that's about it. It's always uncomfortable to pick up roots and start over in a new place, but it's kind of exciting, too.

INTERVIEWER: All right, good. Now let's take a look at the other option you're considering, to move for this new job. What would be the advantages of that?

CLIENT: (*Laughs.*) The first thing that occurs to me is that I'd be far away from my ex. The divorce was pretty ugly, and in a way I'd like to leave all that behind and start over. It's silly, I guess, but somehow I think that moving would give me more of a feeling of starting a new life, without all of the constant reminders.

INTERVIEWER: Funny that that's the first thing you think of.

CLIENT: Well, it would be getting away from unpleasant memories here. They are offering me a much better salary, too. I haven't even told my boss here that I'm thinking about moving. It might be a better work environment, but it's hard to tell. The people I met seem to enjoy working there. I'd have a little more responsibility in my new position, as well.

INTERVIEWER: The new job itself has some real attractions for you: better pay, better colleagues, a more responsible position . . .

CLIENT: Not better colleagues, really. I like the people I work with now, but it's a more pleasant building. It has big windows and doesn't feel so cramped. I guess they need big windows, though, because it rains there all the time.

INTERVIEWER: Nice windows, not such nice weather.

CLIENT: The cost of living is higher there, too, but it's a bigger city and has a lot to offer.

INTERVIEWER: For example . . .

CLIENT: They have more museums and concerts and things, and a really good zoo. I think the schools are better.

INTERVIEWER: Which might be better for Alison, and there would be more for you to do in your free time.

CLIENT: I guess so.

INTERVIEWER: What else?

CLIENT: I don't really know that much else about it. Mainly it's a way to get away from here and start over.

INTERVIEWER: OK, so here we go with the big picture. Let me know if I leave something out. The advantages of staying here are that you're settled in and it's familiar. Moving to a new place always involves a certain amount of disruption. You know your job here, and while it's not perfect, you know what to expect and how to do it. You have good friends here, and particularly important is your synagogue and the community you have there. You like the weather here, and Alison would prefer to stay here and finish school. Perhaps the biggest factor in favor of moving is your feeling of having a fresh new start. It would get you away from your ex, and painful reminders, and would give you a new lease on life. The job is more responsible and the pay is better, in the context of a somewhat higher cost of living. The building where you would work is nicer, and the weather isn't. There is more to do there, and the schools might be better for Alison. How's that?

CLIENT: Excellent—but it doesn't help me much. I still feel confused.

INTERVIEWER: Of course you do. There's not one clear right answer here. Did anything else occur to you as I was talking?

CLIENT: I realize I can tell my boss about the possibility of moving and see what happens. If she gets angry, that might help me decide to go. Or she might offer me a raise if she wants to keep me.

INTERVIEWER: You're not really sure which way it would go.

CLIENT: I think probably she'd try to keep me. She seems to like my work. So that wouldn't make the decision for me, either.

INTERVIEWER: It might only remove one of the differences, the pay difference, and it sounds like that's not one of the most important for you.

CLIENT: Well, it's important. I'd like to have a better salary, but it's not the whole picture by any means.

INTERVIEWER: Then let me ask you this: What is most important to you?

CLIENT: In my job?

INTERVIEWER: No, in life. What do you care most about? What do you value? What do you want to do with your life?

CLIENT: Big question! I care about Alison. I'm not just saying that because I'm supposed to. I really want the very best for her.

INTERVIEWER: Specifically . . .

CLIENT: I want her to be happy. I don't particularly care what she decides she wants to do in life. If she decides she wants more education, she'll get it.

INTERVIEWER: You love her very much.

CLIENT: I do. We're very close.

INTERVIEWER: What else is important to you in life?

CLIENT: I'm a very spiritual person. I know there is more to life than what we can see. I feel like a kindergartner when it comes to religion, but I want to keep growing spiritually.

INTERVIEWER: In what ways?

CLIENT: I don't know how to explain it exactly, but there is a path that I'm meant to walk, and I want to be sure I'm on it. I keep a Jewish home, and that's important to me.

INTERVIEWER: So that's part of the question here, too. One of these two possibilities is on the right path for you, but which one?

CLIENT: Yes. It seems like it ought to be clear, but it's not.

INTERVIEWER: Alison, spiritual growth . . . What else is top priority for you?

CLIENT: I want to be with someone again, probably to be married again. I don't want to live out my life alone. I have Alison, but she'll need to have her own life.

INTERVIEWER: What about the things you cherish most in life?

CLIENT: I love being outdoors, in nature. I love music; I'm not a musician, but I love listening to classical music. And my friends are important to me— having at least a few good, close friends who share everyday life with me.

INTERVIEWER: What about your work?

CLIENT: I don't think I'm going to change the world. Work is a job. I enjoy doing it, but when I go home, then I'm home. I'm much more a people person.

INTERVIEWER: What you've mentioned so far, as the things in life that really matter to you, are your daughter, your faith, being married again or at least having a life partner, nature, and music, and having close friends. How might these values fit in with staying here or moving?

CLIENT: It sounds like moving just for a new job doesn't make much sense. That's not really what this is about. I have friends, and synagogue, and a life here, and Alison wants to stay. There are some attractive things there, but really it's this feeling of needing a new start, wanting to break free.

INTERVIEWER: And a move would do that.

CLIENT: You know, I'm not even sure about that. It's more a feeling I have . . .

Without pushing in one direction or the other, the counselor helps the client explore both sides of the ambivalence and to evaluate them in relation to important personal values. At the end of this example the client seems to be moving toward resolution without the counselor having tried to influence its direction. This exemplifies how motivational interviewing can be used to resolve ambivalence when the counselor has no personal commitment to a particular outcome.

Without the directive aspect, isn't this just client-centered counseling? In many ways, yes it is. The fundamental skills being used are methods described well by Rogers, and the goal is to be nondirective as well as client-centered. An important refinement, we believe, is being consciously nondirective. As an evolution of client-centered counseling, motivational interviewing brings into clearer focus when, how, and why this method can be directive. By understanding when and how client-centered skills can be used directively, one is also, we hope, more prepared to maintain equipoise when appropriate.

SUMMARY

The client-centered methods of motivational interviewing can be used either directively or nondirectively. The difference is in how one responds to change talk and (as we shall see in Chapter 8) to resistance relative to a particular direction of change. When used directively, motivational interviewing involves selectively elaborating, reflecting, summarizing, and affirming change talk. In a nondirective application, the approach is much closer to the original method of client-centered counseling, but with clearer consciousness of how to maintain a neutral balance.

CHAPTER 8

Responding to Resistance

> You're kind of young yet, and we don't know if you've had enough.
>
> —Dr. Bob to Clarence S., quoted in Ernest Kurtz,
> *Not-God: A History of Alcoholics Anonymous*

REFLECTIONS ON RESISTANCE

Some people believe that resistance occurs because of a client's character armor. Some psychodynamic theories, for example, construe resistance as symptomatic of unconscious conflicts and psychological defenses that are established during early childhood. Primitive defense mechanisms such as denial were once believed to be an inherent part of, even diagnostic of, alcoholism. In this way of thinking, resistance walks through the door with the client.

We question this view, which attributes resistance primarily to the client. Instead, we emphasize that, to a significant extent, resistance arises from the interpersonal interaction between counselor and client. In most psychotherapeutic writing, in fact, it is a phenomenon that occurs only in the context of psychotherapy. Research clearly demonstrates that a change in counseling style can directly affect the level of client resistance, driving it upward or downward (Chapter 1). This suggests a practical, here-and-now view of resistance. It means that it is not fixed and that there is something you can do about it.

Yet what is resistance? Clearly it is observable client behavior that occurs within the context of treatment (Chapter 4), and it represents an important signal of dissonance within the counseling process (Chapter 5). In a way, it is a signal that the person is not keeping up with you; it is the client's way of saying, "Wait a minute; I'm not with you; I don't agree." Your general task when this occurs is to double back, understand the reason for resistance behavior and for dissonance in the counseling relationship, and address it. To do this, you need to be able to recognize resistance behavior as a signal, a subject that was addressed in Chapter 5. It is also worth a reminder here that resistance, like change talk, is specific to a particular kind of change. A given client, for example, may be resistant to quitting marijuana use but quite motivated to give up cocaine.

Resistance behavior is more than just interesting information about the process of counseling. Resistance early in treatment is associated with dropout, and the more a person resists during brief counseling, the less likely it is that behavior change will occur.

Yet resistant responses are normal during counseling, and their appearance is not reason for concern. In medicine, in fact, resistance is a term associated with a healthy immune system. Resistance and change talk are like traffic signals that tell you to go ahead, proceed with caution, slow down, or stop what you are doing. You also have the means to change these signals. The occurrence of a red light is normal and helpful (unless you're in too much of a hurry). It is a problem only if the red light stays on, if resistance responses persist or escalate as the client's general pattern throughout a session or a course of treatment.

What happens thereafter, however, is importantly influenced by your own counseling style. It is how you *respond* to client resistance that makes the difference, and that distinguishes motivational interviewing from other approaches. If resistance is increasing during counseling, it is very likely in response to something that you are doing.

Implicit in this argument is another working assumption of motivational interviewing: persistent resistance is not a client problem, but a counselor skill issue. Perhaps this seems an overstatement. For example, some clients may be highly resistant, no matter what therapeutic approach is taken; there are exceptions to every rule. We also recognize that people enter counseling with widely differing initial levels of resistance. Some enter treatment quite angry and defensive, and there is evidence that motivational interviewing can be particularly effective with such clients.[1] Agency-referred clients have been reported to show more initial resistance than self-referred clients.[2] Nevertheless, research clearly demonstrates that the extent to which clients "resist" is powerfully determined by counseling style. The lesson here is that counselors can change their style in ways that will decrease (or increase) client resistance, and it is desirable to decrease client resistance because this pattern is associated with long-term change. This also means, as discussed in Chapter 5, that you can judge your effectiveness in motivational interviewing, in part, from clients' responses during counseling.

In sum, how you respond to resistance matters. In this chapter we discuss some general methods that can be used to diminish resistance by rolling with it. These methods can be useful both in Phase 1, when building motivation for change, and also in Phase 2, when commitment is being strengthened and a change plan is being negotiated (Chapter 9). The skillful handling of resistance is important, in fact, throughout the course of counseling.

We organize methods for responding to resistance into two categories. The first category consists of variations on reflective listening statements: simple reflection, amplified reflection, and double-sided reflection. The second category contains five other responses that move beyond reflection: shifting focus, reframing, agreeing with a twist, emphasizing personal choice and control, and coming alongside.

REFLECTIVE RESPONSES

Simple Reflection

A good general principle is to respond to resistance with nonresistance. A simple acknowledgment of the person's disagreement, feeling, or perception can permit further exploration rather than continued defensiveness, thus avoiding the trap of taking sides. A reflective listening statement will often suffice for this purpose. Sometimes a small shift in emphasis can also be accomplished through reflection. Here are some examples.

CLIENT: I'm trying! If my probation officer would just get off my back, I could focus on getting my life in order.

INTERVIEWER: You're working hard on the changes you need to make.

or

INTERVIEWER: It's frustrating to have a probation officer looking over your shoulder.

CLIENT: Who are you to be giving me advice? What do you know about drugs? You've probably never even smoked a joint!

INTERVIEWER: It's hard to imagine how I could possibly understand.

or

INTERVIEWER: Sounds like you're pretty angry at me.

CLIENT: I just don't want to take pills. I ought to be able to handle this on my own.

INTERVIEWER: You don't think that medication would work for you.

or

INTERVIEWER: You don't want to rely on a drug. It seems to you like a crutch.

CLIENT: I couldn't keep the weight off even if I lost it.

INTERVIEWER: You can't see any way that would work for you.

or

INTERVIEWER: You're rather discouraged about trying again.

Amplified Reflection

A related and quite useful response is to reflect back what the person has said in an amplified or exaggerated form—to state it in an even more extreme fashion. If successful, this will encourage the person to back off a bit and will elicit the other side of ambivalence. This must be done empathically, because any sarcastic tone or too extreme an overstatement may itself elicit a hostile or otherwise resistant reaction:

CLIENT: I couldn't just give up drinking. What would my friends think?

INTERVIEWER: You couldn't handle your friends' reaction if you quit.

CLIENT: I can take care of myself. I don't need my parents always checking up on me.

INTERVIEWER: So you might be better off, really, without parents.

CLIENT: My wife is always exaggerating. I haven't ever been that bad.

INTERVIEWER: It seems to you she has no reason for concern.

CLIENT: Those studies about cancer don't really prove anything anyway.

INTERVIEWER: It seems to you that lung cancer doesn't really have anything to do with smoking. It just happens.

We emphasize again that such reflections must be made in a straightforward, supportive, matter-of-fact manner. Any vocal hint of sarcasm, irony, incredulity, or impatience can quickly recast your response as hostile and thus elicit client resistance.

Double-Sided Reflection

Another approach within the realm of reflective listening is to capture both sides of ambivalence. If the person's recent statement manifests only the resistant side of the argument, a double-sided reflection acknowledges what the client has said and adds to it the other side of his or her own ambivalence (not yours). This requires the use of material that the client has offered previously, perhaps not even in the same session. Here again we encourage use of the conjunction "and" rather than "but" in order to maintain balance of emphasis Here are some examples:

CLIENT: I know it makes sense, but you don't seem to understand how bad the pain is. When I even try to get out of bed, let alone exercise, the pain in my back is terrible. I hurt all the time.

INTERVIEWER: You think that in the long run exercise is likely to help you decrease your pain, and at the same time you're suffering quite a lot, and that makes it hard to get started walking or even to think about it.

CLIENT: I know that what you're trying to do is help me, but I'm just not going to do that!

INTERVIEWER: On the one hand, you know that there are some real problems here I'm trying to help with, and, on the other, what I suggested is just not acceptable to you.

CLIENT: Look, I don't smoke any more than most of my friends. What's wrong with having a joint now and then?

INTERVIEWER: I can see how this is confusing for you. You've told me how you're concerned about your smoking and how it affects you, and also it seems like you're not using any more than your friends do. Hard to sort it out!

CLIENT: OK, maybe I've got some problems with gambling, but it's not like I'm addicted to it.

INTERVIEWER: You see that your gambling is causing problems for you and your family, and it's also important that people not think of you as some kind of addict.

OTHER RESPONSES BEYOND REFLECTION

There are other helpful ways to respond to resistance, besides variations on reflective listening. The intent behind them all is to defuse the underlying dissonance and thereby diminish resistance.

Shifting Focus

One approach is to shift the person's attention away from what seems to be a stumbling block in the way of progress. This amounts to going around barriers rather than trying to climb over them. Such detouring can be a good way to address or at least postpone dissonance when encountering a particularly difficult issue. The general structure of a shifting focus response is to first defuse the initial concern and then direct attention to a more readily workable issue.

CLIENT: You're probably going to give me a diet that I need to stick to, and tell me I have to get some of these exercise machines or go to a gym every day

INTERVIEWER: Hey, slow down! We're just sitting down at the beginning of the game, and you're already worrying about the final score! I'm certainly not ready to jump to any conclusions at this point. What is it that you want to do?

CLIENT: Well now that we're both here, I guess you're going to tell us which one of us is at fault.

INTERVIEWER: That's not the issue at all, and I don't want you worrying about it. It's not going to help to place blame. I am worried, though, that there have been some rather painful things happening between you, that are hurtful to you both and to your relationship. Tell me a little more about . . .

CLIENT: OK, the judge said I had to come here, so tell me what I have to do.

INTERVIEWER: I don't know enough about you yet for us to even start talking about what it makes sense for you to do. What we need to do right now is . . .

Reframing

Another response to resistance behavior is to reframe what the client is offering. This approach acknowledges the validity of the person's raw observations but offers a new meaning or interpretation for them. The client's information is recast into a new form and viewed in a new light that is more likely to be helpful and to support change.

A particularly good example of a reframing opportunity is provided by the phenomenon of alcohol tolerance among heavy drinkers. It is quite common for heavy drinkers to report that they are less affected by alcohol than other people. They can drink large and medically hazardous quantities without feeling or showing the degree of intoxication that would normally be expected. Over a career of heavy drinking, this capacity tends to increase (at least up to the point where liver damage becomes significant, and metabolic tolerance drops). Mostly, tolerance amounts to a failure to feel or show the high level of alcohol that is actually in the bloodstream. The drinker may regularly consume quantities of alcohol that are large enough to do substantial damage to the body but will not feel or show evidence of intoxication. In essence, the person lacks the normal warning system that protects most people from drinking to excess. Here, then, is the opportunity for reframing in medical or counseling consultation. Many heavy drinkers regard the ability to "hold their liquor" as a sign that they are safe, more able to drink with impunity than most people. The truth is exactly the opposite: alcohol tolerance is a risk factor for alcohol problems. Here is an extended example of such educational reframing.

INTERVIEWER: So something you've noticed about your drinking is that you can really hold your liquor, so to speak. You can drink a lot more than most people without feeling or looking drunk. You've even been able to fool people, so that they can't tell how much you've had to drink.

CLIENT: That's right. I've always been like that.

INTERVIEWER: I don't know whether you're aware of this or not—many people aren't—but that is actually a reason for concern. You see, ordinary people will have one or two drinks, and then they start to feel the effects and something happens. They don't want any more. Something tells them that they've had enough. Other people, unfortunately, have a high tolerance. They don't have the normal built-in warning systems. Maybe they're born without them, maybe they lose them or ignore them. Whatever the cause, the result is that they damage themselves without realizing it.

CLIENT: But if I'm not feeling anything, how can I be drunk?

INTERVIEWER: Imagine this: Suddenly you lose all sense of pain. Never again in your life will you feel any physical pain. The sensation is gone. Is that good or bad?

CLIENT: Sounds great!

INTERVIEWER: Many people think that would be wonderful, an incredible blessing, but if you think about it, actually it would be a curse. Your health and your life would be in great danger. The first warning you would have that your hand is resting on a hot stove would be the smell of the smoke. You could strain or break your limbs and go on using and damaging them, because you wouldn't realize what was happening. You wouldn't feel the pains that are early warnings of tooth decay or illness, and by the time you discovered the problem it could be too late to do anything about it. People with a high tolerance for alcohol are like that. They drink large amounts of alcohol, enough to do serious damage to their bodies, but don't feel or show their intoxication. The people around them can't see it as easily, because they don't look drunk. They damage themselves because they're missing the normal warning signs. What you're talking about, "being able to hold your liquor," is not your body's ability to get rid of alcohol at superhuman speed. The alcohol is there, doing its damage. What you're talking about is tolerance, the lack of this warning system, and that's a reason for concern.

This excerpt shows how reframing can involve some detailed teaching—the communication of new information that the person needs in order to understand his or her situation in a new light. Often reframing is much simpler than this, however, and can be accomplished with a few sentences, even one or two. Here are three more examples:

CLIENT: I've tried so many times to change, and failed.

INTERVIEWER: You're very persistent, even in the face of discouragement. This change must really be important to you.

CLIENT: My husband is always nagging me about taking my medicine. He's always reminding me to take my insulin and telling me to watch what I eat.

INTERVIEWER: It sounds like he really cares about you, and is concerned for you. I guess he expresses it in a way that you're angry about, and maybe we can help him learn to tell you in a better way that he loves you and is worried about you.

CLIENT: I've tried to quit smoking three times now and failed every time. I don't think I can do it.

INTERVIEWER: What strikes me is that you've given it three good tries already. You remember that wheel of change we talked about? Every time you give it a good try, you're one turn closer to getting off the wheel. In fact, the average number of tries before people quit is four, so don't give up now!

Agreeing with a Twist

A related way of rolling with resistance is to offer initial agreement, but with a slight twist or change of direction. This retains a sense of consonance between you and the client, while allowing you to continue influencing the direction and momentum of change. Agreement with a twist is basically a reflection followed by a reframe:

CLIENT: Nobody can tell me how to raise my kids. You don't live in my house. You don't know how it is.

INTERVIEWER: The truth is that it really is up to you how your kids are raised and what they learn. You're in the best position to know which ideas are likely to work and which aren't, and I can't just be prescribing things for you. You need to be a full partner in this process.

CLIENT: Why are you and my wife ganging up on me about my temper? What about all her problems? You'd blow up, too, if your family were aggravating you all the time.

INTERVIEWER: You've got a good point there, and that's important. There is a bigger picture here, and maybe I haven't been paying enough attention to that. Conflict isn't as simple as one person's problem, and I agree with you that it's not a matter of placing blame. Temper problems like this do involve and affect the whole family. I think you're absolutely right.

CLIENT: You're probably going to give me a diet that I need to stick to, and tell me I have to get some of these exercise machines or go to a gym every day. I just get so discouraged by that kind of advice!

INTERVIEWER: If I were to tell you a whole lot of things that you have to do, it would immobilize you even further. It's ironic, isn't it? When you feel like you have to do something, it actually prevents you from doing what you want to do.

Emphasizing Personal Choice and Control

Resistance sometimes arises from the phenomenon of psychological reactance.[3] When people perceive that their freedom of choice is being threatened, they tend to react by asserting their liberty (e.g., "I'll show you; nobody tells me what to do!"). It is a common and natural reaction to a threatening loss of choice. Probably the best antidote for this reaction is to assure the person of what is surely the truth: in the end, it is the client who determines what happens. An early assurance of this kind can diminish reactance. Here are some examples:

CLIENT: Why are you giving me this booklet? Are you telling me I have to use condoms?

INTERVIEWER: It's just information. What you do with it is completely up to you. Naturally, no one can make you use condoms.

CLIENT: I don't like the idea of blood pressure medicine. I hear it can have some bad side effects.

INTERVIEWER: And it really is your decision. All I can do is tell you the advantages and disadvantages for you, and give you my opinion. If you decide you don't want to take medication, then you won't. If you do want to, it's available. It's up to you.

CLIENT: What if I tell you I like smoking and don't want to quit?

INTERVIEWER: You're a free person, and it's your choice. I couldn't make the decision for you, even if I wanted to.

CLIENT: The judge told me that I have to come here. I don't have any choice about it.

INTERVIEWER: Actually you do, in several ways. You chose to come here instead of taking your chances with the judge. Also, if you find that you don't want to come here, I can work with you and the court to find a different program for you, one you might like better.

Coming Alongside

If taking up one side of the argument causes an ambivalent person to defend the other, then the process ought to work both ways. When a counselor advocates for change, the ambivalent person argues against it, but what happens if the counselor defends the other side, the counterchange side?

Much has been written about this as a general strategy in psychotherapy. Variations on this theme have been called "reverse psychology" and "therapeutic paradox."[4] Within strategic family therapy, it is used to place the client in a position where opposition or resistance to the counselor results in movement in a desired direction. Another familiar variation is "prescribing the problem." If all change efforts are met with opposition, the counselor recommends that the client should continue on as before, without changing, or should even increase the behavior in question. This is not done in an angry, exasperated, "I give up" manner. Most often it is done in a calm and matter-of-fact way. A detailed rationale may even be given for why the person should not change.

Although this method fits well with the ambivalence model described in earlier chapters, we confess some serious discomfort with the ways in which therapeutic paradox has sometimes been described. There is often the sense of paradox being a clever way of duping people into doing things for their own good. In some writings on paradox, one senses almost a glee in finding innovative ways to trick people without their realizing what is happening. Such cleverness lacks the respectful and collaborative tone that we understand to be fundamental to the dialectical process of motivational interviewing. We do not mean to imply that motivational interviewing is value-neutral or free from concerns about manipulation. We have devoted Chapter 12 to a consideration of such ethical issues.

What, then, is the role of this method of coming alongside? In a way, it is a special case of amplified reflection. It is a straightforward extension of the conceptual model of ambivalence that is presented in Chapters 2 through 5. Motivational interviewing is essentially a dialogue about the client's ambivalence, and the interviewer explores both sides. By the nature of ambivalence, when the counselor raises only one side the client is inclined to explore the other. Because of principles of self-perception theory,[5] it is important for the counselor to be mindful of this process, because a person who is caused to defend one side of the dialogue can be influenced (inadvertently or intentionally) to move in that direction.

Knowing this, it follows that siding with the counterchange perspective should elicit change talk from the client. We postulate nothing more elaborate than this linguistic attribute of ambivalence. We do not conceptualize resistance as strategic or defensive on the client's part; consequently, we have moved away from the chess-match concept of paradox as counterstrategic outsmarting. Coming alongside as the client argues against change is just another way of defusing the argument and eliciting change talk. There is a clear and immediate test of whether this response is having the desired effect: Does it decrease resistance and evoke change talk?

CLIENT: I don't think this is going to work for me, either. I feel pretty hopeless.

INTERVIEWER: It's certainly possible that after giving it another try, you still won't be any better off, and so it might be better not to try at all. What's your inclination?

CLIENT: That's about it, really. I probably drink too much sometimes, and I don't like the hangovers, but I don't think it's that much of a concern, really.

INTERVIEWER: It may just be worth it to you to keep on drinking as you have, even though it causes some problems. It's worth the cost.

CLIENT: I'm not sure if I want to do this program or not. It sounds like it takes a lot of time.

INTERVIEWER: And that's something that concerns me. A program like this does require a lot of motivation and effort. We don't really want to start working with somebody until they're serious about wanting to change, and, frankly, I'm not sure how ready you are. As I listen to you, I'm not convinced that you're motivated enough to carry through.

There is no reason why the client has to be kept in the dark about the dialogue. Consistent with the example of exploring one side of ambivalence at a time (Chapter 7), one can set up a direct debate in which the client defends the need for change. In this case, the counselor simply takes over the counterchange side of the argument:

"One thing that I find is helpful is to clarify the real reasons for change. I've heard from you some of the reasons you are reluctant to think about making a change, and now I have a suggestion. I want to have a little debate with you. I'll defend the position that you don't really have a problem and don't need to change, and I'd like you to do your best to convince me otherwise. Do you understand? I'm going to be you, arguing that I don't need to change, and your job is to persuade me that there really is a problem here that I need to examine and do something about. OK?"

Clients sometimes need extra encouragement to get rolling with a contrived dialogue of this kind. Have the client speak in "you" language, while you as the counselor speak in "I" language and voice the client's prior counterchange arguments. Here's how it might go:

INTERVIEWER: Look, I just can't see the point in all this jumping up and down exercise stuff. I'd rather just relax when I have the time. That's good for my health, too.

CLIENT: Well, I've been putting on some weight . . .

INTERVIEWER: (*Interrupting.*) Sorry. Use "you" instead of "I" when you talk to me. Try it again.

CLIENT: Well, you've been putting on a good bit of weight these last few years, and relaxing isn't going to help you there.

INTERVIEWER: I'm not that overweight, really. I feel pretty good.

CLIENT: But remember that the doctor told you your blood pressure is up, and there aren't really any symptoms with high blood pressure. [out of role] Am I doing OK?

INTERVIEWER: [out of role] You're doing great. Don't go so easy on me, though. Don't let me get away with anything. [in role] You only live once, after all. Besides, I've heard that exercise doesn't really make you live any longer . . . it just makes it seem like you do.

CLIENT: Nonsense! You know you felt better when you weren't so over-weight. And getting some fresh air would be good for you.

Over time, the counselor allows the person to persuade him or her that there is reason for concern and change. This technique is not appropriate for every client, but it can be an appealing, even entertaining way to externalize and examine ambivalence. At the same time, it can elicit quite a lot of change talk from the client, as he or she defends the need for change.

THE DRAMA OF CHANGE

Resistance is a key to successful treatment if you can recognize it for what it is: an opportunity. In expressing resistance, the client is probably rehearsing a script that has been played out many times before. There is an expected role for you to play—one that has been acted out by others in the past. Your lines are predictable. If you speak these same lines, as others have done, the script will come to the same conclusion as before.

But you can rewrite your own role. Your part in the play need not be the dry predictable lines that the client is expecting. In a way, counseling is like improvisational theater. No two sessions run exactly the same way. If one actor changes role, the plot is headed off in a new direction.

Resistance is often the life of the play. It is the twist that adds drama and excitement to the plot. Viewing resistance as a perverse character flaw is a sad mistake. Resistance lies at the very heart of human change. It arises from the motives and struggles of the actors. It foreshadows certain ends to which the play may or may not lead. The true art of a counselor is tested in the recognition and handling of resistance. It is on this stage that the drama of change unfolds.

NOTES

1. Project MATCH Research Group (1997b).
2. Chamberlain, Patterson, Reid, Kavanagh, and Forgatch (1984).
3. Brehm and Brehm (1981).
4. For example, Frankl (1963), Haley (1963), and Stanton, Todd, and Associates (1982).
5. Bem (1967, 1972).

CHAPTER 9

Enhancing Confidence

Things do not change: We change.
—HENRY DAVID THOREAU, *Walden*

Much of the foregoing discussion has focused on increasing the perceived importance of change, on the situation in which a person is ambivalent about wanting to change. As discussed in Chapter 1, however, importance is only one of the three natural language components of motivation for change, the "willing" in "ready, willing, and able." A person can strongly desire change (be willing) but perceive that it is beyond reach. "Confidence" is the term we use to describe the extent to which a person feels able to change.

In general, people cannot be ready to change until they perceive both that they want to (importance) and are able to do so (confidence). We would love to play Grieg's piano concerto and would willingly do so, but we lack the ability. Both importance and confidence, therefore, are Phase 1 issues, and they can interact in complex ways. Sometimes people are reluctant to consider the importance of change if they see no possibility of it happening. If change is beyond reach, then what's the point even in thinking about it? Often, however, it seems to go the other way. Importance increases first, and then the person begins searching for ways in which change might be accomplished. In any event, both importance and confidence are needed in sufficient quantity before moving on to a change plan (Phase 2).

Using just these two constructs—importance and confidence—one can imagine several reasons for low motivation for change, as discussed in Chapter 6. (The third issue of readiness is discussed in Chapter 10.) One might be "unmotivated" because:

> Importance is low, but confidence is high.
> Importance is high, but confidence is low.
> Both importance and confidence are low.

When importance is low (whether with high or low confidence), we generally recommend working first on enhancing the perceived importance of change by developing discrepancy. If low confidence is an obstacle to increasing importance, it will become apparent soon enough.

What about the situation in which importance is high—the person wants to change—but confidence is low? How can motivational interviewing be applied then? That is the focus of this chapter: enhancing confidence for change. The methods described here can also be used, of course, when both importance and confidence are low. Confidence is again treated as an ambivalence issue. It is unlikely that the person feels totally unable to change. There are within the person confidence arguments for why he or she could change, as well as arguments for why it cannot happen. A motivational interviewing approach seeks to elicit and strengthen the former.

A further clarification is warranted here. The discussion in this chapter is directed to the problem of low self-efficacy and not to more generalized confidence problems such as depression, low self-esteem, and learned helplessness. The methods described here are not remedies for these broader confidence problems, for which other effective treatment approaches are available.

CONFIDENCE TRAPS

Just as there are traps to avoid when beginning motivational interviewing to enhance the importance of change, there are also a few to avoid in building confidence.

"I'll Take Over Now, Thank You"

One temptation is to abandon a motivational approach once the person seems to perceive the importance of change. "Now that's behind us, and we can get on with real counseling." The approach to confidence building that we are suggesting here is consonant with the importance-enhancing style described earlier and with motivational interviewing more generally. It continues to be collaborative in spirit, drawing on the person's own resources. It remains reflective and evocative rather than prescriptive. This first trap, then, is to meet low confidence with a prescription: "Here's how you can do it." Falling into this trap involves taking responsibility for the "can" side of the confidence argument, leaving the person to defend the "can't" side. This is not to say that the counselor withholds ideas, only that prescription is not the primary line of response.

"There, There, You'll Be Fine"

Another potential trap is not taking the confidence issue seriously enough. A bald assurance that "I'm sure you can do it" is unlikely to address a genuine lack of self-efficacy. It is also another form of taking up the "can" side of the argument, inviting a "can-not, can-too" struggle.

Gloom à Deux

Still another trap is to fall into and share the person's perception of helplessness or hopelessness. At least one person in the room needs to be optimistic, focused on problem solving rather than despair. Of course, there are things that genuinely cannot be changed, and we are not advocating delusional optimism. Most often, however, some form of change is feasible, and clients need to be able to borrow hope from the counselor until they have their own.[1] Trust that the client has inner resources and creativity to draw on in pursuing change.

ELICITING AND STRENGTHENING CONFIDENCE TALK

Evocative Questions

One of the four categories of change talk described in Chapter 3 is optimism about ability to change—in other words, self-efficacy. Confidence talk is one kind of change talk. Consistent with the style of motivational interviewing, one approach is to elicit the person's own ideas, experiences, and perceptions that are consistent with ability to change. For example, open questions can be used to evoke confidence talk:

> "How might you go about making this change?"
> "What would be a good first step?"
> "What obstacles do you foresee, and how might you deal with them?"
> "What gives you some confidence that you can do this?"

Confidence Ruler

The ruler introduced in Chapter 6 can be used in a similar manner to elicit confidence talk.

> How confident are you that you could _____? On a scale from 0 to 10, where 0 is not at all confident and 10 is extremely confident, where would you say you are?"

0	1	2	3	4	5	6	7	8	9	10
Not at all confident										Extremely confident

The same follow-up questions discussed in Chapter 6 are then used to elicit the client's perspectives of confidence:

"Why are you at a _____ and not 0?"
"What would it take for you to go from _____ to [a higher number]?"

The answers to these questions will be confidence talk. As before, remember not to reverse the questions and ask, "Why are you at _____ and not 10?"

Reviewing Past Successes

Another resource to tap in enhancing confidence is the client's past successes.

"When in your life have you made up your mind to do something, and did it? It might be something new you learned, or a habit that you quit, or some other significant change that you made in your life. When have you done something like that?"

What you are looking for are changes that the client made on their own initiative (rather than being coerced), particularly those that he or she seems pleased about. Look for several examples ("When else?") and then explore them in some depth. What did the client do that worked? Was there specific preparation for change? You are looking in particular for personal skills or strengths that might be generalized and applied in the current situation. Instead of just asking, "Tell me how you did it," it can be useful to have the client go through in some detail what change occurred and how it came about. What did the person do to initiate and maintain change? What obstacles were there, and how did he or she surmount them? Ask to what the client attributes his or her success, and explore what that may mean about his or her resources, skills, and strengths. Remember that you want the client rather than yourself to be making the arguments for confidence.

Personal Strengths and Supports

Another route to confidence talk is ask about more general personal strengths and resources that may be helpful in making the desired change. What you're looking for here are positive personal characteristics that, from an attributional perspective, are stable, internal traits.

"What is there about you, what strong points do you have that could help you succeed in making this change?"

Sometimes it is useful to prompt the client with a list of positive attributes that can help people make changes. One such list is reproduced in Box 9.1, from which almost anyone could find at least a few personal strengths with which he or she can identify.[2]

When the client identifies a personal strength, ask for elaboration. In what ways is this characteristic of the person? Ask for examples, and follow with reflective listening.

It can also be useful to explore here what sources of social support the client has for pursuing change. Are there others on whom he or she could call for support? in what ways? Who else could help with change?

Brainstorming

A classic approach for problem solving is brainstorming, which involves freely generating as many ideas as possible for how a change might be accomplished. The list is generated without critique—all ideas are acceptable, no matter how silly or unrealistic they might seem. The purpose is to stimulate creative, divergent thinking about how change could be achieved. It's OK to suggest ideas

---

BOX 9.1. Some Characteristics of Successful Changers

Accepting	Committed	Flexible	Persevering	Stubborn
Active	Competent	Focused	Persistent	Thankful
Adaptable	Concerned	Forgiving	Positive	Thorough
Adventuresome	Confident	Forward-looking	Powerful	Thoughtful
Affectionate	Considerate	Free	Prayerful	Tough
Affirmative	Courageous	Happy	Quick	Trusting
Alert	Creative	Healthy	Reasonable	Trustworthy
Alive	Decisive	Hopeful	Receptive	Truthful
Ambitious	Dedicated	Imaginative	Relaxed	Understanding
Anchored	Determined	Ingenious	Reliable	Unique
Assertive	Die-hard	Intelligent	Resourceful	Unstoppable
Assured	Diligent	Knowledgeable	Responsible	Vigorous
Attentive	Doer	Loving	Sensible	Visionary
Bold	Eager	Mature	Skillful	Whole
Brave	Earnest	Open	Solid	Willing
Bright	Effective	Optimistic	Spiritual	Winning
Capable	Energetic	Orderly	Stable	Wise
Careful	Experienced	Organized	Steady	Worthy
Cheerful	Faithful	Patient	Straight	Zealous
Clever	Fearless	Perceptive	Strong	Zestful

here, but mostly you should rely on the client's creativity to generate possibilities. Write them down.

Once a list has been generated, ask the client which ideas on the list seem most promising or acceptable, and why. Don't forget that through all of these methods there runs the common theme of eliciting and reinforcing confidence talk by the client. Within the context of motivational interviewing, brainstorming is not only a method for generating ideas but also another format for eliciting confidence talk.

Giving Information and Advice

It is not necessary, of course, for the client to have all the ideas. It is perfectly appropriate to provide information and advice that could be helpful in bolstering confidence. The danger is taking sides: you advocate for a change solution, and the client explains why it won't work.

This issue is discussed in more detail in Chapter 10, but the basic approach is to provide information and advice within a motivational interviewing–consistent context when the client desires it and thus feels free to take or leave it. One such context is when the client asks for your input. It is also possible to ask permission to provide information or advice that may be helpful. Specific methods for doing the latter are found in Chapter 10.

Reframing

Sometimes a person bogs down in attributions of failure, and a process of reframing or reattribution can be helpful. A common theme is "I've tried several times, and each time I failed." The general method here is to reframe "failure" in a way that encourages rather than blocks further change attempts.

The concept of "try" is helpful here. Often the client will use the word (as above) in describing reasons for perceived failure. It is a short step to recast "failures" as "tries." One need not resort to platitudes ("If at first you don't succeed, try, try again") to discuss what the client has done in the past as successive tries toward a goal. Some knowledge of change research can be helpful here. For example, dependent smokers usually do not succeed in quitting on their first try. On average, it requires between three and four serious tries before a smoker permanently escapes the grip of tobacco dependence. Whereas a "failure" sounds like a shameful thing, a "try" is laudable. If one has tried several times without success, it may only mean that one has not yet tried the right approach. Even the same approach may work if tried again. "Try again later" is the message one receives when attempting to log onto an Internet service if no line is available. Gamblers are notoriously persistent in trying their luck. "Trying" is a routine and necessary step toward winning, toward successful change.

Other reframes can facilitate confidence. Explanations of "failure" as being due to internal, stable factors (like inability: "I can't do it") can be reattributed to external and unstable factors like effort or luck: "The time wasn't right." "I haven't done it yet." "I wasn't quite ready." "I was unlucky that time." "I didn't try hard enough, or long enough." Take a lesson from the gambler: Maybe next time is my time.

Hypothetical Change

If the person is struggling with practicalities, it may be helpful to leap into hypo-space, to think in the hypothetical. Subjunctive syntax is useful here:

> "Suppose that you did succeed and are looking back on it now: What most likely is it that worked? How did it happen?"
>
> "Suppose that this one big obstacle weren't there. If that obstacle were removed, then how might you go about making this change?"
>
> "Clearly you are feeling very discouraged, even demoralized about this. So use your imagination: if you were to try again, what might be the best way to try?"

Responding to Confidence Talk

A common purpose that runs through all the methods just outlined is for the client to talk about ways in which change can occur, about confidence: why and how he or she can succeed with change. Consistent with the overall motivational interviewing perspective, it is useful for the client to make these arguments. When such confidence talk occurs, it is important to respond in a manner that reinforces and consolidates it. The same principles outlined in Chapter 7 apply here, for this is just a special case of responding to change talk (in this case, confidence talk).

Reflective listening remains a central skill here. Listen for themes, experiences, ideas, and perceptions that imply confidence, that bespeak the person's ability to make the desired change. Reflect these preferentially, both immediately as they occur and in subsequent reflective summaries. Appropriately affirm the client's expressions of confidence.

As confidence talk emerges, it can also be useful to raise possible problems and challenges that may be encountered, asking the client for solutions:

> "What might you do if . . . ?"
>
> "How could you respond if . . . ?"
>
> "What do you think would happen if . . . ?"

In turn, this elicits further change talk. In fact, it is exactly the opposite of proposing solutions and having the client point out their limitations. Your role here is not to refute the client's change talk but to stimulate further thought and specificity. Asking for examples and elaboration is likewise appropriate.

It is also common to encounter some resistance behavior when discussing issues of confidence, even when importance seems to be high. This occurs most often when a client takes up the counterchange side of ambivalence. Although the content of resistance may be focused on the ability to or feasibility of change, there are no special methods here beyond those discussed in the preceding Chapter 8. The nonoppositional style of rolling with resistance remains the same.

Radical Change

Finally, there are times when the desired change is not circumscribed but involves a number of interrelated problems that are unlikely to respond to a simple solution. For a complex example, consider the situation of a polydrug-dependent commercial sex worker in a city where prostitution is illegal. Like many such women, she may place high importance on escaping from her conundrum but see no possible way of doing so. Complex though it may be, this is a confidence issue. Change might require escaping from dangerous and resourceful associates; finding temporary food and shelter, geographic relocation, and polydrug detoxification and treatment; resolving legal problems; developing new job skills; and finding employment, child care, and housing. To talk about change in any one of these problems (such as drug dependence) without addressing the others is clearly unrealistic, and low confidence is understandable.

In such situations, the only avenue in which a person can have confidence might be one involving radical change that simultaneously addresses multiple problems. Without underestimating complexity, it is possible to discuss how such radical change might occur. Rather than trying to modify a particular behavior, this requires thinking about the big picture of change.

CLINICAL EXAMPLE

The following clinical dialogue illustrates a motivational interviewing approach to enhancing confidence, using the radical change scenario just described. We debated whether so complex a situation would be optimal—as opposed to a single-behavior confidence issue that would have the advantage (and disadvantage) of greater simplicity. The greater complexity, however, lent itself to illustrating the use of a broader range of confidence-enhancing methods. The dialogue begins after a period of discussion about the importance of change, which the client summarizes so concisely that there is no need for the interviewer to do so. The challenge now, before a concrete change plan can be addressed, is very low confidence.

CLIENT: I just can't do this work much longer. *On the importance ruler,* It's too dangerous, and I'm going to end *she rates herself at a 9.* up dead. I have my daughter to think of,

too. I don't want her to have the same
kind of life I've had. I'm a wreck as a
mother—shooting up in the bathroom
so she doesn't see me, out half the night.
Now the social worker is threatening to
take her away from me again, and I
don't blame him. I can't go on like this.

INTERVIEWER: It's a desperate situation
you're in, and you really want out.

CLIENT: I came close to getting out the
other night, but not the way I want
to—in a box.

INTERVIEWER: You were nearly killed.

CLIENT: I've come close before, but
that one really scared me—the
guy I told you about.

INTERVIEWER: So what's the next step?
How do you get out?

CLIENT: That's just it. What can I do? . . .   *An invitation to provide*
solutions. . .

INTERVIEWER: You feel stuck, with   *. . . which the interviewer*
no way out.   *simply reflects.*

CLIENT: No shit! I have no money. I'm   *One can anticipate here*
on probation. CC watches me like   *the likely result of making*
a hawk, and beats me up and cuts off   *suggestions or prescribing*
my drugs if he even thinks I'm   *tasks ("Well, how*
holding out on him. We live in a   *about . . . ?").*
cheap motel room. What am I
supposed to do?

INTERVIEWER: That's exactly the question   *Again the interviewer*
you're faced with. You want out, but   *reflects instead of jumping*
how in the world can you overcome   *in with answers.*
so many incredible obstacles?

CLIENT: I just don't see a way.
Otherwise I'd be out of here.   *Confidence ruler = 1 or 2.*

INTERVIEWER: I certainly don't have the
answers for you, but I have a lot
of confidence that you do, and that
working together we can find a way out.   *Lending hope.*

CLIENT: What do you mean?

INTERVIEWER: Well, for one thing, you're an amazing survivor. I can't believe how strong you are, to have gone through all you've been through and even be alive, let alone sitting here and talking to me about what you want your life to be like in the future. I don't think I could have survived what you've been through.

Utterly genuine affirmation and reframe.

CLIENT: You do what you have to.

INTERVIEWER: How have you come this far and still have the amount of love and compassion that I see in you—not only for your daughter, but for the women you work with, and for other people as well? How do you do it?

Affirmation and open question.

CLIENT: Just one day at a time, like they say. I don't know. I just go way inside, like when I'm doing some john. I don't let myself get hurt. I take care of myself.

INTERVIEWER: Like you take care of your daughter.

Linking reflection.

CLIENT: I hope I take better care of her than I do of myself. But yeah, I take care of myself. Nobody else does.

INTERVIEWER: So you have this amazing inner strength, a solid core inside you where you can't be hurt.

CLIENT: Or don't let myself be hurt.

INTERVIEWER: Oh, right! It's not that you can't feel anything, because you do. You have a way of preserving that loving woman inside you, keeping her safe. So one thing you are is strong. How else might you describe yourself? What other qualities do you have that make you a survivor?

Asking for personal strengths.

CLIENT: I think I'm pretty smart. I mean, you wouldn't know it to look at me, but I can see what's going on around me, and I don't miss much.

Confidence talk begins.

INTERVIEWER: You're a strong and loving woman, and pretty smart. What else?

A collecting summary.

CLIENT: I don't know.

INTERVIEWER: What might someone else say about you, someone who knows you well? What good qualities might they see in you, that could help you make the changes you want?

CLIENT: Persistent. I'm downright bullheaded when I want something.

INTERVIEWER: Nothing stops you when you make up your mind, like a bull.

CLIENT: I do keep going when I want something.

INTERVIEWER: Strong and loving, smart, persistent. Sounds like you have a lot of what it takes to handle tough changes. How about this? Give me an example of a time when you really wanted something, and you went after it.

Reviewing past successes.

CLIENT: You won't like it.

INTERVIEWER: Try me.

CLIENT: I was out of shit last week, and I really wanted it something bad. CC thought I was cheating him, keeping money and not telling him, and so he cut me off. I asked around and nobody had any to give me. It was the afternoon and nothing was happening on the street. So I took my daughter and went over to the freeway entrance. I had to wait until CC went for dinner. I made up this sign that said, "Hungry. Will work for food." In an hour I had enough to get what I needed, and some food for us, too. CC never found out about it.

INTERVIEWER: It's all the things you said. You had to time it all carefully, but you're so aware of what's happening around you that you could do it. You think quickly, and came up with a solution. You stuck with it, and made it happen. How did you make the sign?

CLIENT: Cardboard I found in the motel dumpster, and I borrowed a marker at the desk.

INTERVIEWER: They seem like little things, but I'm impressed at how quickly you solved this one. I'm sad, of course, that all this creativity was spent on getting drugs, but it's just one example of how you can make things happen when you put your mind to it.

CLIENT: Now that's another thing. What do I do about being hooked? The withdrawals are bad.

INTERVIEWER: You've been through them before, then.

CLIENT: Sure. In jail, on the street, even in a detox once, but I don't want to go through it again.

INTERVIEWER: Tell me about the detox. When was that?

CLIENT: Last year. I got real sick and they took me to the emergency room, and from there they took me to detox. I stayed about five days, but I got high right afterward.

INTERVIEWER: But what was the detox like for you?

CLIENT: It was OK. They were nice to me, and they gave me drugs so that I didn't feel uncomfortable. As soon as I hit the street, though, I wanted a fix.

INTERVIEWER: So it was possible, at least, for you to get through the withdrawal process comfortably. The problem came when you went back out. Now let me ask you this. Imagine that you're off the street—like magic. You're through withdrawals and away from the street, out of CC's reach, somewhere else completely. Don't worry for the moment about how you got there— we'll come back to that—but you're free, just you and your daughter. What would you do? What kind of life would you choose?

Using the hypothetical.

CLIENT: I'd need to find a real job. Maybe I'd go back to school and then get a good job. I'd like to get out of the city—live in a little place out in the country somewhere.

Change talk.

INTERVIEWER: A complete change of scenery.

CLIENT: That's what it would take.

INTERVIEWER: And you can imagine it, a new life somewhere with your daughter.

CLIENT: I can imagine it, yes. But how could I get there?

INTERVIEWER: It's such a big change, with so many obstacles, that you don't think you could do it.

CLIENT: I don't know. I might be able to. I just haven't thought about it for a long time.

Confidence ruler = 3 or 4?

INTERVIEWER: Maybe, just maybe, with all your strength and smarts and creativity and stubborn persistence, you could find a way to pull it off. It's what you want, is it?

CLIENT: Yeah, it would be great, getting off the street.

INTERVIEWER: Is this just a pipe dream here, or do you think you might actually be able to do it?

CLIENT: It seems kind of unrealistic, for me at least.

INTERVIEWER: For you. But it might be possible for . . .

CLIENT: I guess I was thinking of my daughter. Or maybe some other women I know, but then I think I'd have as good a chance as they would.

INTERVIEWER: Good! You can imagine you doing it, just like others might. Let me just ask you to do one more thing, then, before we get any more specific. Let's think about what it would take for you to get from the street to that place you imagined. And let's be creative. Let's think of any way at all that it might happen, as many different ways as possible. They can be completely unrealistic or unlikely, no matter. What we want is a lot of ideas. OK?

Introducing the idea of brainstorming.

CLIENT: Sure, why not.

INTERVIEWER: So how might it happen?

CLIENT: I could meet a sugar daddy, like that girl in the *Pretty Woman* movie.

INTERVIEWER: OK, good. That's one. What else?

CLIENT: There could be a miracle. (*Laughs.*)

INTERVIEWER: Right. One miracle coming up. What else?

CLIENT: I could talk my mom into bailing me out again. If she thought I was really serious this time, she might do it.

INTERVIEWER: So your mom could help get you out of here, with money.

CLIENT: She's worried about her granddaughter, I know. We might even be able to live with her for a while, but I don't know if she'll ever trust me again.

Confidence talk is gradually emerging over the course of this 10-minute segment, and there are the beginnings of a possible change plan. Rather than jumping straight to a how-to-do-it discussion with this high-importance/low-confidence woman, the interviewer spends some time in eliciting confidence in her broader adaptive abilities. This paves the way for later development of and commitment to a specific change plan.

SUMMARY

A motivational interviewing approach for enhancing confidence differs from traditional advice-giving or skill-building strategies. While it is not at all incompatible with giving advice or teaching new skills, a motivational interviewing method places its main bets on the person's own resourcefulness. The overall view is that confidence (like the importance aspect of motivation for change) is not something to be imposed but, rather, is evoked from the person, literally called (voiced) forth in the person's own words and ideas. Although there are some special issues and adaptations, the methods used to elicit and reinforce confidence are similar to those discussed in earlier chapters with regard to change talk more generally. Finding hope and confidence for change is a collaborative process in which the counselor is privileged to participate.

NOTES

1. Yahne and Miller (1999).
2. This list was developed by Shelby Steen for Miller (in press).

CHAPTER 10

Phase 2

Strengthening Commitment to Change

It takes two to speak truth—One to speak, and another to hear.
—HENRY DAVID THOREAU,
A Week on the Concord and Merrimack Rivers

RECOGNIZING READINESS

The first phase of motivational interviewing involves building intrinsic motivation for change. This takes much longer with some people than with others. Some come to counseling having given little or no thought to a need for change. Others are in the firm grip of ambivalence, and still others come already voicing the intention to change and needing relatively little motivation building.

There comes a point when it is time to shift approach—when the goal changes from enhancing importance and confidence (Phase 1) to strengthening commitment to a change plan (Phase 2). At the typical point for this transition, the person is willing and able to change and is on the brink of readiness. Salespeople recognize a comparable point in selling: when the customer has privately decided to make a purchase, and they shift strategies toward closing the sale. A leading sales trainer once told us that this is the most critical period in a sale and that the main task at this point is to help the person confirm and justify the decision that has been made. Knowing exactly when to shift strategies is one of the skills that separates successful from unsuccessful salespeople.

Similarly, in cooking there are crucial timing judgments to be made: when the liquid has boiled sufficiently, how long to knead the dough and let it rise before baking, or when the candy is hot enough to set before it burns. Proceeding either too soon or too late can spoil the recipe.

Don't worry about this too much. We doubt that there is often an exact, ideal moment for the transition from Phase 1 to Phase 2. We do believe, though, that once a person has reached a point of readiness, there is a certain window of time during which change should be initiated. How long this window stays open will vary widely, but the recognition of an important discrepancy is just too uncomfortable to sustain forever. If change isn't begun, the person is likely to start using cognitive defensive strategies to decrease the discomfort (rationalizing, minimizing, denying, forgetting, projecting, etc.). It is important to recognize when the window is open, so that you can help the person start stepping through it—and to make sure that it's on the ground level.

What are the signs of an open window? Good research is needed here. At present, we can offer some of the cues that we have used in intuiting when to shift from Phase 1 to Phase 2 (see Box 10.1). Not all of these will happen in all or even most cases, but they are some indicators of readiness for change.

BOX 10.1. Signs of Readiness for Change

1. *Decreased resistance.* The wind seems to have gone out of the sails of resistance. Dissonance in the counseling relationship diminishes, and resistance decreases.

2. *Decreased discussion about the problem.* The client seems to have talked enough about the area of concern. If the client has been asking questions about the problem area, these stop. There is a feeling of at least partial completion, of waiting for the next step.

3. *Resolve.* The client appears to have reached some kind of resolution, and may seem more peaceful, relaxed, calm, unburdened, or settled. This can also have a tone of loss, tearfulness, or resignation.

4. *Change talk.* Whereas resistance diminishes, change talk increases. The client makes direct change statements (see Chapter 5), reflecting disadvantages of the status quo, advantages of change, optimism about change, and/or intention to change.

5. *Questions about change.* The client may begin to ask what he or she could do about the problem, how people change once they decide to, or the like.

6. *Envisioning.* The client talks about how life might be after a change. This can be mistaken for resistance, in that looking ahead to change often causes a person to anticipate difficulties if a change were made. Of course, the client may also envision positive outcomes of change.

7. *Experimenting.* If the client has had time between sessions, he or she may have begun experimenting with possible change actions since the last session.

When there are such signs of readiness, it may be time to shift direction to the new goal of strengthening commitment. This can be a useful process even if a person is entering treatment apparently having already decided to change. The methods presented in this chapter are appropriate for strengthening commitment to change, once a person perceives sufficient importance and confidence to be ready to move on toward action.

Don't expect "Eureka!" experiences to occur at a magical moment of readiness. Typically the signs of readiness for change emerge gradually and subtly. When people do have Eureka! moments, it is most often outside the consulting room.[1]

This is often quite an enjoyable part of counseling. Phase 1 can be slow and hard work—a bit like slogging up a mountain in snowshoes. Once this hard work is done, Phase 2 may proceed much more easily—like skiing down the other side. To be sure, there are hazards on the way down, and we begin by discussing a few of these. Nevertheless, the going tends to be faster and more pleasant. There is a sense of companionship with the client, like the feeling of sitting next to someone on the ski lift, looking over the trails and sorting out which way to go, then pushing off together.

At the top of the mountain, the main task is to persuade the client to come with you down the other side, rather than staying there and ultimately deciding to go back down the way you came. When you reach Phase 2, most of the hard work of motivational interviewing is done. It remains for the client to put on the skis, pick an appropriate slope, make that fateful decision to push off, and enjoy the journey down while avoiding its rocks, moguls, and chasms. As the counselor, you can be a guide throughout this process, or the client may decide to ski on alone.

PHASE 2 HAZARDS

There certainly are a few hazards to watch for in negotiating the slopes of Phase 2. Here are three to beware.

Underestimating Ambivalence

It is quite tempting to assume that once the client is showing signs of readiness for change (see Box 10.1), the decision has been made and it's all downhill from there on. This confuses the commitment-strengthening process with a Eureka! decision. Most decisions to change are not made suddenly, once and for all. People often begin action toward change while still feeling a good bit of ambivalence. They take their first tentative steps over the crest of the hill, still unsure which way it is they want to go, and as they look down the slope they may begin to rethink whether they want to go at all. Sometimes they seem to have progressed well into the journey, only to turn around and double back. There is a substantial risk, then, of becoming overeager at the first signs of a shift toward change. In our alpine analogy, the client in this situation may be like the reluctant student who has finally built up the courage to get to the top, only to be coaxed by the instructor to the edge of what seems the steepest and most menacing slope. The same care and style that characterizes Phase 1 should be maintained during Phase 2 and, indeed, throughout the entire counseling process. Ambivalence does not disappear just because the change process has begun.

Overprescription

Another danger in Phase 2 is to prescribe a plan that is unacceptable to the client. There can be a tendency to say, "Now that you're ready to change, here's what you need to do." This violates the collaborative tone of motivational interviewing and runs the risk of undoing what progress has been made. There is no point in carefully eliciting a person's motivation, only to offer a change plan that is unacceptable. Sometimes one can run into difficulty even when making what seems to be a simple suggestion. The client responds, "Yes, but that won't work because . . . " and adopts the passive role of someone who is waiting for solutions to be provided—a reincarnation of the expert trap. The Phase 1 emphasis on personal responsibility and choice extends to Phase 2 and the negotiation of change strategies.

Insufficient Direction

The opposite risk is to provide the client with too little help. The question "What can I do?" is better answered in Phase 2 by a menu of alternatives than by reflective listening. If a wholly nondirective approach is sustained in Phase 2, the person may flounder. Imagine a novice skier accelerating down a challenging slope and asking for direction, while the instructor reflects, "So you're wondering what it is that you should do next." The methods that we describe in this chapter are meant to guide you between the two extremes of overprescription and insufficient direction. The goals are to channel intrinsic motivation into a negotiated, workable plan for change and to strengthen the client's commitment for carrying out that plan.

INITIATING PHASE 2

Recapitulation

A good first step in making the transition to Phase 2 is to summarize once again the client's current situation, as reflected in your conversations thus far. This is meant to have the effect of drawing Phase 1 to a close. The length of your summary will depend on the complexity of the client's situation. It is usually appropriate to begin this transitional summary with a statement announcing that you are attempting to draw together what has been discussed thus far, for the purpose of evaluating what to do next. Your recapitulation could include the following elements:

1. A summary of the client's own perceptions of the problem, as reflected in his or her change talk
2. A summing-up of the client's ambivalence, including some acknowledgment of what remains positive or attractive about the status quo
3. A review of any objective evidence you may have that is relevant to the importance of change
4. A restatement of any indications the client has offered of wanting, intending, or planning to change, and of his or her confidence talk
5. Your own assessment of the client's situation, particularly at points where it converges with the client's own concerns

The purpose of this summary is to draw together as many reasons for change as possible, while simultaneously acknowledging the client's reluctance or ambivalence. The recapitulation is used as a final preparation for the transition to commitment and leads directly to a key question.

Key Questions

Consistent with the spirit of motivational interviewing, Phase 2 does not involve telling people what they must do but, rather, eliciting what they want and plan to do. That is the purpose of a key question, which ordinarily follows directly from a recapitulation of Phase 1.

Key questions are always open questions. They cannot be answered with a simple "Yes" or "No," and their purpose is to start a person thinking and talking about change. Their basic theme is the question: What is the next step? Though the first key question normally follows the recapitulation, they can be useful throughout Phase 2. There are many variations, but here are some examples of key questions:

"What do you think you will do? What are you thinking at this point about _____?"
"What changes, if any, are you thinking about making?"
"At this point, after reviewing all of this, what's the next step for you?"
"What could you do? What are your options?"
"It sounds like things can't stay the way they are now. What do you think you might do?"
"Of the things we have talked about, which ones concern you the most? What do you want to do at this point?"
"What happens next?"
"Where do we go from here?"
"How would you like things to turn out for you now, ideally?"
"What would be some of the good things about making a change?"

The client's answers to such key questions are met, as usual, with reflective listening. This serves to clarify the client's thoughts and plans and to encourage further exploration. Reflection can also be used selectively to reinforce change talk that is offered (Chapter 6) and to diminish resistance that may arise (Chapter 8). Personal responsibility, freedom, and choice can be emphasized again during this process. Be careful not to shift wholly into a problem-solving mode. The methods from earlier chapters continue to be useful during Phase 2.

Giving Information and Advice

Because of its client-centered roots, motivational interviewing is sometimes assumed to be incompatible with giving information and advice. In fact, it is quite possible and appropriate, within the spirit and principles of motivational interviewing, to share one's expertise with clients. It is the context within which such information and advice are given that determines consistency with the overall clinical method.

This is not license to dispense professional advice or information whenever it crosses one's mind. There are two circumstances under which such expertise is offered in motivational interviewing: when a person requests it, or with the person's permission. In the latter case, it is the clinician who initiates the advice or information giving, and some further guidelines are appropriate here. Ask yourself the following questions before you initiate advice or information giving:

"Have I elicited the client's own ideas and knowledge on this subject?"

and

"Is what I am going to convey important to the client's safety, or likely to enhance the client's motivation for change?"

When the answer to both questions is "Yes," proceed with the client's permission.

What, then, constitutes permission? It is, in essence, some form of acknowledging a person's choice to take or not take the advice you will offer, to hear or not hear the information you want to provide. It may be (but is not always) a direct asking for permission. When you do make such a direct request, it could sound like one of these:

"Would it be all right if I told you a concern that I have about what you're proposing to do?"
"I have an idea here that may or may not be relevant. Do you want to hear it?"
"I think I understand your perspective on this. I wonder if it would be

> OK for me to tell you a few things that occur to me as I listen to you, which you might want to consider."
>
> "I don't know if this will matter to you, or even make sense, but I am a little worried about your plan. Would you mind if I explained why?"
>
> "There are a few things that may or may not be important to you here, and I want to make sure that you know them before we go on. You probably already know some of these, but I want to make sure. Would that be all right with you?"

Asking permission in this way honors the person's autonomy and makes it easier for him or her to hear and consider what you have to say. People almost always give permission for you to continue, but still it's important to ask because of what the asking process communicates: respect, choice, and collaboration.

There are also indirect forms of asking permission. Such language does not request a direct approval from the client. Instead, qualifiers are added that acknowledge the client's freedom to listen or not, and to heed or not:

> "I don't know if this would work for you or not, but I can give you an idea of what some other people have done in your situation."
>
> "This may or may not make sense to you, but it's one possibility. You'll have to judge whether it applies to you."
>
> "I can give you an idea, but I think you'd have to try it out to see if it would work for you."
>
> "All I can give you, of course, is my own opinion. You're really the one who has to find what works for you."

Often during Phase 2, a person will ask you for information or ideas. It is entirely appropriate in this circumstance to offer your own best advice. It is important, however, to guard against falling into the "Yes, but . . . " pattern, which is really a variation on the trap of taking sides. In this script, the counselor gives information and the client says what is wrong with it, or the counselor offers an idea and the client responds by saying why it will not work. A few rounds of this can establish an unhelpful pattern.

There are several ways to guard against this. First, don't be too eager to offer advice. Wait for a direct invitation or request for information. Perhaps even be a bit reluctant to give advice, evoking from the person additional requests and permission for your advice:

> "I'll be happy to give you some ideas, but I don't want to get in the way of your own creative thinking, and you're the expert on you. I'm not sure if you really want or need my advice. Maybe you have some ideas of your own about what to do."
>
> "Of course I can tell you what I think, if you really want to know. But I

don't want you to feel like I'm telling you what you have to do. Does my opinion really make that much difference to you?"

Another useful approach is to offer not one, but a cluster of options. There is evidence that when people choose a course of action from among alternatives, they are more likely to adhere to it and succeed. This further avoids the easy "Yes, but . . . " pattern in which the person rejects suggestions one at a time:

> "Well, there really isn't any one way that works for everybody. I can tell you about some approaches that other people have used successfully, and you can see which of those might fit you best."
> "Let me describe a number of possibilities, and you tell me which of these makes the most sense for you."

It is also possible to solicit requests from the person for information and advice. This can be done, for example, in Phase 2 after offering a closing summary. You might say something like this:

> "We've talked over quite a bit of material here, and you seem to have been giving this a lot of thought. I wonder if there is anything you'd like to ask me now, or that you've been wondering about."

This may evoke requests for more information about material discussed in Phase 1 or for advice about change options. If you are asked something that you do not know, feel free to say that you don't know but will find out.

A common-sense qualification is in order here. This is the general style of motivational interviewing in Phase 2, but as indicated, if you see the person charging down a slippery ski slope headed straight for a tree, politeness may have to wait.

NEGOTIATING A CHANGE PLAN

Through the client's responses to key questions and your own provision of information and advice, a plan for change can begin to emerge. The development of this plan is a process of shared decision making and negotiation that involves (1) setting goals, (2) considering change options, (3) arriving at a plan, and (4) eliciting commitment.

1. Setting Goals

Motivation is driven by a discrepancy between a person's goals and his or her perceived present state. A first step in instigating change, then, is to have clear goals toward which to move. Key questions in this regard might be as follows:

"How would you like for things to be different?"

"What is it that you want to change?"

"If you were completely successful in accomplishing what you want now, what would be changed?"

"Let's take things one step at a time. What do you think is the first step?"

This brings us to the probability that the client's goals may not correspond with your own. For example, you may aspire for a particular person to swear off alcohol and all other psychoactive drugs for the rest of her life, whereas she may be more concerned about improving her marriage and, at most, reducing her drinking to a moderate level. How could you handle this situation?

The fact is that you cannot impose your own goals on another person. In fact, your own goals probably have very little relevance to most clients. You can offer your best advice, but the client is always free to accept or disregard it. Further arguing and insisting would likely evoke defensiveness rather than agreement. It makes little sense to work within a motivational interviewing method throughout Phase 1, only to alienate the client with a rigidly prescriptive style in Phase 2. It is far better, we believe, to maintain a strong working alliance with the client, and to start with the goals toward which he or she is most eager to make progress. If these goals are misguided, it will become apparent soon enough.

Remember to keep a broad view in discussing goals. Although there may appear to be a focal problem, the client also has wider goals and values that are important to consider. Sometimes a person's presenting problem turns out to be entangled with a much deeper issue of values or with broader life goals. Awareness of these larger goals and values can be helpful in building motivation for change (see Chapter 19 for a more thorough discussion of values and motivational interviewing). You may also want to suggest (with permission) additional goals that you believe are important to the client's welfare and change efforts.

Another important consideration is whether a goal is realistic. Too large a gap between present and desired behavior can be demoralizing rather than motivating. There are various ways to evaluate whether a particular goal is achievable, beyond your own judgment on the matter. One is to ask for a confidence rating (Chapter 9). Another is to ask the client to consider what consequences might follow from taking this particular course of action. A person may well have concerns that have not been expressed. Some other possible questions are the following:

"How would your life be different if you pursued this goal and reached it?"

"So that's your goal. What can you think of that might go wrong with this plan?"

"What might be good, and what might be not so good, about reaching this goal?"

Also keep in mind that there are almost always multiple goals along with multiple and interrelated areas of concern. It can therefore be necessary to prioritize goals through a process of shared decision making regarding which are most urgent or important (see the discussion of agenda setting in Chapter 6).

Goal setting leads naturally to the second step: considering how the person might go about achieving the goal. Sometimes all it takes to trigger change is the decision to have a goal, but usually there are things that a person can do to increase the chances of success. Before proceeding, however, make sure the goal seems right. If the client is expressing serious importance or confidence concerns about the goal, there is more work to do before proceeding.

2. Considering Change Options

Once a person's relevant goals have been clarified, the next step is to consider possible methods for achieving the chosen goals. Involve the client directly in this process of brainstorming and evaluating possible change strategies, drawing on his or her own ideas. Remember that there are almost always multiple ways to achieve a behavior change goal. One option is formal treatment, and within it there is often a range of alternative approaches with reasonable evidence of efficacy. A central focus in motivational interviewing, however, is to draw on a person's own internal resources and natural social support. Once people are willing, able, and ready to change, they often go ahead and do so on their own.

The discussion in Chapter 9 of brainstorming is relevant here. It can be useful to generate a range of options, even far-fetched ones, before moving toward a plan. This process can be a pooling of the client's ideas and your own. Introduce this as a creative brainstorming phase, with evaluation temporarily suspended—no discussion of how realistic or acceptable or effective each option might be. This allows the person to suggest ideas without being blocked by their shortcomings and also provides a context within which you can suggest options without immediate resistance. If an option that you add to the list yields a resistant response, reflect the concern, reminding the client that this is only a creative list of options and that you will come back later to evaluate and compare them.

When suggesting change options, it is often good to provide a menu of strategies rather than one at a time. Suggesting one possibility invites a person to say what's wrong with it, essentially voicing counterchange arguments. Offering a menu gives a person a different mental set. In essence, you say:

"Here is a variety of possibilities that people have used successfully. Which of these do you prefer? Which do you think might work best for you?"

The client's task becomes one of choosing rather than refuting.

3. Arriving at a Plan

This discussion leads directly toward the negotiation of a plan for change. As much as possible, elicit this plan by having the person voice it. Key (open) questions are useful here:

> "So what is it specifically that you plan to do?"
> "What do you think is the first step?"
> "How will you go about it?"

It can be useful with some people to fill in a written change plan, summarizing what it is that the client plans to do. One possible format is shown in Box 10.2.

What you are working toward in Phase 2 is a clearly stated plan of action. On the basis of your discussion, summarize the plan that you have developed together, which seems to fit the client's goals, needs, intentions, and beliefs. This is best done in "you" language. Here are two examples:

> "What you want to do, then, is to work on getting your weight and blood pressure down through diet and exercise. You prefer this to going on medication, although if it doesn't work you know that there is medication that can help. You want to give this a try for at least 2 months, and you'll make an appointment for a month from now just to check in. There is a health club near your house, and you plan to go join today or tomorrow and have them help you develop a realistic exercise plan. You want to stay away from restaurants for a while, and I've given you some guidelines for food preparation, and you want to find a class you can take on healthy cooking that is also good-tasting. You plan to weigh yourself every second day in the morning, and keep a chart, and you'll get a blood pressure monitor so you can also check that every other day. Have I missed anything?"

> "Let me see if I can accurately summarize where you are, then. You wanted to know about different ways that people can change their drinking, and we've talked about a number of possibilities. You're thinking that you may need to quit completely in the long run, but you're really not ready to do that without first giving moderation a good try. You considered different options and decided that you'd like to work on your own with the self-control materials I showed you. We should be able to tell in 6 to 8 weeks whether that is going to work for you, and that should tell us what you want to know. Even if you decide then that what you want to do is quit, cutting down is a reasonable step on the way. So what you are going to do is read this material I've given you, begin keeping daily records, and come back in 2 weeks to let me know how you're

BOX 10.2. A Change Plan Worksheet

The most important reasons why I want to make this change are:

My main goals for myself in making this change are:

I plan to do these things in order to accomplish my goals:

Specific action   When?

Other people could help me with change in these ways:

Person   Possible ways to help

These are some possible obstacles to change, and how I could handle them:

Possible obstacle to change   How to respond

I will know that my plan is working when I see these results:

doing. We also discussed bringing Jan along to that session, and you thought that would be a good idea. You're still a little nervous about this plan, I think, but you do see that you need to make a change, and this sounds like the one you've chosen. Do I have it right?"

4. Eliciting Commitment

Ideally, this plan summary brings you to the point of commitment. You are looking for the client's approval of and assent to the plan. The simplest way to get such commitment is to ask for it. The basic question is: "Is this what you want to do?" The answer you hope for is: "Yes."

Getting to a "Yes" may require a few more steps. The client may want to amend the plan as you have stated it. If the response you get indicates a low level of commitment (e.g., "I guess so" or "I'll think about it"), you still have some work to do. Explore what reluctance the client still has about this plan, using Phase 1 methods to resolve ambivalence.

Commitment to a plan can be enhanced by making it public. If a spouse or other loved one is present in the session, the commitment is made with that person's knowledge and consent. You can suggest that the client visit, write, or telephone other people to let them know about the decision and to ask for their help. Such a telephone call can even be made during the counseling session. If the client has had positive contact with other staff members within the clinic, you may ask permission to share his or her plan with them, or you may call them into the session to have the client describe it. The more the client verbalizes the plan to others, the more commitment is strengthened. There is also the very real social support benefit of recruiting the help and support of others. If it appears that telling others may be difficult or risky, rehearse this with the client during the session.

The point is to arrive at a clear plan, to obtain the client's verbal decision to follow the plan, and to reinforce the client's decision. It can be useful to agree on and initiate some immediate steps for implementing the plan.

If a person is not quite ready to make a commitment, do not press, for to do so would be to fall into the taking-sides trap at the very last step. One option is to come alongside the reluctance:

> "If you're not quite ready, then I don't want you to make a commitment yet. This is too important, and you don't have to make up your mind this minute. Go home and think about it, and we can talk about it more next time."

In this case, do follow up with the person and maintain contact to keep the door open. When checking back, avoid closed questions like, "Have you decided yet?" and instead ask what the person is thinking at this point or what's been happening with regard to his or her plan for change.

TRANSITION

The commitment to a change plan completes the formal cycle of motivational interviewing. Sometimes people proceed with change on their own from here. It can also work well, however, to transition from this initial motivational consultation into action-focused counseling if the person so chooses. Furthermore, the general style of motivational interviewing can be used to facilitate change throughout the process of counseling. Ambivalence, after all, rarely disappears on the first step of a journey.

NOTE

1. See Miller and C'de Baca (2001).

CHAPTER 11

A Practical Case Example

> We found that . . . drinkers would not take pressure in any form,
> excepting from John Barleycorn himself. They always had to be
> led, not pushed. . . . We found we had to make haste slowly.
> —BILL WILSON, 1955, quoted in Ernest Kurtz,
> *Not-God: A History of Alcoholics Anonymous*

The practice of motivational interviewing involves a creative integration of the methods we have outlined. There are no standard scripts that can be followed. Each person is unique and poses different challenges.

For this reason, we have hesitated about offering a case example from start to finish. There is a limited amount that can be learned from observing any single clinical example. No particular case can demonstrate the rich variety of situations and problems you will face or the range of ways in which these challenges can be met. Still, we have thought it helpful to provide a detailed example of how motivational interviewing proceeds. The exact counseling approach reflected here may not be well suited to other individuals, but it does illustrate how motivational interviewing methods are interwoven in actual practice.

The case to be described is that of a 38-year-old photographer who came for consultation about his drinking. He had never sought help for alcohol problems before, and he certainly was not ready or willing to quit drinking. He was not at all certain that he even needed help or change, but two events had precipitated his coming. The first was a check-up by his physician, in response to some stomach pains he had been having. Based on this examination, the physician had told him that both his complaints and his memory blackouts indicated he was drinking too much, and he recommended that he see a specialist. Second, when he discussed this with his wife, she to his surprise voiced her own concern that his drinking was getting out of hand. The combination of these comments was just enough to prompt him to make an appointment.

INTERVIEWER: Good morning. Please have a seat here. I believe you wanted to talk about some concerns with your drinking. We have about 45 minutes today, and mainly I want to hear about your situation and your concerns. I'll need to get some specific information from you later, but right now perhaps you could start by telling me what your concerns are.

The interviewer begins with a brief structuring statement and an open question.

CLIENT: Well, to tell you the truth, I'm not really sure that there's anything to be concerned about. My wife seems to think that I drink too much. My doctor did some blood tests, and he told me those showed I am probably drinking too much. "Probably," he said, but ever since I told my wife about that, she's been worried about my drinking. So I told her I would come here, but I'm not really sure if I should be here.

The client immediately expresses ambivalence that could easily be understood as defensiveness.

INTERVIEWER: So at least two other people, your wife and your doctor, have been worried that maybe alcohol is harming you. But I wonder: What have you noticed yourself? Is there anything that you have observed about your drinking over the years that might be reason for concern? Tell me something about your drinking.

A simple reflection.

It would have been easy here to fall into the question–answer trap, by asking a series of specific questions. Instead the counselor asks a cluster of open questions.

CLIENT: I guess maybe I drink more than I used to. My wife says I've been drinking more over the past few years.

Change talk: The client acknowledges a possible reason for concern.

INTERVIEWER: So one thing you've noticed is that you are drinking more now than you used to. What else?

Reflection and "What else?"

CLIENT: I can't really think of anything else. It doesn't really affect me much. I don't get drunk very often.

INTERVIEWER: Although you know that your drinking has gone up over the past few years, it doesn't really seem to affect you any more than before.

Reflection, slightly amplified.

CLIENT: Right. I can drink all night and it doesn't make me drunk. Other guys have trouble keeping up with me.

INTERVIEWER: That's interesting. What do you make of that?

Open question.

CLIENT: I think it runs in my family. My dad was like that. He could drink most guys under the table, and it never seemed to bother him.

INTERVIEWER: He was like you. Is he still *living?*

Reflection and closed question.

CLIENT: No, he died of a heart attack a few years ago. But that was after he had stopped drinking.

A hint of defensiveness in this response.

INTERVIEWER: Why did he stop?

An open question, and useful information, but a risk of too many questions in a row.

CLIENT: My mother wanted him to. He used to tell people that he quit for his health—that he wanted to lose some weight, and beer contains a lot of calories.

INTERVIEWER: So you think your drinking has been increasing over the years, and you've noticed that, as with your dad, alcohol doesn't seem to affect you as much as it does other people. And you think that since you father was like that, it might be something that runs in the family.

A linking summary of change talk offered thus far, picking up a possible motivational theme related to the father's drinking.

CLIENT: Is that possible?

INTERVIEWER: Yes, it is, and that may be important. What else have you noticed?

Because it is a bit early for information giving, the

What about other ways in which your drinking seems like your father's?

counselor gives a short answer and returns to eliciting change talk.

CLIENT: Lately, there have been some times when I can't remember things that happened. I'll be drinking at a party, and the next morning I can't remember getting home. It's not too pleasant to wake up and have no idea where you left your car.

More change talk—disadvantages of status quo.

INTERVIEWER: That can be scary, especially the first few times it happens. Give me an example.

The counselor reflects feeling, then asks for elaboration of the change talk.

CLIENT: About 2 weeks ago, I was out with Bob, and I guess I drank a little more than usual. We were playing billiards, with loser buying rounds. When I woke up in the morning, I couldn't think of where my car was, and I remembered starting this one game but I couldn't remember how it ended. I looked out the window and my car was in the driveway, so I guess I drove it there. I felt terrible.

INTERVIEWER: In what ways?

Again, asking for elaboration.

CLIENT: Well, I wondered if I had done anything stupid. I guess I could wake up in jail.

More change talk.

INTERVIEWER: For driving while intoxicated.

Continuing the paragraph.

CLIENT: I don't usually get that drunk, but probably that time I was.

INTERVIEWER: What else bothered you that morning?

Asking for elaboration.

CLIENT: I know that happened to my dad, too. He told me about it.

INTERVIEWER: It worries you that the same thing is happening to you. What do you think it means?

The counselor stays with reflection of feeling, with open question for elaboration.

CLIENT: I don't know. I haven't really

thought that much about it. I
remember he'd get up in the morning
looking pretty shaky and needing
a drink.

INTERVIEWER: You feel that way yourself
sometimes.

*A guess—continuing the
paragraph.*

CLIENT: No, I don't think I ever feel like I
need a drink. But I have felt pretty bad
some mornings. I don't usually drink in
the morning, though.

INTERVIEWER: That's a rule you've kept for
yourself.

CLIENT: Yes, except on rare occasions. I
don't think it's good to drink in the
morning.

INTERVIEWER: Why is that?

CLIENT: I've noticed that I feel better; it gets
rid of the hangover. That could get to be
a bad habit. I usually just tough it out
and it goes away.

INTERVIEWER: When you stop to think about
it, then, there are several things you've
noticed. Your drinking seems to be going
up over the years, and you know that
you've driven sometimes when you've had
too much. Your wife is concerned about
you, as your mother was about your father,
and your doctor has told you that it's
affecting your health. You've noticed that,
like your father, you can drink quite a bit
without feeling intoxicated, and you've
been having these problems with your
memory. You've had some bad hangovers,
and you notice that if you drink some
more in the morning you feel better.
Which of these things concern you
the most?

*A collecting summary,
drawing together the
change-talk themes that
have emerged.*

CLIENT: My health, I suppose.

INTERVIEWER: So if you thought that you
were harming your health, that would
worry you. What else concerns you?

CLIENT: I don't like not remembering things.

INTERVIEWER: That doesn't seem normal to you.

Reflection, continuing the paragraph.

CLIENT: No. But I don't think I'm an alcoholic. I've know some alcoholics, and I'm not like that.

Resistance, perhaps in response to the reference to "normal." The labeling trap opens up.

INTERVIEWER: Your situation doesn't seem so bad to you.

Reflection.

CLIENT: No, it doesn't. I've quit drinking for weeks at a time with no problem. And I can have a couple of drinks and leave it alone. I have a good job and family. How could I be an alcoholic?

INTERVIEWER: That must be confusing to you, as you think about it. On the one hand, you can see some warning signs that you are drinking too much, like your father did, and it worries you. On the other hand, you don't really fit your picture of an alcoholic.

Reflection of feeling, and a double-sided reflection.

CLIENT: Right. I mean I've got some problems, but I'm not a drunk.

The client responds by acknowledging both sides of the ambivalence.

INTERVIEWER: And that's why thus far it hasn't seemed like you needed to do anything. But now you're here. Why now?

Reflection by continuing the paragraph then an open question.

CLIENT: It just seemed like I ought to talk to somebody. I don't want to ignore this. I saw what happened to my dad, and I don't want that to happen to me and my family.

Change talk.

INTERVIEWER: Your family is really important to you.

Reflection, reinforcing an important value.

CLIENT: I love my wife and my son.

INTERVIEWER: And it sounds like they love you, too. Your wife cared enough to tell you how worried she is about your drinking. And though you don't see yourself as an alcoholic, you're a little worried yourself.

Reframe and reflection.

CLIENT: Yes, I guess so.

INTERVIEWER: It must have been a difficult thing for you to decide to come here. You must care quite a bit about yourself and your family, and I respect you for being so open here. It's not an easy thing that you did, coming here.

Affirmation.

CLIENT: I didn't really want to come. Do you think I'm an alcoholic?

Labeling trap yawns again.

INTERVIEWER: That's a term that means many things to different people. What matters, really, is that we take a good close look at what's going on here. I can see why you're concerned, and I'd like to help you get clear on what risk you're facing, and then what, if anything, you want to do about it.

A simple "yes" here would likely have led to disso- nance and resistance. In- stead the counselor reframed the issue and shifted the focus back to the task at hand: exploring his drinking and its effects.

CLIENT: What do you think I should do?

Commentary. This is an example of the Phase 1 process of eliciting change talk as a means for building intrinsic motivation for change. Most of the counselor's responses up to this point were in the form of open questions to elicit change talk, or they indicated reflective listening and summaries to re- inforce motivational themes. At many points where it might have been tempt- ing to begin confronting, the counselor retained a generally empathic stance and avoided argumentation. Clients are often surprised and relieved at this; instead of resisting, they tend to be willing to continue the self-evaluation pro- cess.

At this point, the client asks an important question: "What do you think I should do?" The counselor has to make a decision here. Is there enough of a motivational base to begin discussing strategies for change? If this had been an office consultation with a physician, where time was quite limited, or if this had been a one-time opportunity, it might have been best to try strengthening commitment and negotiating a plan (Phase 2). The risk, however, is that not enough Phase 1 work has been done, and the counselor could be put in the role of making suggestions that the client would then reject (a form of the trap of taking sides). In this case, the client is consulting a specialist, and it is there- fore possible to engage him in a longer counseling process. One option is to continue the present interview with Phase 1 methods, accumulating further change talk that could be used to develop discrepancy. Another is to use the limited rapport base that has been established to involve the client in a more detailed evaluation, which, in turn, would provide more material to discuss. The counselor chose the latter route and offered a transition to structured assessment. Such assessment is not an essential part of motivational interviewing, but the following illustrates how assessment results can be integrated into the motivational interviewing process.

CLIENT: What do you think I should do?

INTERVIEWER: There are quite a few possibilities, and I could help you think about your options right now if you like. But if you want my opinion, I think that first we ought to get a better picture of your present situation. What you have told me so far raises a few concerns, but we really don't know enough yet to make good decisions. What I would suggest, then, is that we take some time for a good check-up. There are some questionnaires you could answer, and I'd also like to spend a couple of hours with you getting more helpful information. After that, when we have a clearer picture of exactly what is happening in your life, we can focus on your options. What do you think? Are you interested enough to spend a couple of hours finding out more about yourself?

The client completed several questionnaires at home, and in this case the counselor administered an assessment about drinking practices. It is possible, of course, to conduct a simpler assessment or to do motivational interviewing without special assessment. This material is included here to illustrate how the style of motivational interviewing can be used to provide assessment feedback.[1] Here is a portion of the subsequent interview, in which this feedback was provided. The client was given a written report to follow as the counselor reviewed the findings.

INTERVIEWER: I appreciate the time and care that you took with these tests. What I want us to do now is to review the results together. First, you remember that we went through a typical week and added up your drinking, That came out to about 53 standard drinks a week, with one "drink" here being a regular glass of either beer or wine or about an

This typifies the motivational interviewing style for presenting results. The client's score is explained, relative to normative data. Rather than being told what to think or how to feel about the result, the

ounce of liquor. If we compare that to the whole population, you're drinking more than 95% of adults. How does that sound to you?

person is asked for reactions, which are then reflected.

CLIENT: It sounds like a lot. I never really added it up before, but I don't think of myself as a heavy drinker.

INTERVIEWER: You're surprised.

Instead of confronting, the counselor uses simple reflection.

CLIENT: Yes! I know that when you were asking me about how much I drink usually, it sounded like a lot. But I drink about the same as most of my friends do.

INTERVIEWER: So this is confusing for you. On the one hand, you can see that it's a lot, and this says it's more than 95% of adults drink. Yet it seems about normal among your friends. How could both things be true?

Double-sided reflection.

CLIENT: I guess I can drink with the top 5%.

INTERVIEWER: Your friends are pretty heavy drinkers.

The counselor would have done better to understate this reflection.

CLIENT: I don't know about "heavy." I guess we drink more than our share.

INTERVIEWER: We also have a computer program that estimates blood alcohol levels based on drinking patterns. Most drinkers stop somewhere between 20 and 50 on this scale. Fifty here is the same as 0.05, which is enough to impair driving. Our estimate is that you get up around 179 units, or 0.179, in the course of a typical week of drinking. That's over three times the upper limit for most drinkers and far into the legal intoxication range for impaired driving.

CLIENT: You mean every week?

INTERVIEWER: From what you told me, yes, that's right. I believe you said there are three nights a week when you get up around this level.

CLIENT: That can't be right. I never even feel drunk. I drive home all the time, and I've never had a problem.

Resistance: Challenging.

INTERVIEWER: It seems to you that something must be wrong with the computer.

Amplified reflection, without a hint of irony or sarcasm in the voice.

CLIENT: Well, no, but I don't ever feel that drunk.

The client backs down a bit.

INTERVIEWER: You can't see how you possibly could have that much alcohol in your body without feeling it.

Agreement with a twist.

CLIENT: Is that possible?

INTERVIEWER: Not only that, it's common among heavy drinkers. It's called "tolerance," although most people call it "being able to hold your liquor." We talked about that the first time I saw you.

Giving information.

CLIENT: So I can drink a lot and not feel it?

INTERVIEWER: That's right. You can have a fairly high blood alcohol level—enough to make driving unsafe and even do damage to your internal organs—but not feel like you're intoxicated.

CLIENT: So I'm driving around legally drunk three times a week?

INTERVIEWER: That's how it looks. What do you make of that?

CLIENT: I guess I've been lucky.

INTERVIEWER: Now this score is for those heavier drinking times we talked about. On one of those weekends, we estimate, you get up as high as 220 units, or 0.22. That makes sense, because that's the range in which memory blackouts can occur.

CLIENT: Wow!

INTERVIEWER: That seems high to you.   *Simple reflection.*

CLIENT: I just . . . I never thought about it.

INTERVIEWER: Well, that's why we're doing
this, and I appreciate how honestly you   *Affirmation.*
answered these questions. I can see,
though, that this is hard for you. I've
been through this with a lot of people,
and it's tough to look at yourself in the
mirror like this. Do you want to go on?   *Asking permission.*

CLIENT: It's OK.

INTERVIEWER: This next one is a rough mea-   *Giving information.*
sure of alcohol's effects in your life, the
number of places it has caused problems.
Your score of 18 falls in the middle of
the range that we call "significant problems"—not quite severe, but more than
just mild or moderate effects. Does that
make sense to you?

CLIENT: About right, I guess.

INTERVIEWER: OK. I don't know what you'll   *Giving information.*
make of this next result. This reflects the
degree to which you are depending on
alcohol, becoming dependent on it. Your
score here is at the bottom of the range
we call "definite and significant symptoms of dependence." Roughly, that
means that you are starting to show
some of the common signs of alcohol dependence, although you still have a way
to go before getting into severe problems.

CLIENT: You mean I'm addicted?

INTERVIEWER: It's not as simple as either you   *Giving information*
are or you aren't addicted. Dependence is
something that happens gradually, in
steps or degrees. This tells you about
how far along that path you've gone. It
says there is definitely something happening here, that you are starting to show
early signs of dependence on alcohol.

CLIENT: I don't like that at all.

INTERVIEWER: You don't like the idea of being dependent on alcohol.

CLIENT: On anything!

INTERVIEWER: You like to be in charge of yourself, in control.

CLIENT: Yes.

INTERVIEWER: Well, we're not talking about *severe* problems yet. Dependence increases over the years, sometimes at a fast rate, sometimes more slowly. You're just in the middle range now. But it looks like that one really concerns you.

Here the counselor takes up the status quo side, voicing the "maybe it's not so bad" side of the person's ambivalence, and then ending with a reflection.

CLIENT: (*Silent for some time.*) Let's go on to the next one.

INTERVIEWER: I'm worried that I'm giving you too much new information here. This is difficult, and I don't want to give you too much at once. Do you want some more time to take this in or talk about it?

The counselor offers support and some personal choice about how to proceed.

CLIENT: No, it's OK. Let's go ahead.

Commentary. This feedback process can be difficult for a person, and counselor empathy is needed throughout this phase. Feedback of this kind can be quite useful in developing discrepancy and the perception that a change is needed. Resistance is commonly encountered in response to some results and should be responded to empathically rather than opposed (see Chapter 8). At the conclusion of this process, the counselor invites any questions, then summarizes the feedback and integrates it with the person's own stated concerns. This recapitulation prepares the way for asking key questions (Chapter 10).

INTERVIEWER: We've covered a lot of ground. I wonder if there's anything you'd like to ask me—anything you've wondered about so far, or something else you'd like to know.

An invitation to receive information and advice.

CLIENT: Well, yes. Is this something I could have inherited from my father?

INTERVIEWER: There is good evidence that people can inherit a predisposition to alcohol problems. It's not quite as simple as inheriting a condition called "alcoholism." It's a bit more like hereditary risk for high blood pressure or heart disease. Your blood pressure is determined in part by genetics, but it is also influenced by your diet and exercise, your stress level, your use of salt, and so on. Drinking is like that, too. Men who have biological relatives with drinking problems seem to have a higher risk themselves. And tolerance is also a risk factor.

CLIENT: So I have a higher risk, then.

INTERVIEWER: That's it, really. You have more reason than most people to be careful about your drinking. Anything else you're wondering about?

CLIENT: I guess not.

INTERVIEWER: Then let me try to summarize where we are, and you can tell me if I've left anything out. You came here partly at the urging of your wife, partly because of your doctor, and partly because you were concerned about your own drinking, though you hadn't really thought that much about it before. You were aware that your drinking has been going up over the years, and now it's over 50 drinks in a typical week. You were also aware that you drink more than other people, and you seem to have a substantial tolerance for alcohol. You can drink a lot of it without feeling drunk, even though—as we discussed today—you have enough alcohol in your bloodstream to affect you and do some damage. You want to take care of yourself, and you are concerned for your own health. The blood tests that your physician did suggest that your body is being damaged by your drinking. You've already piled up some problems related to drinking, and there are some indications

In recapitulation, the counselor collects the change-talk themes that emerged throughout the two interviews.

that you are becoming dependent on alcohol, particularly when you want to so-
cialize or change how you feel. At the
same time, you don't think of yourself as
an alcoholic, and in the past you've assumed that if you're not an alcoholic you
have nothing to worry about in regard to
drinking. You don't like the idea of being dependent on anything. You've had
some bad hangovers, and you're concerned about alcohol's effects on your
memory. I know you've thought about
how your drinking is looking like your
father's in some ways, and that's a
worry. We talked about your family history, and how you probably have a
higher risk than most people for being
harmed by alcohol. You especially want
to make sure that your drinking doesn't
hurt your family, because you know
firsthand what that hurt is like. Is that a
fair summary?

CLIENT: Yes, except that I didn't really think
when I came here that I was drinking
more than other people.

INTERVIEWER: Right—I forgot that. It had   *Amplified reflection.*
seemed to you that your drinking was
perfectly normal.

CLIENT: Well, maybe not normal, but not abnormal, either. I just hadn't thought
about it.

INTERVIEWER: And now you are thinking
about it. I've given you a lot of informa-
tion, and some of it is fairly new. What   *Key question.*
are you thinking at this point? What do
you make of all this?

CLIENT: It's kind of depressing. I really didn't
think I had a problem, at least not this
bad.

INTERVIEWER: This isn't what you expected   *Reflection.*
to hear, and I can see how it must be
distressing for you. Let me put this in
perspective, though. On all of these

measures, you are roughly in a twilight zone, a border region. The good news is that you realized what was happening before any of these troubles became severe. People who discover what is happening and do something about it in time can head off serious damage. Other people wait until they have done severe or irreversible damage. You didn't wait. It's like so many other problems: the earlier you catch it, the better your chances are of turning it around and staying healthy.

Reframing.

Supporting self-efficacy.

CLIENT: What would I do on the weekend if I gave up alcohol? (*Grins.*)

Envisioning.

INTERVIEWER: It's hard to imagine how different your life might be.

Commentary. Here is another choice point: The counselor has to decide whether to press on toward setting goals, negotiating a plan for change, and obtaining commitment. It would have been possible to continue with Phase 1 methods, perhaps by constructing a decisional balance sheet with the pros and cons of change. The question is this: How ready is this person for change? Several of the signs listed in Box 10.1 (Chapter 10) are evident. There is little resistance, and the client is asking few questions about the problem. He is offering some change talk, although the counselor could at this point seek to elicit more (e.g., "What do you think are the most important reasons for concern here? Of the things we've talked about, what are the most important reasons for making a change? What do you think will happen if you don't change your drinking?"). There is an indication of the client's envisioning how life might be without alcohol. The client's nonverbal cues at this point might suggest a kind of surrender, a sad resignation. The counselor decides to test the waters with a key question about change.

INTERVIEWER: So what does this mean about your drinking? What happens now?

Key question.

CLIENT: Well, I want to do something. I don't want to just let this go on.

Change talk.

INTERVIEWER: And what are the possibilities on that "do something" list? What's the next step?

Key question.

CLIENT: I guess I have to do something about my drinking—either cut it down or give it up.

The client opens up the negotiation process by discussing goals.

INTERVIEWER: One or the other.

CLIENT: Well, I can't just let it go! If I keep drinking, won't all of this get worse?

Change talk.

INTERVIEWER: Probably.

CLIENT: Then something's got to change. I either cut down or quit.

INTERVIEWER: What do you think about these two possibilities?

CLIENT: If I had my choice, I would prefer to just cut down. I'd like to drink sometimes.

INTERVIEWER: Drinking is important to you.

Amplified reflection.

Envisioning.

CLIENT: Not important, really. It's just that I enjoy a drink, and I might feel strange sitting there sipping a soft drink while everybody else is drinking.

INTERVIEWER: It might be uncomfortable for you; you'd feel out of place.

CLIENT: Yes. That's not too serious, I guess. I'd just rather not give it up if I don't have to.

INTERVIEWER: But if it were clear to you that you had to quit altogether, then you could.

Supporting self-efficacy.

CLIENT: Sure. If I knew I had to.

INTERVIEWER: How can you find out?

The counselor continues to leave solutions and decision making to the client.

CLIENT: I guess I try something and see if it works.

INTERVIEWER: How much help would you want?

CLIENT: What kind of help?

INTERVIEWER: I mean help from other people—support, counseling, ideas, that sort of thing. How much would you try it on your own, and how much would it help to have some support?

CLIENT: I don't know. I've never tried. I like to handle things myself, and I think I could do it, but maybe it would help to talk to somebody else about it, too.

INTERVIEWER: So you might be open to some support if you decide to change your drinking.

CLIENT: I think so, yes.

INTERVIEWER: What do you think you will do?   *Key question.*

CLIENT: You're the expert. What can I do?   *A reasonable request, but beware the expert trap.*

INTERVIEWER: I can tell you some things that other people have tried successfully, but you're the expert on you. All I can do is give you ideas. Maybe some of them will make sense to you; maybe none of them will. You're the one who has to decide what to do. Do you want some ideas?

Introducing the "menu" concept.

Emphasizing personal control.

Requesting permission to give advice.

CLIENT: Sure.

INTERVIEWER: First of all, there's your decision about cutting down versus quitting. Some people do succeed in getting their drinking reduced to a point that it no longer causes them problems. Others find it's necessary or easier to abstain. You're not sure which way to go.

CLIENT: No. What do you think?

INTERVIEWER: This has to be your decision; I can't make it for you, but I can tell you what I think.

Emphasizing personal control, and renewing permission.

CLIENT: Please. I don't have to do it just because you say it.

INTERVIEWER: OK. I guess if I were in your place, I think I'd be concerned about things getting worse, including the health effects the doctor talked about. The surest way to reverse those problems and get them back toward normal is a period of total abstinence, if you can handle it.   *Personal challenge.*

CLIENT: Oh, I can handle it all right. How long do you think I ought to go on the wagon?

INTERVIEWER: That's hard to say. At least long enough for your body to get back to normal. I'd say that 3 months would be a good start. It might be a good idea to repeat some of these tests after that to see how you are doing.

CLIENT: And if I keep drinking, I won't get better?

INTERVIEWER: I can't say for sure. You could take your chances. But I do think that the surest and quickest way to repair this damage would be to take a vacation from alcohol. That's my opinion. I don't know how that sounds to you.

CLIENT: Then when I am healthy again, I can start drinking again if I want to?

INTERVIEWER: The fact is that you *can* start drinking any time you want to. Nobody can stop you. It's not a question of whether you *can*. The real question is what would happen. As I told you, some people are careful with their drinking and they manage. The danger, of course, is falling back into old habits and starting to drink in a way that endangers your health and your family again. But you don't need to make that decision now. You can decide that after you've had your vacation. You might even find that you *like* not drinking!

Emphasizing personal control.

Delaying a decision.

CLIENT: But for now I have to quit.

A hint of externalizing the decision.

INTERVIEWER: You asked me what I think. I didn't tell you that you have to, only that it's what I think would be best. What you do is up to you. What do you think you'll do?

The counselor avoids taking responsibility for the change side of the client's ambivalence, and reemphasizes personal control.

CLIENT: That seems like the safest thing to do.

INTERVIEWER: Then let me ask you this: What still stands in the way of your quitting? If you have decided to let go of alcohol, at least for a period of time, what might make that hard?

CLIENT: My friends. A lot of the time I spend with them is drinking, and I don't know how I would handle that.

INTERVIEWER: What could you do?

CLIENT: Maybe I spend more time with my friends who don't drink, or stay away from the bars and see them when they're not drinking.

INTERVIEWER: Can you manage that?

Personal challenge.

CLIENT: I think so, yes.

INTERVIEWER: What else would be hard?

CLIENT: I like to drink. But I guess that's not a big problem. I just have to remind myself that quitting is important.

INTERVIEWER: Let me ask you this: What do you think might happen if you don't change your drinking? What would be happening 5 or 10 years down the line if you keep on drinking as you have been?

The counselor assumes that there is continuing ambivalence, and uses this opportunity to reinforce motivation by looking ahead.

CLIENT: I guess all of those things we talked about could get worse—my liver, my memory. And I think my family would have a hard time —I don't like to think about losing them. Maybe even lose my job if it got bad enough. It's not very pleasant to think about.

INTERVIEWER: How do you feel about drinking right this minute?

CLIENT: It doesn't seem very appealing.

INTERVIEWER: One more thing. Usually there's a bigger picture than just drinking. How else would you like for things to be different? What other changes you would like to see?

CLIENT: I'd like to get along better with my wife.

INTERVIEWER: So it might be good for the

two of you to talk to somebody together,
to work on your relationship. Would
both of you be willing to do that?

CLIENT: I think so.

Commentary. At this point, the counselor reviews with the person a range of options available to help him in carrying out his plan. The client expressed a preference to "do it on my own," but shows some interest in coming back for follow-up sessions with his wife. The counselor proceeds with a plan summary.

INTERVIEWER: Let me make sure I understand what you want to do, then. You've decided that what you want is to take a break from alcohol for a period of at least 3 months, and you're going to go home and explain it to your wife. You think it would be a good idea for the two of you to come back together and to be able to check in with me on how you're doing. You like the idea of being able to accomplish this on your own, so for now you don't want to try other kinds of support. You did, say, though, that if it doesn't work out and you take up drinking again in the next 3 months, then we would talk about some additional support. You're going to come back next Thursday with your wife, so we can go over this plan with her, and then we'll decide what to do from there. Is that what you want to do?

CLIENT: Yes, I guess so.

INTERVIEWER: You sound a little reluctant still, and I guess that's understandable. This is a big change for you. What is there about this plan that you're nervous about? Have I missed something?

Reflecting the ambivalence.

CLIENT: I'm not really "nervous" about it. No, it's OK. I was just thinking about some of the good times I have had.

INTERVIEWER: And it's hard because you're weighing those against your health and

your family and the good times to come. *Reflection (continuing the*
It's hard to let go. *paragraph).*

CLIENT: But it's what I have to do.

INTERVIEWER: No, you don't have to. It hap-   *Emphasizing personal*
pens only if it's what you *choose* to do,   *control.*
if you want it enough. Is this what you
want?

CLIENT: Yes. It is.

INTERVIEWER: Then I'll see you and your
wife on Thursday.

This is just one example of how motivational interviewing flows in practice. There are many different approaches through which the basic principles
of motivational interviewing can be pursued. This case is illustrative of some
of the choice points that arise, and how a skilled counselor might proceed.
The challenge for your creativity is in applying the general principles with
each individual person.

NOTE

1. For more detail on how to combine motivational interviewing and assessment feedback, see Miller, Zweben, DiClemente, and Rychtarik (1992).

CHAPTER 12

Ethical Considerations

I have not the right to want to change another if I am not open to be changed.
                                                                    —MARTIN BUBER

ETHICAL ITCHES IN MOTIVATIONAL INTERVIEWING

Yes, "itches." These are issues gone awry. Ethical issues often have to do with the use of influence, and in this way they apply not only to all forms of counseling and psychotherapy but also to nearly all spheres of human interaction. Ethical concerns are quite central when one is coercing people to do what they don't (or otherwise wouldn't) want to do.

Somehow such issues are particularly salient with motivational interviewing. Although we place strong emphasis on principles of respect, benevolence, and autonomy, the issue of undue influence (manipulation) invariably arises in discussions and training. It arises in part because motivational interviewing is about changing what a person wants. The individual's wishes are normally one standard against which ethical practice is judged, but what about methods that seek to alter the person's wishes themselves?

It is not an uncommon situation, of course. Virtually all of marketing and advertising are directly focused on causing people to want certain things, most of which they do not really need. Religions, schools, and "motivational speakers" are partially about the business of instilling certain values, causing people to prefer and choose one option over another. There are many who want you to want what they have to offer, and who will do what they can to increase its perceived importance in your eyes.

Counselors and psychotherapists sometimes regard what they do to be value-free, or at least directed toward the client's values rather than their own. Intentionally altering what people want and value can therefore be an ethically itchy area. It raises interesting questions, discomforts, and concerns.

There is nothing wrong with that. In fact, we worry if someone practices motivational interviewing without feeling ethical itches or if he or she sees such concerns as nonissues. Just as addictive behaviors provide a particularly clear lens through which to study processes of human volition and change, so motivational interviewing seems to bring into clearer focus ethical issues of influence in counseling.

Aspirations of the Client

A primary consideration is what the client wants and hopes for from counseling. Sometimes this is clear, or at least implicit from the context. A person asking for help from an accountant or a consumer credit counseling service most likely wants to get some financial affairs in order. A person walking through the door of the "Center on Alcoholism, Substance Abuse, and Addictions" is not left wondering what topics may be discussed in consultation.

Even in what seem like rather focused specialist settings, however, what clients want from treatment and what they use it for can be quite diverse.[1] On a 17-item questionnaire regarding "What I want from treatment,"[2] clients seeking help from an alcohol dependence treatment program evidenced wide variation in their hopes; furthermore, better treatment outcomes (on drinking measures) at follow-up were associated with the extent to which they reported (at the end of treatment) that they had received those services which they had indicated, at intake, that they wanted. Said more simply: When people get what they want from treatment, they are more likely to show positive change.

Although much discussion is focused on clients' change goals for themselves, it is also the case that people want and ask for particular things from health professionals. A common frustration of physicians is patients who come asking for or demanding certain medical services that the doctor does not regard as warranted: the drug-seeking patient who wants analgesics or sleeping medication, or the mother who is convinced that her sick child needs antibiotics. It is thus appropriate to ask clients not only what they want but, more specifically, "What do you want from me?"

Aspirations of the Counselor: Compassion, Opinion, and Investment

Clients are not the only people with aspirations. Start with the prototypic case for which motivational interviewing was designed. The client stands at a crossroads, looking down at least two different paths and ambivalent about which to take. We will consider here some different kinds of aspirations that a counselor might have regarding a client.

To say that the counselor in a given case is indifferent to which path the client chooses could have at least three different meanings. First, it could mean that the counselor simply has no compassion for the client and doesn't care about the outcome. The counselor might anticipate very different outcomes, depending on which path is taken, but be uninterested in what the specific client chooses to do. We will assume for purposes of discussion that this is not the meaning, and we will take it for granted that the counselor is genuinely interested in the client's welfare. If a counselor comes to the place, through burnout or otherwise, where this kind of indifference is present and counseling becomes a rote or intellectual exercise, it is time to find another line of work.

Second, it might mean that the counselor is compassionate and has the client's best interests at heart but really has no opinion as to which would be the better course for the client to take. In this case—which is called equipoise in Chapter 7—the counselor has no professional advice to give. From the counselor's perspective, the two paths appear likely to lead to similar outcomes for the client. The counselor may still be helpful to the person in the process of making the choice, as illustrated in the description of nondirective motivational interviewing at the end of Chapter 7.

Third, it might mean that the counselor has no particular investment, no vested interest, in the person's choice of paths. The outcomes for the counselor are similar, no matter which path the client chooses. The counselor may be of the opinion that very different outcomes will result for the client from choosing one path versus another and may compassionately wish the best outcomes for the client but be disinterested from the perspective of any personal loss or gain.

For purposes of the present discussion, we refer to these three forms of interest as compassion, opinion, and investment. Any one of them can be present without the others.

Compassion is loving, selfless concern for the person's welfare. A compassionate person has the other's best interests at heart. It is what Erich Fromm described in his classic, *The Art of Loving*.[3]

Opinion is a judgment as to which choice serves the client's best interests. The judgment is, one hopes, well-informed and professional, although opinions about the relative merits of choices can have many origins. Clients often ask for a professional opinion and may even seek a second opinion. The question here is: What does the counselor anticipate that the outcomes would be for the client in resolving the ambivalence in one direction versus another?

Investment involves differential gain or loss to the counselor, depending on which choice the client makes. The interest may be material. Salespeople, for example, are invested in outcome because they gain or lose a sale (and associated profit), depending on whether a customer decides to buy. A recruiter for the armed forces can advise potential recruits on the advantages of enlisting but also has a tangible interest in their decision in that the recruiter's job performance evaluation is based in part on the rate of enlistment. An intake worker in a for-profit treatment program is likely to have a similarly vested interest in persuading potential clients to enter treatment.

For others, the investment is more symbolic. A counselor who is recovering from the same problem being presented by a client may overidentify with the person (particularly early in the counselor's recovery process) and zealously promote particular choices. Professionals who equate client outcomes with their personal worth and competence are likely to be overinvested in choices that their clients make. By virtue of deeply held values, there may be particular outcomes that counselors hope for when working in planned parenthood centers, marital and domestic abuse counseling centers, or prenatal care clinics that serve women who are using alcohol and other drugs.

Investment can also arise by virtue of relationship. Family members are not disinterested parties; a client's choices and outcomes may affect them directly in many ways. Psychotherapists ordinarily avoid the entanglements of treating people with whom they have some other personal or professional relationship.

We find these three types of counselor interest in client outcomes—compassion, opinion, and investment—to be quite helpful in sorting out some of the ethical dilemmas that one encounters in relation to motivational interviewing. These dilemmas are by no means unique to motivational interviewing; they are important for any helping professional to ponder.

Meeting of Aspirations

Needless to say, clients' and counselors' aspirations do not always match. Consonance is greatest when both are working toward the same goals. When aspirations are dissonant, however, there arises the question of how to set goals and agenda for counseling.

It is here that ethical principles of benevolence and autonomy can come into conflict. Most counselors believe in the client's right to make choices and to at least influence, if not set, the goals of counseling. What a client initially wants from the counselor and counseling, however, may be discrepant with the counselor's opinion as to what is in the best interests of the client. A few examples will suffice:

A doctor is concerned about a patient's high blood pressure and wants to prescribe medication; the patient does not want to take medication and prefers to try managing blood pressure with diet and exercise.

A couple seek counseling for marital conflict. The counselor's personal faith is inconsistent with divorce, and he also places strong value on marital fidelity. One partner privately confides an ongoing extramarital affair and a desire to continue it while seeing whether marital therapy "works out." It is the counselor's opinion that this is not in the best interest of either partner or their relationship.

A person convicted of driving while intoxicated (DWI) is referred to treatment and wants to pursue a goal of controlled drinking; the counselor believes, given the severity of alcohol dependence, that this goal is not only unrealistic but dangerous for the client, and wishes for the client to abstain totally from alcohol.

A client's aspirations can conflict not only with the counselor's professional opinion as to what is in the client's best interest, but also with issues of counselor investment. This is apparent in the last two scenarios above. The DWI counselor, for example, may not only believe that abstinence is in the client's best interest but may be concerned about the program's legal liability if the client were to pursue a controlled drinking goal and then injure or kill someone in a subsequent DWI incident. Here are a few other examples of conflict between client aspirations and counselor investment:

A woman who seeks consultation about hormone replacement therapy turns out to be more eager to discuss her marital problems. The nurse doesn't want to get involved in marital counseling and needs to get on with this consultation to attend to the queue of other patients in the waiting room.

A counselor in private practice has a low caseload at present, wants more clients, and is interviewing a person who needs to be treated for obsessive–compulsive disorder. Although the counselor has had some experience in this area and believes she could provide reasonably competent treatment, she knows a colleague with excellent training and experience specifically in the treatment of this disorder. The client, however, expresses reluctance to be referred once again to another professional and says he likes this counselor.

A patient is concerned about persistent pain and wants the doctor to order a series of expensive tests to rule out what are possible but somewhat unlikely disorders. The doctor is employed by a managed care organization in which physicians receive salary bonuses for maintaining low utilization of expensive tests.

The last two examples also illustrate a still more complex issue in which the counselor's personal investment may directly conflict not only with the client's wishes but also with the counselor's own sense of what is in the best interest of the client.

Power and Its Use

Now let us add one more complexity, before we examine how motivational interviewing interacts with these ethical dilemmas. There is variability, from one counseling context to another, in the degree of power that the counselor holds to influence client behavior and outcomes. At the low extreme, a counselor has just met the client and is offering only consultation with regard to the client's problems. There is always a power differential in counseling, of course, and the counselor will presumably be able to exert some influence over the client's behavior; that is assumed in the role. Nevertheless, the complications of power do not exceed those inherent in all counseling. At the other extreme, consider a counselor who works with offenders on parole and probation and who has the power at any time to revoke that status and order incarceration.

The presence of special influence in the counseling relationship further complicates the overall ethical picture. The counselor now may have not only an opinion as to what is best for the client, and a personal stake in the client's choices and outcomes, but also coercive power to act on such opinion and investment. A counselor who holds such power must further choose whether to use it to persuade the client to move in a desired direction.

ETHICAL COMPLEXITY AND MOTIVATIONAL INTERVIEWING

How do these complexities interact with the particular nature of motivational interviewing? If our conception of the method is correct, it has the potential, within limits, to influence a person's willingness, confidence, and readiness to change in one way or another. Thus one concern is raised by the potential that the method can be effective in altering motivation and volition, as well as related behavior. This is not of particular concern when the client's aspirations are consonant with those of the counselor. When there is dissonance between counselor and client aspirations, however, ethical consideration should be given to any methods that are effective in changing client aspirations to more closely match those of the counselor. This issue is further complicated when the counselor's "client" (the one desiring change) is not the person who is seated in the consultation room but is another party—such as a court system, parent, or school—asking for change in the person.

When a client's aspirations differ from those of the counselor, it is also the case that interventions designed to alter motivation for change are done without the person's permission, at least to some extent. One can point to contextual factors that may mitigate this concern somewhat. A person voluntarily seeking counseling at an addiction treatment program may profess no desire to change his or her use of drug A (although motivation might be high to stop using drug B), but will not be surprised that a counselor in this context may seek to enhance the person's motivation to stop drug A as well. Those being seen at a religiously based counseling service may expect, or even desire, that the counselor advocates values that conflict with their current behavior and aspirations. Nevertheless, one cannot entirely dodge the point that in seeking to alter what it is that a person desires, one is in some sense doing so without the person's direct assent or request.

This issue of assent is related to a further concern, which is that a method like motivational interviewing may succeed in altering what someone desires without the person being aware of the process and how it works. Subliminal advertising in movie theaters is banned on this basis, although advertising more generally is designed to enhance motivation without needing the person's direct consent or awareness of the underlying psychological processes.

In sum, three potential ethical concerns about motivational interventions are (1) that they may work, (2) that they may work without the person's direct assent, and (3) that they may work without the person's awareness.[4] We regard these as legitimate issues for ethical consideration, and in the following section we offer some guidelines for the use of motivational interviewing, in particular, in relation to these complexities.

Before moving on to these guidelines, however, some discussion of the issue of coerciveness in motivational interviewing is needed. This is related to the question implied by the ability of motivational interviewing within limits to alter one's being ready, willing, and able to act in a particular way. What are those limits? For example, can a client be caused, through motivational interviewing, to behave in a manner directly contradictory to the person's intrinsic core values? We believe that the answer to this question is no, in part because of our understanding of how the method works. To the extent that we are correct in asserting that developing internal discrepancy is a key process in motivational interviewing, the question arises: Discrepancy with what? The answer must be the person's own goals and values. *We believe that unless a current "problem" behavior is in conflict with something that the person values more highly, there is no basis for motivational interviewing to work.* The focus is on intrinsic motivation for change. It is irrelevant whether the client's behavior is discrepant with someone else's values, unless, of course, it is someone highly regarded and valued by the client, in which case intrinsic value discrepancy is again operating. That being the case, motivational interviewing will not induce behavior change unless the client perceives that such change serves a higher intrinsic value and is thereby in his or her own best interest.

This protective condition of consistency with intrinsic values is not present for coercive methods. People can sometimes be coerced to behave in ways that violate values they hold dear. This is one intention behind torture and brainwashing, and it is also why institutional review boards exist to protect research participants from coercive conditions such as enticingly high payment to be exposed to risk. Within the realm of counseling, a method known as "constructive coercion" uses the contingent power of an employer to motivate employees into treatment they might otherwise refuse.[5] "The intervention" propounded by the Johnson Institute[6] typically involves a planned and rehearsed surprise group confrontation by family members (and sometimes others such as friends or employers) of a person perceived to have a problem (usually with alcohol or other drugs). In addition to expressing compassionate concern, members of the group may also announce negative consequences that will ensue if the person does not comply with the group's aspiration, which is often for the person to enter a private treatment program. Such interventions are clearly undertaken without the person's knowledge or desire, with the ethical principle of benevolence being given greater importance than autonomy, at least temporarily.

It is our assertion that motivational interviewing, by virtue of its reliance on discrepancy with intrinsic values, cannot work in violation of a person's autonomy. It may cause a person to want to do something, but for the reason that the anticipated change is ultimately consistent with important intrinsic goals and values. In this way, it differs from coercive strategies, which are explicitly designed to override what a person wants.

Within this context, we can now address the ethical relationship between motivational interviewing and aspirations of the counselor and client. From the preceding discussion we identify three conditions under which the use of motivational interviewing warrants special care. The more combinations of these complicating conditions that are present in a given case, the more caution is required, and under certain conditions we believe that the use of motivational interviewing is ethically inappropriate. We specifically do not limit this discussion to the counselor–client relationship, because applications of motivational interviewing are being considered in other contexts. Consequently in this discourse we refer only to the "interviewer" and the "person," wherein the interviewer might be a counselor, salesperson, physician, police officer, parent, employer, or other interested party. The three ethical complexities are as follows:

1. When the person's aspirations are dissonant with the interviewer's opinion as to what is in the person's best interest
2. When the interviewer has a personal investment in which direction the person takes
3. When the nature of the relationship includes coercive power of the interviewer to influence the direction the person takes

Dissonance of aspirations is not uncommon in motivational interviewing. Although things are simplest when aspirations are consonant, there are many circumstances in which motivational interviewing is ethically appropriate, despite initially dissonant aspirations. The ethical principle of benevolence is preeminent here, but it does rely on the assumption that there is independent objective value in the interviewer's judgment as to what is in the person's best interest.

Things become considerably more cloudy when the interviewer has a personal stake in what the person does. Under this condition, the independent objective value of the interviewer's opinion begins to come into question because of conflict of interest. The greater the interviewer's investment in a particular action or outcome for a specific person, the more serious the concern. A special case occurs when the interviewer's investment is contrary to what is in the person's best interest (as judged by the interviewer's opinion, or by a reasonable observer). This is one case in which we unreservedly advise that motivational interviewing is ethically inappropriate. We do so despite our belief that motivational interviewing does not violate the principle of autonomy. If, for example, either of two alternatives could be judged to be in the person's interest and consistent with the person's values, but one of them serves the interviewer's interest whereas the other does not, we believe it is inappropriate to use motivational interviewing to tip the balance in the direction of a resolution consistent with the interviewer's investment.

Ethical complexities are further increased when the interviewer has power to coerce or enforce contingencies on the person's behavior. Of course, the interviewer can decide not to use such power, but there is reason for ethical concern because the potential for use of such power can itself be coercive when aspirations are dissonant. We therefore assert that motivational interviewing warrants particular caution when the interviewer holds special influence (beyond an ordinary professional relationship) over the person's behavior and outcomes. We address those precautions in the guidelines and case examples that follow.

Finally, when both coercive power and personal investment are present, we regard the use of motivational interviewing to be inappropriate. Examples include an employer interviewing a prospective employee and a detective interviewing a suspect (although in both of these situations, good reflective listening skills alone can be very appropriately used).

We summarize these points in Box 12.1, illustrating from left to right the increasing degrees of ethical complexity and contraindication to the use of motivational interviewing. There are, of course, other combinations than those shown.

SOME GUIDELINES FOR ETHICAL PRACTICE

We conclude by offering a few guidelines that follow from the preceding discussion. The broader guidelines of ethical professional practice also apply, of course, and when you feel an ethical itch, pay attention to it and explore it. (If you don't feel any ethical itches when doing motivational interviewing, worry!) We have focused in these guidelines on issues that are particularly salient in motivational interviewing. With each, we also offer what we hope are illustrative case examples. Although we think primarily of the counselor–client context in offering these guidelines, they do apply to the use of this clinical method more generally.

Guideline 1: When you sense dissonance in the relationship or an area of ethical discomfort, clarify the person's aspirations and your own.

Example 1. A young woman came to see me (Rollnick), distressed by panic attacks that were leaving her more and more fearful and restricted. Motivational commitment is a significant issue in treating panic attacks and ago-

BOX 12.1. Ethical Complexity and Motivational Interviewing

Ethical complexity	Very low						Very high
Do you have a clear opinion as to which direction is in the person's best interest?	No	Yes	Yes	Yes	Yes	Yes	Yes
Are your aspirations (both opinion and investment) consonant with the person's aspirations?	NA	Yes	No	No	No	No	No
Do you have a personal investment in which direction the person takes?	No	No	No	No	Yes	Yes	Yes
Is your personal investment in conflict with what is in the person's best interest?	NA	NA	NA	NA	No	Yes	Yes
Do you have power to influence which direction the person takes?	No	No	No	Yes	No	No	Yes
Is motivational interviewing appropriate?	Yes	Yes	With care	With care	With care	No	No

Note. Grey boxes denote, within rows, conditions of greater ethical complexity; black boxes denote, within columns, combinations of conditions under which the authors regard the use of motivational interviewing to be ethically questionable.

raphobia, and I have had much experience and some encouraging success in this area. We began behavioral treatment of the panic attacks right away and also developed a list of agenda items that included smoking cessation and shyness, both of which turned out to be tied in with her panic attacks. Each session, she seemed to have a new concern to discuss. In one she revealed that she suffered from anorexia and that she used smoking to curb her appetite. During the next session she described being attracted to a woman coworker and wanted to explore sexual identity issues. That issue was gone the following week, and we discussed her shyness around men. I felt growing discomfort that we were wandering around in the desert, and that I wouldn't be of much help to her unless we focused on her main concern, but what was it? Clearly she enjoyed coming to see me and might be generating new concerns in order to continue. My own aspiration was still to help her with the panic attacks, because she had presented that as a quite disabling concern, but her own goals for counseling had become unclear to me.

I decided to express my dilemma directly. "I'm a bit confused here," I said. "I had the impression that you were particularly concerned about your panic attacks, with which I would be glad to help you, but is that what you want? I feel like we're losing the thread, so I need to understand what it is that you want from counseling now." We agreed, through a process of motivational interviewing and agenda setting, to focus on two issues of particular concern to her, one of which was her panic attacks. We set specific goals, and over the next few sessions she made excellent progress in managing her fear of fear, so that her panic attacks subsided.

Guideline 2: When your opinion as to what is in the person's best interests is dissonant with what the person wants, reconsider and negotiate your agenda, making clear your own concerns and aspirations for the person.

Example 2a. A middle-aged woman came to see me (Rollnick) with concerns about problematic gambling. She had been spending large amounts of time in gambling establishments and losing substantial sums of money. Her request was to be given strategies for managing her gambling problem. When I asked her, as a simple device, for an importance rating, she said 9, and her confidence rating was 3, quite consistent with her request for behavior change strategies. Yet I felt an itch; something bothered me, and it was my hunch that the solution to her problem lay not in teaching her skills to manage her gambling but in exploring the motivation for her gambling.

Consequently I asked her permission to discuss how we would spend our time, and I explained my hunch. I agreed to spend time toward the end of our first session giving her some concrete behavioral strategies, and I hoped she would be willing to spend some time exploring the reasons for her gambling. She agreed.

"So why are you at a 9 on the importance scale, and not a 2?" I asked. "My husband," she said; "he's threatened to leave me because of my gambling." It turned out that 9 was her husband's rating of importance, and her own interest in stopping gambling was at 2. It emerged that this woman, who had been the manager of a large store, was terribly bored with her life as a housewife, and gambling filled her time and eased her boredom and loneliness. "So," I summarized halfway through our session, "your husband has threatened to divorce you because of your gambling. Your life feels quite empty to you, and you're bored silly with it. You feel lonely, and going to the casino helps to fill your time. What you'd like from me is to give you some self-management strategies to control your gambling." She burst into tears.

We spent the rest of that session and the next discussing ways in which she could have more meaning and activity in her life, to address her boredom and loneliness directly rather than through gambling. By the second session, she was unconcerned about changing her gambling, saying that it would sort itself out, and she thanked me for helping her. "I've got what I need," she said. I set up a 6-month follow-up visit with her, at which time she had implemented a number of important changes in her life, and the gambling problem had resolved.

Example 2b. He was a cartoonist who had to come up with a new idea every day for his newspaper strip. He had used various forms of meditation to stimulate his creativity, but lately he had been troubled during meditation by intrusive and distressing visual images of the face of a man with whom he had had significant conflict. Whereas he normally could clear his mind and allow creative ideas to arise, he found himself unable to stop this intrusive image, and it was seriously hindering his work. "I think hypnosis might help me," he said.

Although I (Miller) had been trained in clinical hypnosis, I was uncomfortable with his idea because the outcome literature on obsessive–intrusive thoughts showed little efficacy for hypnosis and pointed instead toward cognitive–behavioral management methods. I explained this to him, and he agreed to try what I had in mind. Several sessions later, the intrusion problem was still getting worse, despite his faithful practice of the skills I had been teaching him. So we renegotiated, and I agreed to try hypnosis with him in that session.

I hypnotized him just once. The obsessive imagery vanished, and he was not troubled by it again.

It taught me something about listening to what clients want.

Guideline 3: *The greater your personal investment in a particular client outcome, the more inappropriate it is to use the method of motivational interviewing. It is clearly inappropriate when your personal investment may be dissonant with what is in the client's best interests.*

Example 3a. I (Miller) was sitting in on a transcontinental flight, a situation in which I ordinarily keep to myself and certainly don't talk to the person next to me about what I do for a living. This woman was particularly persistent, however, and I learned that her job was to sell private jet aircraft to executives, most of whom didn't really need them. She explained that the key is to convince them that a private jet offers much greater prestige and convenience than using commercial flights, and that owning one was therefore in their best interests. I became engaged, and asked her in some detail about her methods for motivating and closing sales. In the course of our conversation, some of my own interests emerged, and I explained a few parallels between the methods she was describing and the approach I was using to help people decide to make changes in their health behavior. Then she became engaged and wanted to know in great detail all about motivational interviewing. Suddenly I was feeling not just ethical itches but smoke alarms, and I politely shut myself up in my laptop. I also did not purchase an aircraft.

Example 3b. We (Miller) were running a bit behind in recruitment into a clinical trial. Patients who might benefit from the treatments we were testing were declining to participate for a variety of reasons. "How about if we try motivational interviewing?" someone suggested. While one might have argued that participating in this particular clinical trial was in the patients' best interest (all experimental groups included an active treatment that could reasonably be expected to yield benefit), there is no way to untangle this judgment from the investigator's clear investment in recruitment into the study. We therefore regard it as unethical to use motivational interviewing to enhance consent to participate in research.

Example 3c. An attorney contacted me (Rollnick), representing a woman whose leg had been paralyzed in an automobile accident. Could I, as a psychologist, speak to her about how this injury had affected her life? Specifically, the attorney asked me to persuade her, via motivational interviewing, that some ambiguous areas in her life had actually been impaired by the accidental injury (for example, not being employed, not having a second child), even though the woman herself currently saw no relationship between these facts and her injury. The outcome would affect the amount of damages to be requested in a civil lawsuit against the other driver. In this case, the strong investment in a particular outcome was not my own, but her attorney's, who stood to benefit financially from a larger award, an investment that, in my opinion, did not necessarily serve the woman's best interests. I refused.

Guideline 4: *The more your role includes coercive power to influence the person's behavior and outcomes, the more caution is warranted in the use of motivational interviewing. When coercive power is combined with a personal investment in the person's behavior and outcomes, the use of motivational interviewing is inappropriate.*

Example 4a. An attorney contacted me (Rollnick) to ask how she could learn motivational interviewing to help her clients resolve ambivalence around issues on which she was representing them. Often, she indicated, it was not a particular decision that was needed, as much as a clear resolution so that legal matters could proceed. "Often my clients go back and forth on important issues about which they feel ambivalent, and use up large amounts of my time for which I have to bill them, just because they're not clear what they want. If I could help them decide what they want, it would benefit us all." We trained her, with the additional advice that it would be inappropriate for her to use this method in interviewing clients of opposing counsel, where her investment would typically be contrary to the interviewee's interests.

Example 4b. During a workshop on motivational interviewing that we (Miller) offered for probation officers, there was much discussion of how this method would mesh with the legal power they held over their clients. Our advice was to be straightforward about their own aspirations for clients, and specifically to explain the purpose of this type of counseling. For example:

"I have two different roles here, and it is sometimes tricky for me to put them together. One of them is as a representative of the court, to ensure that you keep the conditions of probation that the judge set for you, and I have to honor that role. The other is to be your counselor, to help you make changes in your life that we agree would be beneficial. There are also likely to be some areas we'll discover, where I am hoping to see a change that you're not sure you want to make. What I hope is that by talking together here every week, we can resolve some of those differences and are able to find areas of change we can agree on. I'm sure I'll be asking you to consider some changes that right now don't sound very good to you, and that's normal. We'll keep exploring those issues during our time together, and see if we can come to some agreement. How does that sound to you?"

We offer one more example of a very common problem to which motivational interviewing has been applied: medication compliance. While we don't resonate to the power relationship implied in the term "compliance," it is nevertheless a common and important problem. It is a useful example, because changes in investment and power have important ethical implications for the appropriateness of motivational interviewing in addressing this problem.

Example 5a. A man is being treated for newly diagnosed schizophrenia, and the psychiatrist is explaining to him how the prescribed medication works and how important it is to take it regularly. Having conveyed this information, the psychiatrist talks with him, using the style of motivational interviewing, about the advantages and disadvantages of taking the medication as prescribed.
Our opinion: The application is entirely appropriate.

Example 5b. The same man has been seen in crisis units several times, each time shortly after he discontinued taking his medication. Consequently, he receives regular home visits from a community nurse. The nurse has some investment in his medication adherence for several reasons. When he does not take it, she is likely to be called in the middle of the night to deal with crises. She must also do extra paperwork and reporting, and she must involve several other health professionals if he discontinues taking his medicine. If he is rehospitalized, it also reflects badly on her performance. Nevertheless, her investment is judged to be consistent with the best interests of the patient, despite his own ambivalence, and she does not have any significant coercive power over the patient.
Our opinion: It is appropriate for her to use motivational interviewing to encourage the patient to take his medication regularly.

Example 5c. The same man has been admitted involuntarily to a forensic unit in the hospital after a psychotic episode during which he committed several minor crimes and jeopardized his own life in a confrontation with police. All beds in the unit are full, and there is a substantial waiting list, with pressure from the courts to admit those who are waiting. He has been in the unit for 3 weeks and is stabilized as an inpatient. The principal obstacle to discharge is his continuing reluctance to take his medication. A social worker trained in motivational interviewing is asked by the physician in charge of the unit to persuade him to agree to take his medicine, so that he can be discharged to make room for another patient.

Our opinion: We regard this to be an unethical application of motivational interviewing because of the simultaneous presence of decisional power and substantial investment in a particular outcome. It is irrelevant whether the staff's investment in an empty bed is judged to be consistent or inconsistent with the patient's best interests, because the simultaneous presence of power and investment is itself sufficient ethical contraindication for the use of motivational interviewing.

NOTES

1. Yates (1984).
2. Brown and Miller (1993); Miller (1999a).
3. Fromm (1956).
4. For a more detailed discussion of these three issues in motivational interviewing, see Miller (1994).
5. Smart (1974); Trice and Beyer (1983).
6. Johnson (1986).

PART III

Learning Motivational Interviewing

CHAPTER 13

Reflections on Learning

There is no such thing as teaching; there is only learning.
—MONTY ROBERTS

How do people learn the interpersonal style of motivational interviewing? What makes a counselor more effective in enhancing people's motivation for change? Are skillful motivational interviewers born or made? What experiences are most helpful in learning motivational interviewing?

These are questions that both fascinate and concern us. Over the years, as interest in motivational interviewing has grown, the focus of our own time and effort has shifted—first from treating clients to teaching health professionals and conducting research about the method, and then to training trainers and studying how best to help people learn motivational interviewing.

In this chapter we offer some reflections on the process of learning motivational interviewing, in hopes that these will be useful to readers who want to strengthen their own counseling skills in this area. In the first edition, this chapter presented a series of exercises for teaching motivational interviewing. This time we have shifted our focus from teaching to learning, believing that fundamentally they are different terms for the same process. In some languages, in fact, "to teach" and "to learn" are the same verb. We realize in retrospect that the life of Carl Rogers reflects a similar transition, from a focus on technique and training to an exploration of the phenomenological processes of learning and change.

To begin, we point out that neither of us learned motivational interviewing through traditional training. There were no books, no training videotapes, no workshops or courses or supervisors to show us how to do it. No one, in fact, was doing it, at least not formally (if, indeed, one ever does "formal" motivational interviewing). Within our chosen specialty field, addictive behaviors, treatment was by and large rather confrontational. The doctor or counselor was the acknowledged expert, whose task it was to educate, persuade, cajole, confront, or coerce clients into giving up their favorite habits. There was much emphasis on conditioning, medicating, punishing, training, and humiliating clients into compliance with a program's goals. There had been few studies of client-centered counseling, an approach largely dismissed as ineffective in treating addictions.

Our clients were our teachers, and our students were our trainers. Blissfully ignorant of then-prevalent specialist methods for treating addictions, we started out talking with people who had addiction problems much as we would with any other client. We asked them open questions, curious to learn how their experience had led them into such seemingly self-destructive patterns. We were interested in what they wanted in life, what they valued, what was important and less important to them. We listened a lot, and found the process stimulating, enjoyable, fascinating, often moving. We perceived that these were interesting and resourceful people who had chosen one path but could also choose others. We were puzzled, then, how they had come to make the choices they had made, how they understood their current situation, and where they saw their lives going. Over time, our clients taught us how to help them and others like them.

Now we receive regular requests to come teach others how to do motivational interviewing, so many that we could not begin to respond, and so we started in 1993 to train trainers. We much enjoy training others, but there has always been something disquieting about the process. Eventually we realized what was bothering us: a traditional training format is analogous to the very same expert model that we seek to avoid in our counseling. An expert provides the answers to relatively passive recipients, often without even understanding the questions that brought people to training in the first place. That is why Part III of this book now emphasizes learning instead of teaching.

CLIENTS AS TEACHERS

A first point, then, is that the very same teachers from whom we learned motivational interviewing are also available to you. One of the reasons it is possible to keep on learning and improving one's skills in motivational interviewing is that immediate expert feedback is continuously available. It is available from those you serve.

Accurate feedback is what is needed to acquire and increase any kind of skill. Accuracy in archery is continually shaped by seeing how close arrows fall to the target. It is difficult to learn to play golf in the dark. The reason answers are in the back of math exercise workbooks is so that in practicing one can have immediate corrective feedback about the accuracy of problem solving.

The same information is available to you in learning motivational interviewing. Once you learn what to watch for in your clients, you have an excellent source of immediate corrective feedback. The reason for this is that what people say during motivational interviewing is a reasonably good predictor of behavior change. The goal is to reinforce change talk and decrease resistance, both of which involve increased commitment to change. The more this happens—the more the client's level of commitment language increases during an interview—the greater the chances that behavior change will occur. Change talk is a beacon toward which to steer. Resistance is a signal that you may be veering off course a bit.

We first noticed this in regard to learning reflective listening, the foundational skill upon which motivational interviewing develops. When the counselor offers an effective reflective listening statement, the person keeps talking, even when the counselor's guess about meaning was wrong. When the counselor instead offers a roadblock response, the person stops, or backs up, or heads off in a different direction. The person's response thus provides immediate feedback about one's listening skills.

Furthermore, client responses also give immediate information about the accuracy of reflection. First of all, each reflection tends to be answered with a direct or implicit "Yes" or "No" from the person. That is, the person tells you whether or not you got it right. There is no penalty for missing here. If it was a good but not accurate reflection, the person keeps talking and corrects the bits you missed. Once you realize that clients are your teachers, and you attend to their responses as skill-relevant feedback, every person offers an opportunity to further shape and refine your reflective listening skills.

The same is true of motivational interviewing more generally. Once you learn to differentiate the signals of change talk and resistance statements from the background of client speech, you have the cues you need both to work more effectively with each person and to learn from each person (see Chapter 5). Regardless of the level of readiness at which a person begins a session, you know you're on the right track when your manner enhances client commitment language (increased change talk and decreased resistance). The ultimate criterion, of course, is whether client behavior changes, but clinicians seldom get reliable feedback of long-term behavior change. Furthermore, such feedback is too delayed and nonspecific to be very useful in shaping more effective practice. Because it is linked to behavioral outcomes, the minute-to-minute immediate feedback of client responses during sessions is a more useful guide, and it is continually available at no additional cost.

USING YOUR DISSONANCE DETECTOR

In practicing motivational interviewing, it is helpful to pay attention not only to your client's reactions but also to your own. The consonance–dissonance dimension is palpable. As the counseling process begins to slide into dissonance, both client and counselor can sense it. It may not be consciously registered as dissonance in the relationship, but there is an inner experience you can learn to use as a marker. For some counselors it is an "uh oh" thought. For others it is more a physical or emotional sensation. Attend to your own internal responses to dissonance and learn to notice them as markers.

A further step in self-consciousness is to become aware of how you react, in overt behavior, when you sense dissonance. Some practitioners abruptly change the subject, steering away from conflictual material. We find this to be particularly true with clinicians who work in settings (such as managed health care) where time for consultation is short and needs to be task-focused. In such settings, dissonance can signal a potential time-consuming interaction, from which busy practitioners may simply veer away. There are, of course, other reasons for conflict avoidance, as well.

Other counselors respond differently. American addiction counselors, for example, used to be trained to regard the signals of dissonance as manifestations of robust client defense mechanisms that were pathognomonic of the disease of addiction. The response advocated in many training programs was aggressive confrontation to "break down the client's defenses" and "overcome denial." For counselors with this mental set, client resistance behavior is likely to elicit offensive tactics that are intended to counteract denial. From the perspective offered in this volume, of course, this is precisely backward: the counselor is strongly defending the "good" side of the client's ambivalence, which elicits his or her further resistance behavior and decreases the likelihood of change.

Whatever your reflexive response to dissonance, it is wise to monitor your dissonance detector and consciously choose how you respond. Chapter 9 offers a menu of responses that are designed to diminish dissonance and client resistance.

OTHER AIDS TO LEARNING

Several other sources of practice feedback have been helpful to us in learning and refining our motivational interviewing skills. There is really no substitute for listening to audiotapes or viewing videotapes of practice. It is much easier to perceive what is happening on tape (be it one's own or another's session) than in the midst of doing motivational interviewing. It is also possible, with proper consent, to review tapes with colleagues and discuss the dynamics observed. This further affords the opportunity, unavailable in real time, to stop the tape, rewind, and review what has happened.

It can also be quite instructive to ask clients for their own perspectives on what is happening. One recent learning experience came from smokers who volunteered to help in developing new ideas to be used in training doctors.[1] They were told that the goal was not to give them counseling but to experiment with different ways of talking to them and to learn how they responded. They were interviewed using a one-way mirror and a video camera. The practitioners swapped places whenever necessary, trying out new and old ideas, and then discussing with the smokers afterward what they found useful and why. Our learning took place on two levels. We discovered from the smokers how to ask simple questions that elicited change statements in brief consultations. At a deeper level, we advanced our understanding of the consultation process as a direct result of these encounters. We were using a simple readiness ruler on paper, and we wondered why so many were placing themselves on the central "unsure" part of the line. To find out, we asked them: "Why here (pointing to the center of the line) and not there (the 'not ready' end of the line)?" Besides finding that this question elicited change talk, we were led to the twin concepts of importance and confidence as critical ingredients of readiness for change. These learning experiences subsequently formed the heart of a text on behavior change counseling.[2]

We have also developed various systems for coding motivational interviewing session tapes, allowing for an even finer-grained analysis. A group of motivational interviewing colleagues, for example, developed a detailed coding system to study the extent to which counselors acquire motivational interviewing skillfulness over the course of training. The system involves three separate analyses.[3] The first is a set of global practice ratings of counselor style, client response, and the quality of interaction. The second and most demanding analysis requires the classification of each counselor response (e.g., open question, closed question, reflection, advice, giving information) and client utterance (e.g., change talk, resistance) using a system of mutually exclusive behavior categories. The third pass simply records client and counselor talk time and provides the percentage of talk time occupied by each. We had anticipated that the coding of tapes with this Motivational Interviewing Skill Code (MISC) system would be rather tedious, but, in fact, highly experienced motivational interviewing clinicians and less experienced coders alike found it to be quite engaging and fascinating. It provides an inside analysis of the dynamics of motivational interviewing in a way that simply listening to sessions cannot.

We coded sessions not only for trainees before and after a training workshop but also for senior clinicians who were highly experienced in motivational interviewing. This gave us an idea of the amount of change to expect from a workshop alone (an issue discussed in Chapter 14), as well as some ideal norms to shoot for in training, based on model sessions. Without going into the details of coding, we arrived at the following general practice guidelines:

- Talk less than your client does.
- Offer two to three reflections for every question that you ask.
- Ask twice as many open questions as closed questions.
- When you listen empathically, more than half of the reflections you offer should be deeper, more complex reflections (paraphrase) rather than simpler repetition or rephrasing of what the client offered.

SUMMARY

One substantial advantage in learning motivational interviewing is the extent to which clients provide ongoing and immediate corrective feedback once the essential perspectives and basic skills have been established. After you know what to look for from clients, they become your teachers. Correctly applied methods for eliciting change talk will elicit change talk. Missteps elicit and increase resistance. Well-done reflective listening results in the person continuing to explore openly; roadblocks divert the process of self-exploration. Most reflective listening statements lead to immediate feedback on the correctness of the reflection along with further elaboration, which over time further hones the accuracy of your reflections. A well-timed transition into Phase 2 leads to a commitment to change; a premature press for commitment yields back-pedaling.

The overall point is to pay attention to your clients, with eyes and ears open to the fact that what they say (and how they say it) is not simply arising from within them but is in large measure a dynamic response to your own counseling behavior. Our own clients have been our guides, and it is from them that we learned motivational interviewing. There are no better teachers.

NOTES

1. Rollnick, Butler, and Stott (1997).
2. Rollnick, Mason, and Butler (1999).
3. Miller and Mount (2001).

CHAPTER 14

Facilitating Learning

> Learning is nothing but discovery that something is possible. To
> teach means to show a person that something is possible.
> —FRITZ PERLS, *Gestalt Therapy Verbatim*

To facilitate *in others* the kind of quality learning experiences that are described in Chapter 13 is the subject of this chapter. The scenario is a familiar
one to both recipients and facilitators of training: a group of expectant people
gather, and the learning begins! Yet afterward, in everyday practice, is anything done differently? Often, perhaps, very little really changes.

At other times, though, one hears a report from a counselor like this:
"Things seem different in my day to day work. I do less talking, and it's really
satisfying to see reflective listening working. The whole business seems quieter
and less hurried, yet we make good progress, and the client talks away about
changes and challenges. This is definitely improving my practice."

This chapter is for those who want to facilitate the learning of motivational interviewing by others. It centers on the following question: How do
people learn motivational interviewing when they are given a structured opportunity to do so? If *we* learned it by gradual transformation, as we suspect
most others do as well, how can this learning be harnessed and encouraged in
others? This chapter does not identify recommended content of a course,
workshop, or program but addresses the broader issues and principles that
have a critical effect on how learning experiences can be structured. A first
step is to view this not as something acquired at an event like a workshop but
as an ongoing process, in which counselors might struggle over a period of

months or years, using different learning opportunities to reflect about, reformulate, and refine their clinical practice.

Motivational interviewing involves the integration of a complex set of clinical skills and poses special challenges for facilitators and supervisors. It is not an approach that can be acquired merely by reading, listening to lectures, or watching demonstration videotapes—or, indeed, by attending a single workshop. For novices, it requires learning a set of integrated therapeutic skills and the development of judgment about when and how to use them. For experienced clinicians, it may also involve unlearning familiar styles and habits in dealing with clients.

SOME GUIDING PRINCIPLES

Teaching motivational interviewing is like doing it. When facilitation is going well, it often has to do with the facilitator's attitude and spirit—a respect for and curiosity about the learning needs and perspectives of others. Together, facilitator and learners become engaged in a process that has a collaborative, exploratory feeling.

The principles outlined in this chapter are merely some that we have learned in the course of everyday practice in helping others learn motivational interviewing. If things are not going quite right in facilitation, it is tempting to blame the learners for being resistant or to search for some teaching technique to fix the problem, but we have learned instead to check on whether we might be violating the principles of facilitation that we now describe.

Practice What You Preach

Certainly, it is common sense that to facilitate the learning of motivational interviewing in others, you ought to have a high level of skillfulness in the style yourself. This means having had substantial experience in applying motivational interviewing with a range of clients, preferably with supervision and feedback. The facilitator should be ready, willing, and able, when asked, to sit down and skillfully show how it's done.

The very same qualities that make an effective motivational counselor are also helpful in facilitating learning in others. This requires respect for individual differences, tolerance for disagreement and ambivalence, patience with gradual approximations, and a genuine caring for and interest in the people you serve. The facilitator communicates enthusiasm and commitment in teaching this approach but takes no offense at those who disagree and prefer other approaches. Motivational interviewing is not for everyone, and some counselors find that it does not fit their own style and skills. Good facilitation, like good counseling, respects personal choice, with the attitude of "Take what you want and leave the rest." The skills and qualities of motivational interviewing can be demonstrated by the very manner in which you deal with your trainees. There is a certain integrity to showing, in your own training manner, the very style you wish to impart.

Listen to the Learners

Learning to listen is a challenge on both sides of the educational process. It is important to listen to the experiences, concerns, and expectations of those you are serving—a guideline that can be hard to follow when you have your workshop all planned out. It can mean, for example, abandoning a carefully worked-out plan midway through a training event, taking on board some constructive criticism and allowing people to have quite a big say about how they would like to proceed.

One good approach that can prevent some painful experiences is for the facilitator to do some listening *in advance* about the specific needs, hopes, and desires of those who are to learn. Groups of learners, like clients, come in many varieties. We have had the pleasure of working with groups who have been studying, practicing, and discussing motivational interviewing and eagerly await a further opportunity to learn. We have also walked into workshops where the participants had been told, "You're going to learn motivational interviewing and do it whether you like it or not." These are quite different starting points. Often there are particular examples and situations that are common to the learners' workplace, and these should be incorporated into the learning process in order to enhance its relevance.

Beware the Expert Trap

Clinicians who wish to "get a feel" for a new topic often attend a one-session or one-day workshop and listen across a crowded room to an expert's presentation of the subject. Few would regard this as an exercise in acquisition of skills. Many nevertheless leave satisfied. They return to their working lives, perhaps thinking "I already do that." If a situation jogs their memory they might try out a new response, or at least think a little differently about some of the surrounding issues. Motivational interviewing, cognitive-behavioral therapy and countless other therapeutic methods have been introduced to people in this way. They learn *about* the method, not how to do it.

Although there can be value in an expert-driven, top-down presentation of key concepts and skills, it is difficult to miss the parallel between exhorting motivation in clients and advising clinicians to consider changes to their everyday routines. Tell them, as the expert, that they need to change and why, and how they should go about it, and the result is reasonably predictable: disengagement, resistance, and lack of enduring change in practice. The art of facilitating learning is to find the right balance between inviting new approaches to familiar problems and drawing personally relevant solutions from trainees. Being told what to do by an expert is no more persuasive and inviting to a clinician than it is to a client.

Avoid the Technical Twitch

There is no greater comfort to an expert than delivering technical expertise. Make it neat, clean, logical, straightforward, step-by-step. The learning of motivational interviewing, however, is not just a technical matter. Counselors need not only to feel *able* to change and develop their competency in a new approach but also feel *willing and ready* to do so—they must feel that it is important and helpful to them and that their concerns about its relevance or realism are understood. Complex ethical, professional, cultural, and clinical issues often arise when learning about motivational interviewing. Responding constructively to such broader concerns can be just as important as focusing on more technical matters. Alternatively, learners will become frustrated if the experience bogs down into contemplation and the method itself is not conveyed. A training program is usually best balanced by a healthy mixture of the two.

Get Close to the Learners' Everyday Experiences

The goal of facilitation is to get close to the heart of the counselors' everyday experience, to have an effect on their repetitive routines and more occasional triumphs and disasters. In this respect, facilitating learning in counselors can be easier than pursuing the same goal with clients. A facilitator can come right alongside and discuss experiences soon after they occur. A window can be opened into the counselor's everyday world, through audiotapes or videotapes. One can structure periods of quiet reflection, observe learners in real-life or simulated encounters, offer suggestions (with permission, of course), encourage rehearsal, and so on. In short, one can enter into the counselor's context. To ignore this tremendous advantage is a bit like teaching people to play tennis or golf while sitting in a classroom. To use it constructively requires a keen eye for learning opportunities.

Adapt to Individual Learning Preferences

People have varied preferences for what and how they learn at any given point in time. This seemingly banal observation can be very difficult to respect when working with a group of learners. The tendency is to provide the same opportunities for all, for purely practical reasons. For example, imagine that one person is very ready to discuss the value of listening, while another would like supervised practice, a third wants to watch you do it, and a fourth is convinced she already knows all this. To ignore these differing aspirations would be unfortunate, yet one often seems obliged to do just this in training.

It is possible, however, particularly if one is working with a cofacilitator, to provide more variety for participants. Those who already feel proficient can be asked to serve as models or coaches in small-group practice. Those who want to observe can be engaged in this role within practice groups. In one corner of the room, a cotrainer may offer a demonstration, while others who prefer to practice do so. We once improvised a number of options for a group of primary care professionals with diverse learning needs, so that they effectively moved in sequence through a series of learning "stations." At one point in time, while two of them were observing each others' videos, a third was discussing the impact of her interviewing style with a simulated client; two others were going through new approaches with one of the facilitators, another was in supervision with the second facilitator, and one decided that he needed some time out from learning! It is not always possible to be so flexible with the range of learning opportunities provided, but to bear this in mind as a principle of good practice is certainly worthwhile.

Keep It Simple

Our colleague Steve Berg-Smith has worked as a facilitator for many years, and was once asked, "What is the most useful thing you have learned?" His answer was a single word: "Simplicity." It can be useful to consider the distinction between foreground and background when presenting people with new material. If the initial (foreground) presentation is kept simple, people can then look into the more complex background material at a pace, and to a level of detail, that suits their needs.

Like others who facilitate the learning of this approach, we constantly search for ways to convey the fundamental spirit, principles, and skills of motivational interviewing in simple language that is suited to the learners' context. In working with physicians we seldom are given sufficient time to teach skillful reflective listening, but we find that we can often convey the essence by asking them to offer "simple summaries" of what their patients say to them in a particular context. Learner-appropriate analogies such as "dancing versus wrestling" may quickly convey an aspect of the spirit of this approach. The acronym OARS (Chapter 6) can be a helpful mnemonic for the four microskills that form the client-centered foundation of motivational interviewing. Again, there is a gentle balance between creative simplicity and oversimplification.

SOME PRACTICAL ASPECTS OF FACILITATION

To keep these principles in mind might seem quite difficult, there being so much to think about in a short space of time. One's first inclination is often to get concrete! To serve this learning need, we reflect here on some practicalities of facilitation.

What Topics Should Be Covered?

The first practical issue is one of the most common raised by facilitators, and also one that we do not answer in this book: What should I include in my

training? The answer is almost entirely context-dependent. This context includes the experience of the facilitator, the setting in which the learners work,
their experiences and aspirations, their clients' problems, the time available,
and so on. Trainers have developed a wealth of resources, some of which can
be found on the *www.motivationalinterview.org* website and in the first edition of this book. Creative facilitation involves understanding the needs of the
learners and creating learning opportunities to meet them.

In this sense, thinking about content is not always a fruitful starting
point. Other questions beckon, which arise from the context of the recipients:
What do they want? What experiences have they had that make motivational
interviewing seem important or unimportant? How do they currently cope
with these challenges? Often, once such questions are answered, the topics to
be covered fall into place.

What about Listening Skills?

Empathic listening is a fundamental foundational skill without which motivational interviewing cannot be practiced. The essential spirit of this approach
also involves an interest in and a willingness to listen to a person's inner
world. It is perhaps the facilitator's most important task, therefore, to foster
an interest in this topic, along with the willingness and patience to develop
real skillfulness in reflective listening.

One mistake that we have learned not to make is to assume that learners—including professional psychologists, counselors, pastors, social workers,
and such—are already proficient in reflective listening. Ask a group of these
folks if they are good listeners, and they will tell you that they are, that they
already know how to do client-centered reflection. But sit them down and ask
them to show you good listening, and three or four times out of five (depending on the group) you're likely to see mostly roadblocks, mixed with a few
low-level reflections. Skillful reflective listening is a *difficult* skill to master,
and far more people believe they have it than actually do. As with chess,
empathic skillfulness continues to develop and mature throughout a lifetime
of practice. The message: *Don't* bypass listening skills unless you know for a
fact that your learners are already proficient at this level.

Here, then, is a common challenge for facilitators. Without reflective listening skills, your learners can go no further with motivational interviewing.
It is possible, of course, to teach specific techniques or tools (such as the readiness ruler) through which some of the nature of this approach may be manifested without taking the time to develop clinical skillfulness. If what you are
trying to do is teach the method of motivational interviewing, however, good
reflective listening is fundamental. Yet it is common to encounter learners
who doubt the value of spending time on listening, regarding it to be "just basic counseling skills that I already know how to use." A confrontational trap
is set to spring, in which your opening line is: "No, you really don't know
how to do this, and you need to learn it."

Fortunately, a facilitator of motivational interviewing is likely to have a good understanding of the dynamics of resistance, as well as facility in resolving it. Acknowledge that learners will already have established varying levels of proficiency in this skill. Reflect concerns. Ask participants to describe, with examples, how reflection works effectively for them, or why they enjoy it, and discuss how it is a fundamental starting point for advanced skills in motivational interviewing. Sometimes we construct an imaginary ruler on the floor and have people physically line themselves up at various points along the scale to express their perceived level of proficiency in reflective listening or their level of interest in improving their skillfulness in this area; then we briefly interview people at various points on the scale. These are simply examples to illustrate that the same methods used to respond to resistance in clients can be applied creatively in the process of facilitating the learning of this approach.

How Important Are Practice, Feedback, and Role Play?

A key in acquiring the necessary skills for motivational interviewing (and, indeed, for almost any communication or other complex skill) is practice with feedback. Role play is often considered to be the central device for allowing people to practice, receive feedback, and so on. Facilitators have designed a wide range of creative exercises to ensure that this is a stimulating experience for people. Standardized patient–actors are now widely used in teaching communication skills in health care training institutions.

But the reception of role play by learners and healthcare practitioners does not always match the enthusiasm among trainers. Indeed, the reaction can border on the contemptuous and may be accompanied by stories of bad experiences (which are often the outcome of poorly designed exercises). Discomfort and resistance may be encountered around the "contrived" or "artificial" nature of practice exercises. Ask learners in groups if they want to practice in role play, and the response will often be unenthusiastic; they prefer the passive roles of listening and watching demonstrations. If you accede to this passivity, however, you have an audience instead of a learning experience.

As many facilitators have discovered, it is possible to win over even hardened skeptics with enjoyable and interesting role-play scenarios. If various roles are available within practice exercises (e.g., speaker or client, listener, observer, coder), participants can sort themselves into more comfortable roles. Giving permission or even instruction to experiment with mistakes can ease the pressure. Offering a demonstration first can also facilitate subsequent practice.

Abstract Processes and Everyday Practice

Continuing professional education is sometimes thought of as a kind of time-out from everyday practice—time to step back a bit and reflect on what one is doing and, perhaps, build a more flexible repertoire of clinical skills. Training is often provided on the principles and processes of a new approach in the abstract, decontextualized from the everyday settings in which they are to be applied. For example, a facilitator might choose to emphasize generic application of certain technical skills, such as particular kinds of reflective listening statements. Learners' everyday clinical experience is thus put to one side, leaving integration to the talent of the individual.

A focus on the abstract is quite common in communication training.[1] In undergraduate and initial graduate training this is quite understandable, as trainees are often learning skills before entering the world of everyday practice. Often in teaching motivational interviewing, however, we are working not with relative beginners but with seasoned practitioners. Does it still make sense, with experienced clinicians, to set aside everyday experiences to focus on more general communication principles and techniques?

What if everyday practice were in the foreground rather than the background? In this case, primary focus would be on the practical problems faced in a clinical setting, and aspects of a new approach (such as motivational interviewing) would be called forth only as they apply to that setting. A facilitator who places everyday practice in the foreground might draw on real cases, design exercises to address common challenges in daily practice, make use of recordings or transcriptions of actual interactions, invite real clients to help with training, and so on.

Effective facilitation often involves finding a healthy balance between these two approaches. If the learners' needs and practice settings are diverse, it can be more challenging to tailor training to everyday experience. When working with the staff of a particular program, it may be preferable to place everyday practice in the foreground. We have had good experience in offering a "contextualized" approach to on-site training of clinicians, focusing on the particular challenges of the setting. Communication skills and motivational interviewing techniques are kept in the background and are brought forward only when they may help address a specific problem. We have found that experienced practitioners often prefer this approach to a decontextualized off-site communication skills seminar.

CREATING LEARNING OPPORTUNITIES

Perhaps it is becoming clear why we have not prescribed particular programs, exercises, or structures for training. The learning of motivational interviewing is a process, not a curriculum. The content of a program of learning is best designed to match the personal and professional context of the learners. Once one has an idea of this context, a suitable selection of learning opportunities can be assembled from a menu of options that include individual and group supervision, distance and self-guided learning, and more formally constructed seminars, workshops, and tutorials.

Uses and Limitations of Workshops

Although most continuing professional education is delivered via training workshops, and entire training organizations rely on this format, our experience and research cause us to question whether this is in fact the best approach to learning. To be sure, there are times when it is quite beneficial for people to remove themselves from the stresses of the everyday workplace and attend an off-site workshop. It can be a time to reflect, meet colleagues, observe others, and discuss clinical issues, free from daily duties and distractions. Examining clinical challenges and practicing skills in a set-apart context has its clear uses. Who, after all, first learned to drive in busy traffic? With skill, workshop scenarios can be constructed that are very close to everyday practice.

The disadvantages of this format are worth considering as well, not in order to discard workshops but to encourage the pursuit and development of additional learning opportunities. The issue of detachment from everyday experiences has already been mentioned. The one-time nature of workshops does not match well what is known about learning. One of the oldest questions addressed in the psychology of learning is the value of massed practice (intensively, all at one time) versus spaced practice (spread out over time). Across a wide range of content, spaced practice is usually much more effective in producing behavior change that is maintained, whereas material learned by massed practice (as in cramming for a final examination) is often quickly forgotten. Public self-consciousness is another issue in workshop settings. How many people will *happily* risk new adventure in a simulated encounter in the presence of colleagues and superiors? Finally, in workshops with diverse participants, it can be difficult to find topics or learning exercises that suit everyone because of variations in skill level, learning style, context, and the particular issues that brought them to training.

Toward Tailored and On-Site Learning Opportunities

If gardeners, tennis coaches, and master mechanics teach people mostly in real life settings, under what circumstances should a counselor *not* be trained in a similar manner? The answer to this question is unclear, calling for both creativity and humility in how we encourage learning. Our hunch is that closeness to everyday context might have considerable value.

Simulated Clients

It is standard practice in many healthcare settings to use simulated patients in some form or another. They are ideally suited to facilitating skill acquisition in motivational interviewing. Actors can present the same case scenario to each member of a group, thus providing a common experience to review, or they can adjust the presentation of a case to suit the needs of an individual. In on-site training, a measure of privacy can be provided by allowing each participant to interact with an actor alone, in rotation. Participants can be asked to complete some reaction notes immediately after an encounter, to be reviewed with a colleague or in a larger group. Actors can also be trained to provide specific feedback about motivational interviewing. Furthermore, trained actors lend a degree of realism to practice exercises and avoid the disadvantages of clinicians' role playing with their own colleagues or superiors during training. Interviews with simulated patients can be audiotaped or videotaped for later review by the learner, with or without observation by others.

The use of simulated patient-actors offers an assessment of competence to use motivational interviewing skills. If a learner cannot demonstrate motivational interviewing skills when asked to do so while knowingly interacting with a simulated patient, it is highly unlikely that such skills will be manifest in daily work with actual clients. The ability to demonstrate competent skills on demand, however, does not guarantee the effective use of those skills in everyday practice.

Tapes and Transcripts

If the behavior to be influenced by training is a learner's performance under normal practice conditions, then what better source of information could there be than samples of actual practice dialogue? In some settings (such as supervision of newer therapists or in clinical trials), all sessions are recorded for training or quality-control purposes, with the practitioner not knowing which tapes will be reviewed. In other settings, only certain interactions or sessions are recorded. When the learner self-selects which sessions to tape or present, of course, there may be a bias toward "best behavior." Still others have assessed real-life practice by having simulated patients present unannounced, with feedback provided afterward to the practitioner.

Tapes of actual practice (or transcripts of them) can provide a rich resource for learning when working with a group, whether culled from real or simulated clients. Learners can be asked to bring these along for use in any number of ways: private observation and reflection, discussion with a colleague, a microanalysis of listening skills, and so on. On-site training can be centered around practice tapes. For example, if all participants see the same standardized client a day or two before a seminar, they can be asked to review their own tape or transcript in private immediately before meeting so that they can discuss and compare their experiences. This provides a common recent experience for all participants to examine.

An interesting question is whether the facilitator should provide comments on tapes or transcripts, which is quite a temptation in the face of such excellent raw data. We have found it usually best to give learners time to absorb, reflect on, and even write down what they liked and what they would change about the encounter *before* anyone else (like a trainer or supervisor) comments on it. Being given "expert" comments can actually get in the way of a much more powerful experience: coming face-to-face, in private, with one's own consulting behavior. We have seen counselors' engagement with the subject, their curiosity, and their motivation to change enhanced considerably by this kind of private encounter with their own work. We also find that learners observing their own work frequently come up with many of the same points we would have made had we provided the commentary.

If it is feasible to obtain practice tapes or transcripts in advance of training, this is also an excellent way to understand, as a starting point, the variety of skills currently being used by counselors. People are often happy for the facilitator to analyze transcripts of participants and then discuss with the group the skills observed. Examples of particularly skillful dialogue from colleagues can be a rich source for learning.

Peer Consultation

A shortcoming of engaging an outside trainer is that the trainer is outside. The process of learning motivational interviewing does not occur suddenly as the result of a training event but, rather, over time with practice, feedback, and encouragement. This is one reason that we have encouraged agencies not to send just one clinician for training, but to send at least two people from the same setting or to have a trainer come and work on-site with several staff. Those who are seeking to learn this approach can then work together in various peer consultation or supervision formats, to learn from and encourage each other by discussing cases, reviewing tapes, and practicing skills. An outside trainer can be involved in this process from time to time, perhaps through further on-site consultation or by reviewing and commenting on practice samples. Most of the learning, however, happens within the context of learners working together in peer consultation.

EVALUATING TRAINING

If we seem in this chapter to have discussed training in a somewhat broad, open-ended manner, it is because the research base for training is much thinner than for how to work with clients. Indeed, we believe that far too little attention has been paid to the processes by which practitioners develop proficiency in counseling and psychotherapy more generally. We would not expect to produce long-term change our clients' behavior by having them attend a one-day didactic. Yet that is the method most often relied on to strengthen and update clinical practice.

If we are correct in our assumptions about how motivational interviewing works, it involves artful skills in reflective listening, attending to subtle shifts in tension, and selectively eliciting and reinforcing certain kinds of client speech. It follows that the skillfulness of those who deliver such counseling would be crucial. A shortcoming pointed out in Chapter 16 is that studies to date have rarely included measures to assess and assure the quality of the motivational interviewing being tested. Clients' outcomes can differ substantially, depending on the skill level of the counselor to whom they were assigned.

With better methods becoming available to measure the acquisition and quality of motivational interviewing, it is time to evaluate the effectiveness of training with the same degree of care that is given to evaluating treatment outcomes. The ultimate impact of this (or any) intervention approach will depend on the ability of clinicians to learn and apply it in practice. Those who initiate and provide resources for the training of staff should know the extent to which their staff have acquired the desired skills, in part to know whether (and for whom) additional training may be warranted. That, in turn, requires of us a better understanding of what learning experiences are usually necessary and sufficient to produce competent practice, and what additional experiences to provide when they are not. Research on the effectiveness of training methods would not only strengthen treatment outcome evaluation but also inform trainers how better to meet the needs of the learners they serve.

CULTURE CHANGE

Those who treat people with behavioral health problems know that it is often important to understand and address not only the client but also the social environment in which he or she lives. The same is true when facilitating learning of motivational interviewing. Consider these four successful examples:

> Probation officers were frustrated that their counseling efforts to help clients lead safer and less self-destructive lives were being undermined by the system within which they worked, which tended to generate distrust between them and their clients. One counselor read about motivational interviewing and decided to see whether she could develop a more constructive tone to her meetings with clients. She attended a 2-day practitioner workshop. For the next few months, she struggled with her supervisor and in everyday practice to integrate the roles of counselor and probation officer. Nevertheless, she reported making good progress through the use of what she called "careful listening and selected, pointed reflective listening statements." Her training manager took an interest in her work and encouraged more counselors to attend training. Some of these colleagues returned to their practice unconvinced that they could apply this approach in their work, but a small group started a peer supervision group and later asked an ex-offender to attend one of their meetings to discuss better ways of helping clients with changing their lifestyles.

> The director of a community-based service read about motivational interviewing, went to a practitioner workshop, and began training her staff through reading material and individual supervision. This led her to attend a training for trainers and to offer more intensive on-site workshops

for her staff. Over the next 5 years, other members of the counseling team received training as trainers and began to work with staff from other agencies. The culture in the service changed accordingly, from a loosely structured and eclectic counseling service to one in which motivational interviewing became a shared and basic counseling style, used in combination with various other approaches such as marital counseling and cognitive-behavioral therapy. Collaborating and encouraging each other, the team began to offer regular training experiences around the country and also became a program base for research on motivational interviewing and other treatment methods.

The staff of a specialist service for adolescents with insulin-dependent diabetes had become truly expert in charting the troubled waters of working with young people. Still, their patients too often did not adhere to the demanding regimens (such as regular monitoring, diet, and injecting) needed to manage their serious illness. Review of practice transcripts indicated that the staff knew how to avoid conflict and serious trouble in their interviews, but they felt stuck in how to make positive progress with many of their young patients. Three staff members—a doctor, a nurse, and a psychologist—were encouraged to learn motivational interviewing. They conducted a small research project on how best to integrate motivational interviewing into everyday practice in their clinic, based on interviews with both staff and patients. They analyzed transcripts of consultations. Each new patient was designated to a "key worker," who applied motivational interviewing from the very first meeting onward. They found that, over time, their patients were less estranged from the service and that compliance rates with self-care regimens improved.

A public substance abuse treatment program faced a common problem: many clients who presented for an intake evaluation never returned. Some of the counseling staff had obtained on-site training in motivational interviewing, but they found that the intake system itself made it difficult to use this approach. Clients began lining up after 7:00 A.M. outside a reception window that opened at 8:00, to sign up for a limited number of intake interview slots for the day. The rest were told to come back the following morning (many of whom did not). Furthermore, the standard intake procedure required the completion of 2 hours of paperwork by at least three different administrative and medical staff before the client was scheduled by a secretary to return for an initial session with a counselor, often 2 to 3 weeks later. Many potential clients left before finishing the paperwork, and even among those who completed this phase, many never returned for a first counseling appointment. In turn, counselors were frustrated with the long delay in being able to see clients and with the high no-show rate. Over a period of 6 months, the intake system was redesigned. A more comfortable waiting room was provided, and, instead of being required to come at one fixed time each morning, clients were offered a larger number of intake appointment or walk-in times throughout the day. The increased number of appointments was accommodated by having counselors who had been trained in motivational interviewing provide the intake interviews. The staff considered which paperwork absolutely had to be completed on the first visit, and it turned out to be about 20 minutes' worth, which was moved to the end rather than the beginning of the interview. Thus when clients contacted the agency, the first person they talked to was a clinical counselor who listened to them for half an hour to understand their problems, learn about their needs, and enhance motivation for change before completing the needed paperwork. There was a rapid increase in the number of clients who completed intake, they began counseling more quickly, dropouts decreased, and the waiting list was eliminated. The medical staff felt less harried and became interested in receiving training in motivational interviewing.

What these four real-life examples have in common is that in each case, what happened was something much more than skill-training for isolated staff. Those who learned the method also saw the need for change in the system of care delivery itself, and they took effective steps to bring about culture change, in some cases reaching beyond their own agency.

It is all well and good for an individual counselor to learn how to express empathy, develop discrepancy, roll with resistance, and support self-efficacy. That counselor may be working within a system in which other people or components take an approach that counteracts the counselor's individual efforts, however. The culture may also place practical and interpersonal constraints on the counselor that make it difficult even for him or her to practice motivational interviewing with clients. In such situations, the challenge is systemic: to gradually change the whole culture—office staff, counselors, managers, the physical environment, access barriers—so that clients are consistently treated by the *system* with respect and understanding (autonomy), are listened to rather than confronted (collaboration), and are encouraged and empowered to use their own resources toward change (evocation).

We began our discussion of motivational interviewing by explaining and emphasizing the underlying spirit of the method. That facilitative spirit can characterize not only individuals who practice motivational interviewing but also the systems within which they work. Wise therapists attend not merely to the client sitting in the consulting room but to the client's social environment, which exerts such important influence in the accomplishment and maintenance of change. Similarly, those who would help others learn motivational interviewing are wise to address both the skills of the learners and the context within which those skills are to be applied.

NOTE

1. Rollnick, Kinnersley, and Butler (2002).

PART IV

Applications of
Motivational Interviewing

CHAPTER 15

Motivational Interviewing and the Stages of Change

CARLO C. DiCLEMENTE *and* MARY MARDEN VELASQUEZ

THE TRANSTHEORETICAL MODEL

The notion that behavior change involves a process that occurs in increments and that involves specific and varied tasks is at the heart of the transtheoretical model of intentional human behavior change (TTM; DiClemente & Prochaska, 1985, 1998; Prochaska & DiClemente, 1983, 1994). This model offers an integrative framework for understanding the process of behavior change whether that change involves the initiation, the modification, or the cessation of a particular behavior. The stages of change represent a key component of the TTM and describe a series of stages though which people pass as they change a behavior. In this model change is viewed as a progression from an initial precontemplation stage, where the person is not currently considering change; to contemplation, where the individual undertakes a serious evaluation of considerations for or against change; and then to preparation, where planning and commitment are secured. Successful accomplishment of these initial stage tasks lead to taking action to make the specific behavioral change; if successful, action leads to the final and fifth stage of change, maintenance, in which the person works to maintain and sustain long-term change (DiClemente & Prochaska, 1998; Prochaska, DiClemente, & Norcross,

1992). These stages appear to be applicable to the larger process of behavior change, whether that change occurs with or without the help of a therapist, an intervention, or a treatment program.

Research has isolated the stages of change across a range of health risk and health protective behaviors. Application of these stages and support for the varied aspects of the process of change represented by these stages have been demonstrated in many behavior changes from cessation of smoking, alcohol, and drugs to mammography screening, dietary modification, gambling, exercise adoption, and condom use and pregnancy prevention (Carney & Kivlahan, 1995; DiClemente & Hughes, 1990; DiClemente & Prochaska, 1998; DiClemente, Story, & Murray, 2000; Glanz et al., 1994; Grimley, Riley, Bellis, & Prochaska, 1993; Isenhart, 1994; Marcus, Rossi, Selby, Niaura, & Abrams, 1992; Weinstein, Rothman, & Sutton, 1998; Werch & DiClemente, 1994; Willoughby & Edens, 1996). Thus, although the behavior change targets differ, the structure of the change process appears to be the same. Individuals move from being unaware or unwilling to do anything about the problem to considering the possibility of change, then to becoming determined and prepared to make the change, and finally to taking action and sustaining or maintaining that change over time.

GROWING UP TOGETHER

TTM, in particular the stages of change aspect of the model, has played an integral role in the development of motivational interviewing and brief interventions using a motivational approach (DiClemente, 1999a; Miller & Rollnick, 1991; Rollnick, Mason, & Butler, 1999). The TTM view of behavior change as a series of gradual steps that involve multiple tasks and require different coping activities rather than a single dimension—or an "all or none" process—has led to a significant change in the way behavioral health professionals conceptualize health behavior change (DiClemente, 1999b; Joseph, Breslin, & Skinner, 1999; Shaffer, 1992; Weinstein et al., 1998). However, moving through the stages of change requires effort and energy for thinking, planning, and doing. Motivation is what provides the impetus for the focus, effort, and energy needed to move through the entire process of change (DiClemente, 1999a; Rollnick et al., 1999; Simpson & Joe, 1993). Thus, motivational interviewing can be used to assist individuals to accomplish the various tasks required to transition from the precontemplation stage through the maintenance stage. Although a client's motivation to begin thinking about changing a particular behavior differs somewhat from the motivation to sustain the effort and energy and maintain a behavior change, motivation is needed from the beginning to the end of the process of change (CSAT Treatment Improvement Protocol No. 35).

The most obvious connection between motivational interviewing and the stages of change is that motivational interviewing is an excellent counseling style to use with clients who are in the early stages. Precontemplators do not want to be lectured to or given "action" techniques when they are not ready to change. Likewise, contemplators, who are considering the possibility of making a change but are not quite ready to make a commitment, are resistant to more traditional approaches that encourage (or try to force) them to make changes for which they are not yet ready. Through the use of motivational interviewing strategies, clinicians facilitate clients in examining their own particular situations, considering the pros and cons of changing and making decisions about change. This is done in a nonthreatening and supportive manner that encourages the client to take responsibility for his or her own situation. The motivational interviewing philosophy, approach, and methods are uniquely suited to addressing the tasks and emotional reactions of individuals who are moving through the first two stages of change.

Clinicians have also found motivational interviewing to be a very effective style to use with clients in the later stages as they prepare for change, take action, and maintain the change over time. Miller and Rollnick (1991) have called this Phase 2 of motivational interviewing: at this point, the client has made a decision to change. In this phase, the clinician's job changes from one of motivating the client to one of advising and "coaching" as the client develops a workable change plan, anticipates barriers to change, and identifies potential support systems. Although most change strategies in this phase (the preparation, action, and maintenance stages) are more action-oriented, clients are still more responsive, and ultimately more successful, when the role of continued motivation is not forgotten and they are treated in the empathic, caring style inherent in motivational interviewing. For clients in the action and maintenance stages, motivational interviewing approaches can help increase self-efficacy and reinforce their accomplishments, both of which are important in sustaining long-term change.

As evidenced by the way researchers and clinicians around the world have embraced the two models, it is apparent that motivational interviewing and the stages of change are a "natural fit." Recognizing the parallels and potential synergy of these ways of understanding and treating problem behaviors, professionals have used these models in many diverse areas of behavior change to develop client-centered, personalized, motivational interventions that are sensitive to the process and processes of change (Connors, Donovan, & DiClemente, 2001; DiClemente, Marinilli, Singh, & Bellino, 2001; Miller, Zweben, DiClemente, & Rychtarik, 1992; Prochaska, DiClemente, Velicer, & Rossi, 1993; Velasquez, Maurer, Crouch, & DiClemente, 2001; Velicer et al., 1993). We describe in some detail how motivational interviewing approaches can be linked to each of the stages of change from the transtheoretical model.

TAILORING INTERVENTIONS TO CLIENTS' READINESS TO CHANGE

Individuals can come to the attention of healthcare providers when they are in any one of the stages of change. Sometimes they are there to seek help in negotiating successful passage through the action stage change. At other times they are unwilling to change but are "mandated" to treatment, either by the legal system or by concerned family members, friends, or employers. Often clients arrive with problems or conditions in which there may be multiple behaviors that need changing (DiClemente, Carbonari, & Velasquez, 1992; Prochaska & DiClemente, 1984). Drug abusers with psychiatric disorders, diabetics in health care clinics, and drug-dependent, cigarette-smoking pregnant women are often in different stages of change, depending on which behavior is the focus of attention. For example, a patient who arrives for a clinic visit for hypertension may be in one stage of change for stress-reduction strategies, another stage for adopting regular exercise, and yet another for adherence to antihypertension medication. In each of these situations, the challenge to the clinician is first to understand where the client is in the change cycle and then to offer the appropriate assistance. In this chapter, we describe each stage of change and offer suggestions about overall motivational interviewing style and specific motivational techniques that may be appropriate for each particular stage. While the target behavior, the setting, and the availability of time will influence the choice of strategies, this chapter offers guidance on how best to integrate the use of motivational interviewing and knowledge of the client's individual stage of readiness to change throughout the entire change process.

FACILITATING CHANGE IN PRECONTEMPLATORS

Precontemplation is the earliest stage of change. People in precontemplation are either unaware of problem behavior or are unwilling or discouraged when it comes to changing it. They engage in little activity that could shift their view of problem behavior and can be rather defensive about the targeted problem behavior. Precontemplators are not convinced that the negative aspects of the current or problem behavior outweigh the positive.

In many areas, particularly the addictive behaviors, precontemplators often have been labeled "resistant." As clinicians our challenge is to learn why our client may be resistant to change and to use strategies that diffuse that resistance in a positive way. The stages of change help us think about client resistance as a state that can be influenced. Rather than feeling discouraged when we encounter client resistance, we realize that the client is in an early stage of change, and we try to learn more about his or her reason for being in that state. Through talking to thousands of precontemplators through the years, we have realized that there are many reasons for someone to be in the precontemplation stage. It can be helpful to think about precontemplators' resistance to change in what can best be summarized as the four R's: reluctance, rebellion, resignation, and rationalization. Each of these patterns of thinking, feeling, and reasoning helps keep precontemplators not ready to change. Although most precontemplators use a combination of these patterns, we will describe each pattern as a distinct type.

Reluctant precontemplators are those who, through lack of knowledge or perhaps inertia, do not want to consider change. For these clients, the information or the effect of their problem behavior has not become fully conscious. Rather than being actively resistant, they are actually more passively reluctant to change. It may be that they are fearful of change, or perhaps they are comfortable where they are and don't want to risk the potential discomfort of change. For these clients, careful listening and providing feedback in a sensitive, empathic manner can be very helpful. Motivating this type of precontemplator often takes time, as it did with Harvey, a client Dr. DiClemente saw in his practice:

> Harvey was a very successful businessman who had been promoted to senior vice president from a direct sales position in an advertising company. However, he found that managing others was much more difficult than doing the job himself, because of his problems in being direct with others. During the evaluation visits, we discussed many issues related to the job, the politics of the company, and his personal limitations. I listened carefully and reflected back to Harvey what I heard him describing about his job situations. Using the motivational interviewing strategies of reflective listening, summarizing, and affirmation, I encouraged Harvey to explore his situation. He soon began to see patterns to his behavior. He expressed surprise when he came to the conclusion that he had difficulty being direct when it involved criticism of another. Harvey saw himself as an open, "no-nonsense" person. Eventually Harvey chose to resign his management position rather than work on changing his interpersonal style. He was reluctant to change at that particular time. Although I might have been tempted to encourage him to change, I acknowledged that some precontemplators are OK right where they are for the time being. Once the "seeds" have been planted, precontemplators often need time to let them germinate. I also knew that through our sessions Harvey had begun to consider change. I suspected that he would eventually come to his own decision to make a change. One year later, Harvey returned asking for a referral to work on interpersonal issues. It seemed that the job change had relieved the immediate stress, but he had recently entered a romantic relationship where the problems we had discussed became quite apparent. He returned stating, "You know those problems we discussed last year? I am ready to tackle them now."

Sometimes the reluctant client will progress rapidly once he or she verbalizes the reluctance, feels listened to, and begins to feel the tension between the reluctance to change and the possibility of a different future. At other times, the change may take longer, as in Harvey's case. By allowing clients the freedom to make their own decisions, clinicians facilitate a situation where the possibility of change can be explored in a nonthreatening manner.

Unlike reluctant precontemplators, *rebellious precontemplators* often have a great deal of knowledge about the problem behavior. In fact, they often have a heavy investment in the behavior. They are also invested in making their own decisions. They do not like being told what to do! The rebellion may be a residue of prolonged adolescence or the result of insecurity and fears. No matter what the source, the rebellious precontemplator will appear hostile and resistant to change. It is easy to recognize a rebellious precontemplator; they often argue with the clinician, demonstrate either verbally or nonverbally that they don't want to be there, and provide a host of reasons that they are not going to change. Motivational interviewing provides a way of allowing rebellious precontemplators the freedom to express their strong feelings about change while at the same time directing their energy in a positive direction. For example, when a counselor agrees with the rebellious precontemplator that no one can force them to change, and in fact the counselor wouldn't dream of trying, it often diffuses the strength of their argument.

Providing a menu of options seems to be the best strategy for working with the rebellious precontemplator. Encouraging clients to think about the choices available, including small incremental changes instead of complete and abrupt abstinence, for example, often opens the door to the possibility of change. Keep in mind that the rebellious precontemplator has a lot of energy invested in the problem behavior. The real challenge is helping the client shift some of that energy into contemplating change rather than using it to resist or rebel. Once a rebellious precontemplator decides to change, the energy often shifts to a positive energy of determination to succeed.

Lack of energy and investment, by contrast, is the hallmark of the *resigned precontemplator*. These clients have given up on the possibility of change and seem overwhelmed by the problem. For example, many smoking clients begin by saying how many other attempts they have made to quit. They feel hopelessly addicted to cigarettes and out of control. They see the habit as controlling them, not their own capacity. Often these individuals will tell us that the only way to deal with the smoking problem is to stop young people from starting to smoke in the first place. The clear message is that it is too late for them. One recent study examined a variant of resignation called cessation hopelessness in a sample of smokers in the precontemplation stage. Those precontemplators who were high in a measure of cessation hopelessness had levels of temptation to smoke that were very high and exceeded their confidence to abstain by a greater amount that those who were lower on this measure (Walker Daniels, 1998).

Instilling hope and exploring barriers to change are the most productive strategies for these resigned precontemplators. It is important to help these clients see that relapse is common and not to be viewed as a failure. Many people go through the stages several times before maintaining a change, and each change attempt is a learning opportunity. It is important for all clients to realize that behavior change is difficult, but it is not impossible. Often, the key to working with the resigned precontemplator is to build confidence a bit at a time by assisting them in making the decision to begin with a small change and affirming each success they have, however small. Keep in mind that research shows that the clinician's belief in the client's ability to change is a strong predictor of outcome. Success builds on success, and with each small change the resigned precontemplator builds self-efficacy about making bigger changes.

While the resigned precontemplator often feels that they have none of the answers to their problems, the *rationalizing precontemplator* often appears to have all the answers. These clients are not considering change because they often think they have figured out the odds of personal risk or believe that their behavior is the result of another's problem, not theirs. It is easy to identify the rationalizing client in a session: it is when the clinician begins to feel as though he or she is in a debate, or a session of "point counterpoint." Although it may feel like rebellion, the resistance of the rationalizing client lies much more in their thinking than in their emotions. Prime examples are smokers who are convinced that they are really not at much risk because they started smoking after 21 years of age; are only smoking 15 cigarettes a day; have only smoked for 10 years; or have a 90-year-old grandfather who smokes. The same study that examined cessation hopelessness also evaluated a characteristic labeled "harm minimization" among precontemplating smokers. Those smokers who had higher scores on the harm minimization scale demonstrated significantly lower levels of cognitive processes of change, like consciousness raising and self-reevaluation (Walker Daniels, 1998). Minimizing the harm reduces contemplation activities.

Often the rationalizing precontemplator will want to discuss their rationale. The problem is that the discussion typically only serves to strengthen their side of the argument! Empathy and reflective listening seem to work best with this type of client. Starting with a decisional balance exercise in which the client is asked to tell the "good things" about the behavior is an ideal strategy for the rationalizing precontemplator. They quickly realize that you are not going to argue with them, and that you will actually acknowledge that they have some compelling reasons for their behavior. Once they have talked about the pros of their behavior, clients are often more open to considering that there are also "not so good" things. The skilled motivational interviewing clinician gently reflects both the pros and cons of change and encourages the client to elaborate. Double-sided reflections can be used to reflect any ambivalence about change, and summarizing both sides of the behavior may help the rationalizing precontemplator recognize that some of their rationale may be flawed. A note of caution: it can be very tempting to use the decisional balance "cons" as ammunition in which we use the clients' own words to remind them of all the negative things about their behavior and to argue for change. This defeats the purpose of the exercise. Motivational interviewing is effective in large part because it avoids argumentation and allows the client to hear and assimilate his or her own "change statements" (see Chapter 7). Again, it may be best to summarize the decisional balance and then ask where this leaves the client in terms of thinking about the behavior. The clinician who trusts the process and lets clients come to their own conclusions and change in their own time is often surprised at how frequently this exercise motivates rationalizing precontemplators to reexamine, and change, their behavior.

Before leaving the land of the precontemplator, it is important to mention that there is a myth among clinicians that in dealing with serious health-related, addictive, or other problems, more is always better. We often hear it said that motivational interviewing is a good technique to use in some cases, but when a person is really at risk (like a pregnant smoker or a drug-addicted client) more must be done. Clinicians often believe that more education, more intense treatment, or more confrontation will necessarily produce more change. Nowhere is this less true than with precontemplators. More intensity will often produce fewer results with this group (Heather, Rollnick, & Bell, 1993; Miller, Benefield, & Tonigan, 1993). So it is particularly important to use careful motivational strategies rather than to mount high-intensity programs or efforts that will be ignored by those uninterested in changing the particular problem behavior. It is just as erroneous, however, to believe that precontemplators don't ever change and there is nothing we can do. They can be coaxed, encouraged, informed, and advised. We cannot make precontemplators change, but we can help motivate them to move to contemplation.

CONTEMPLATION: A RISK–REWARD ANALYSIS

In the contemplation stage of change, a person acknowledges that he or she has a problem and begins to think seriously about solving it. Contemplators struggle to understand their problem, to see its causes, and to think about possible solutions. Contemplators may be far from actually making a commitment to action, however. For example, a contemplator might gather a lot of information about treatment programs but not actually enroll. That is often the nature of contemplation. The individual knows where he or she wants to be and maybe even how to get there, but he or she is not quite ready to make a commitment. Although many contemplators move on to the action stage, it is possible to spend many months or years in contemplation (Carbonari, DiClemente, & Sewell, 1999). The clinician's goal when working with a contemplator is to help the client "tip the balance" in favor of change.

Contemplation is often a very paradoxical stage of change. The fact that the client is willing to consider the problem and the possibility of change offers hope for change. Contemplation is the stage when clients are quite open to information about the behavior and to exploring decisional balance considerations. It is also the stage where clients experience the most ambivalence. As clinicians, it is important that we be comfortable with and that we recognize ambivalence as a vital part of the contemplation stage of change. We should also realize that contemplation does not mean commitment.

Clinicians often make the mistake of thinking that a person who is contemplating change is ready to make a commitment; this is not the case. A good example of this confusion is in workplace smoking cessation programs. When surveys are taken in the workplace, large numbers of smokers (up to 70% or even 80%) express interest in quitting. So programs are developed and offered. Typically, these programs are very poorly attended and are lucky to attract 3% to 5% of the smokers. Clearly, thinking about quitting does not equal commitment to quit. Most smokers wish to change or wish that they could stop smoking. Many are considering change in the near future. When confronted by a choice to sign up for a specific cessation program on a specific date, however, they find many reasons why right now is not the right time. What are missing in most of these worksite programs are adequate motivational strategies to assist individuals in moving from contemplation to preparation and being ready to take action (DiClemente & Scott, 1997).

Some studies have found a relationship between contemplation and higher levels of depression (Velasquez, Carbonari, & DiClemente, 1999). It may be that there is a subgroup of contemplators who are in what DiClemente and Prochaska (1998) have called "chronic contemplation." They think about change, often to the point of rumination, but they don't move beyond the contemplation stage. When working with contemplators, it is important to assess how long the person has been considering change and whether they have made past attempts. The key here is to assist the contemplator in thinking through the risks of the behavior and potential benefits of change and to instill hope that change is possible. It is also important for contemplators to receive accurate information about their behavior and personal feedback about the effect the behavior is having on their lives. Although one piece of information will not make the decision for the individual, this type of personally relevant information or feedback can be extremely persuasive. For example, when we talk with groups of smokers, we try to give accurate information about the facts of smoking: for example, there are over 1,000 different gases in cigarette smoke; smoking contributes not only to lung cancer, but also to heart disease and chronic obstructive lung disease; tar coats the cilia of the lungs, making them very inefficient in transferring oxygen. But information alone is not enough. We also try to make this information personally relevant by asking about their smoker's cough, telling them to breathe out the smoke through a white handkerchief in order to see the residue, or discussing the number of colds or respiratory problems they are having.

Other examples of feedback that can help contemplators resolve ambivalence are "reports" based on client assessment such as those used in the motivational enhancement therapy treatment in Project MATCH (Miller et al., 1992). These reports detailed information about the client's level of drinking, a comparison between their drinking levels and those of the American population (gender-specific norms), family risk factors, and other variables. In healthcare settings, blood test results, pulmonary functioning tests, and cholesterol level results can provide important feedback to the contemplator. This information, which is visible and personally relevant, is more powerful in shifting the decisional balance toward action than all the scare tactics, general lectures, and nagging in the world (DiClemente et al., 2001; Kreuter, Strecher, & Glassman, 1999).

In the preceding section, we discussed how the decisional balance exercise can be helpful in assisting the precontemplator to talk about the problem behavior. It is also very useful in the contemplation stage. In fact, research shows that for many different behaviors, contemplation is the stage in which evaluations of the pros and cons of the behavior are more or less equal (Prochaska et al., 1994). The task for the clinician, then, is to help the client move from this balanced state to one that is "tipped" in favor of change. Once this happens, the client is ready to move on to the next stage.

An important strategy with contemplators is to "accentuate the positive." Often individuals considering changing a problem behavior will concentrate on all the negative aspects of the behavior. "I know how bad my drinking is for me," they say. In fact, they can often produce a litany of reasons why what they are doing is bad for them. Clinician and client are often baffled by the fact that even with all these negatives, change does not occur. The reality is that if the behavior were not in some way beneficial to the client, he or she would not be doing it. Until a client acknowledges the "good things" about the behavior, they cannot prepare to combat temptation once they make an attempt to change. The decisional balance helps facilitate this process. Once the client has evaluated the benefits of the behavior, they move to focusing on the "not so good things." The clinician listens for change statements here, which include expressions of concern, problem recognition, optimism about change, or intent to change. Offering periodic summaries, using double-sided reflections, and reflecting and affirming self-motivational statements are ways to help the client get the most from the decisional balance exercise.

Careful listening, summarizing, feedback, double-sided reflections, affirmation, and increasing self-efficacy are powerful facilitators of change when working with contemplators. Overcoming the ambivalence and shifting the decisional balance can take time and requires great patience and persistence on the part of the motivational interviewer.

DEVELOPING A PLAN AND PREPARING FOR ACTION

In the preparation stage, the person is ready to change in the near future. They are on the verge of taking action. People in this stage may have tried and failed to change in the past. Yet, they have often learned valuable lessons from past change attempts. Individuals in this stage of change need to develop a plan that will work for them. Then they need to make firm commitments to follow through on the action option they choose.

The decision to take appropriate steps to stop a problem behavior or to initiate a positive behavior provides access to the preparation stage. Most people in this stage will make a serious attempt at change in the near future. They appear to be ready for and committed to action. The challenge is to help the client develop a change plan that is acceptable, accessible, and effective.

Once clients have committed to action, it would seem to be a simple task to assist them in preparing to move forward. However, commitment to change does not necessarily mean that change is automatic, that change methods used will be efficient, or that the attempt will be successful in the long term. Being prepared for action does not mean that all ambivalence is resolved. In fact, the decision-making process continues throughout the preparation stage.

The first task for the clinician working with the client in preparation is to assess the strength of the client's commitment to change. This is often difficult to assess simply from verbal self-report. Sometimes clients who are adamant about being ready to change are trying to convince themselves as much as they are trying to convince the clinician. For example, Dr. Velasquez recently worked with a woman who was about to be released from a county jail. This client had a history of substance abuse and expressed a strong desire to stay abstinent upon release. She enthusiastically recited all the reasons she was going to change and vowed never to use drugs or alcohol again. Upon discussing the client's plans for change, however, it became clear that she had not given much thought to how she planned to accomplish her goal. In fact, her plans were to return to a relationship with a drug-abusing boyfriend. She had no plans for a job or for filling her free time, and she had not thought about further treatment or how to avoid her substance-abusing friends. In other words, this client said she was ready and determined to make a change, but she lacked the plans for doing so. The task here was to use motivational interviewing to assist the client in making a solid realistic assessment of the difficulties she might encounter upon release, a plan for each of these contingencies, and a way to know when she might need additional help.

Using a motivational interviewing approach, the clinician helps the client think creatively about how to develop the most effective plan. Considering the client's personal life circumstances and drawing on their past experience with change, the clinician guides the client in developing change strategies. Presenting a menu of possible options from which the client can choose is often helpful. The clinician can also draw on his or her own experience with past clients, gently suggesting strategies that have worked for other people. While respecting the client's choices, the clinician can also gently warn against change plan strategies that seem inappropriate or ineffective. While the clinician's tasks are different in this phase, they are no less challenging. A solid, workable change plan is not easy to develop; it takes careful listening, reflection, and incisive intervention on the part of the clinician, as well as the client's careful thought and determination.

ACTION: IMPLEMENTING THE PLAN

In the action stage of change people most overtly modify their behavior. They stop smoking, remove all the desserts from the house, pour the last beer down the drain, or enter a treatment program. In short, they make the move and implement the plan for which they have been preparing. Action is the most obviously busy period and the one that requires the greatest commitment of time and energy. Changes made during the action stage are more visible to others than those made during the other stages and therefore receive the greatest recognition. The danger is that many people, including professional therapists, can erroneously equate action with change, overlooking not only the critical work that prepares people for successful action but the equally important (and often more challenging) efforts to maintain the changes following action.

What do people in action need from a clinician? They have often made a plan and have begun to implement it before we even see them. Often, making an appointment has coincided with other changes they have made. Clients in the action stage have various reasons for consulting a clinician. This might be to make a public commitment to action, to get some external confirmation of the plan, to seek support, to gain greater self-efficacy, or sometimes to create external monitors of their activity. Working with clients in the action stage can be rather easy and quite rewarding for clinicians. In fact, clients at this stage represent many of our "miracle cures" that see us for one session, make significant and long-lasting changes, and tell everyone what great therapists we are! It is important, however, not to assume that once a person has reached the action stage, it is an easy downhill ride. Clients in action may still have some conflicting feelings about the change. They may miss their old lifestyles in some ways and be struggling to fit into this new behavior. Careful listening and affirming clients that they are doing the right thing are important in this stage. It is also important to check with the client to see if he or she has discovered any parts of the change plan that need revision. Some clients in action will discover their change plans need to be revised, and the clinician can be of assistance in this process. Clients also need affirmation for what they have accomplished and assurance that they can continue to make the desired changes.

No matter how much a person wants to change, and regardless of their willingness to take action, if they do not have adequate self-efficacy, they are not likely to experience long-term success. Motivational interviewing can help build clients' self-efficacy as they take action. By focusing on their successful activity, reaffirming their decisions, and helping clients make intrinsic attributions of success, clinicians can bolster clients' self-efficacy evaluations.

MAINTENANCE, RELAPSE, AND RECYCLING

Maintenance is the final stage in the process of change. Sustaining behavior change can be difficult. In the maintenance stage, the person works to consolidate the gains attained during the action stage and struggles to prevent relapse. Although traditional therapy views maintenance as a static stage, the transtheoretical model sees it as a critically important continuation that can last from as little as more than 6 months to as long as a lifetime. Motivation to consolidate the change is needed. Without a strong commitment to maintenance, there will surely be relapse. Often change is not completely established even after 6 months or so of action. This is particularly true if the environment is filled with cues that can trigger the problem behavior. We all know of cases where an individual who has stopped drinking relapses just when everyone thinks the problem is finally resolved. It is important to help individuals in this stage practice an active and intelligent maintenance of the changes they have made (CSAT, 1999).

The TTM model recognizes that relapse is possible (even likely) when moving through the stages of change. People often "recycle" through the stages many different times before reaching success; thus, a "slip" should not be considered an utter failure but, rather, a step back. Many people progress from contemplation through preparation to action and then maintenance, but many will relapse. After a relapse, individuals often regress to an earlier stage and then begin progressing through the stages yet again. Frequently, people who do relapse have a better chance of success during the next cycle. They have often learned new ways to deal with old behaviors, and they now have a history of partial successes to build on.

Relapse can occur for many different reasons. Individuals may experience a particularly strong, unexpected urge or temptation to return to the problem behavior and fail to cope with it successfully. Sometimes relaxing their guard or testing themselves begins the slide back to the former behavior pattern. Often the complete personal cost of the change is not realized until later, and commitment or self-efficacy erodes. Most often relapse does not occur automatically but takes place gradually after an initial slip occurs.

During what Saul Shiffman (1982) calls these "relapse crises," clients may turn to a therapist or other health care provider for help. Either they have slipped and are early into relapse or they are scared and shaken by their desire to go back to smoking or drinking or drugs. They come to the clinician with a weakened self-efficacy and a fear that the old habit may be stronger than they are. They seek reassurance and some way to make sense of the relapse crisis. It is important to help these clients see the crisis as an opportunity to learn rather than a failure. Understanding the cycle of change in a learning context can assist both the clinician and the client. Effective use of the motivational interviewing approach and strategies can help motivate the individual to renew or recommence the journey through the early stages once again, to problem solve the failed plan in order to create a more effective one, and to initiate another change attempt.

CURRENT STATUS AND FUTURE CHALLENGES

It should be quite apparent by now that motivational interviewing strategies can be knit together rather seamlessly with the stages of change model. The philosophical underpinnings of motivational interviewing are consonant with respect to the client's process of change. Motivational interviewing assumes, as does TTM, that change is the responsibility of the individual and occurs in the entire life space of the individual and not simply in the context of any specific intervention. However, identifying a client's status in terms of the stages of change can be very helpful in deciding which motivational strategies to use and when to use them. Motivational interviewing approaches are appropriate for clients in each of the stages of change. The content and strategies will vary, but the objective remains the same (CSAT, 1999; DiClemente, 1999a). Clients often need help to negotiate the passage from one stage to the next in the process of change. The ultimate goal is to help the individual make efficient and effective changes in his or her life, with the assumption being that these changes will be life enhancing and become reinforcing in their own right. At some point, these behaviors will become sustained over time and integrated into his or her lifestyle so that the individual can exit the cycle of change (DiClemente, in press; DiClemente & Prochaska, 1998). Motivational and other types of interventions punctuate and promote the process of change, but that process always extends well beyond any specific intervention.

Although the change processes delineated in the TTM and motivational interviewing approaches are quite compatible and have been integrated, there are continued challenges for understanding and intervening in this process that should be explored. These include understanding how motivational interviewing approaches affect specific client processes of change, applicability of TTM and motivational interviewing cross culturally, and the issue of brief versus more extensive interventions.

In addition to the stages of change, TTM has identified a number of processes of change that have been implicated in movement from one stage to the next and in successful change (Carbonari & DiClemente, 2000; DiClemente & Prochaska, 1998; Prochaska & DiClemente, 1984; Prochaska, Velicer, DiClemente, Guadagnoli, & Rossi, 1991). Cognitive and experiential processes of change appear to be more important in the earlier stages of change, and behavioral processes appear to be more important in the later stages (Perz, DiClemente, & Carbonari, 1996). It is assumed that motivational interviewing approaches influence cognitive and experiential processes like consciousness raising, self-reevaluation, environmental reevaluation, and the like with clients in early stages of change. Alternatively, as clients move forward in the process, motivational interviewing influences efficacy and the behavioral processes of change. These assumptions need to be explored (Joseph et al., 1999). The data from Project MATCH indicate that motivational enhancement therapy (Miller et al., 1992) was as effective as more extensive treatments for the most part (Project MATCH Research Group, 1997b). However, an analysis of the process of change indicated that this treatment did not have a differential effect on process activity, compared to other treatments (DiClemente, Carbonari, Zweben, Morrel, & Lee, 2001). It may be too difficult to capture processes of change and critical transitions in large-scale treatment trials. Experimental trials are needed to examine specifically how various motivational interviewing strategies and approaches affect the different processes of change that have been identified in TTM.

The stages of change have been examined with a number of different behaviors and in a variety of populations in various countries around the world. Motivational interviewing has also been translated into different languages and thus transported into cultures beyond the confines of the United States, Great Britain, and Australia where it was developed. Initial data and reports of application from various parts of the world support the contention that the same basic process of change occurs cross culturally. Contemplation, preparation, action, and maintenance tasks appear to present similar challenges in addiction treatment, for example, in both Western and Eastern cultures. If this is true, the challenge is to understand how to facilitate movement through the stages among various ethnically and culturally diverse populations (Suris, Trapp, DiClemente, & Cousins, 1998). It is clear that the types of considerations, value systems, action strategies, and support systems differ in diverse populations as individuals move from one stage to another. This may mean that the structure of the process of change remains the same, but the content of decisional considerations, the nature of commitment, and the specific strategies in action and maintenance plans would differ. The challenges lie in measuring the stages of change (Carey, Purnine, Maisto, & Carey, 1999) and in understanding which strategies of the motivational interviewing approach can be used cross culturally to promote stage transitions and which need significant adaptation by practitioners in the different cultures in order to be sensitive to their needs, as well as the needs of clients.

Finally, motivational strategies have most often been used in the context of brief or briefer interventions. The process of change as conceptualized in TTM can take a significant amount of time, even years, for an individual to change one single target behavior. When multiple behaviors in various areas of life functioning are involved, the task becomes even more complicated (DiClemente, 1994, 1999b; DiClemente & Prochaska, 1998). How should motivational approaches and strategies be synchronized with the process of change? Are additional types of strategies (cognitive-behavioral interventions) needed in addition to the motivational interviewing intervention for some clients or some types of problems? Some clinical approaches are beginning to use a motivational intervention first and then to switch to a more intensive cognitive-behavioral intervention, as is being evaluated in a large clinical trial of alcoholism treatment called Project COMBINE sponsored by the National Institute on Alcohol and Alcoholism. Other programs are using motivational enhancement as a pretreatment before using more intensive approaches (see Chapter 20). Other approaches have integrated stages into more traditional treatments (Connors et al., 2001) or combined motivational interviewing approaches and processes of change-based strategies into group therapy sessions (Velasquez et al., 2001). How to integrate motivational interviewing strategies with more intensive interventions and whether this combination of approaches is needed for any or all clients are questions that demand additional research.

Although there are continuing questions and challenges related to understanding the interplay between TTM and motivational interviewing, one thing is clear. Health and addiction researchers and clinicians have seen both of these perspectives as helpful. Many have begun to use TTM to broaden their view of the process of change and to extend the scope of potential interventions from precontemplation to maintenance issues. At the same time, they have adopted motivational approaches to intervention to address the critical issue of motivation that most often had been left completely in the domain of the client. Only understanding more fully and intervening more effectively in the process of change will realize the promise of TTM and motivational interviewing.

CHAPTER 16

The Efficacy of Motivational Interviewing and Its Adaptations

What We Know So Far

BRIAN L. BURKE, HAL ARKOWITZ, *and* CHRISTOPHER DUNN

> From a single drop of water, a logician could infer the
> possibility of an Atlantic or a Niagara without having seen or
> heard of one or the other. So all life is a great chain, the nature of
> which is known whenever we are shown a single link of it. Like
> all other arts, the Science of Deduction and Analysis is one which
> can only be acquired by long and patient study, nor is life long
> enough to allow any mortal to attain the highest possible
> perfection in it.
> —SHERLOCK HOLMES, in Sir Arthur Conan Doyle, *A Study in Scarlet*

When the first edition of this book was published in 1991, there was good reason to believe that the authors had put their hands on a promising approach for helping people change their addictive and other troubling behaviors. Yet, at that time, only a handful of studies had been done to evaluate the efficacy of approaches related to motivational interviewing. The past decade, however, has yielded mounting empirical research on these approaches for a wide variety of clinical problems. This chapter will critically review the domain, focusing on controlled trials of individually delivered interventions that incorporate the basic principles of motivational interviewing.

WHAT IS MOTIVATIONAL INTERVIEWING?

In this book, Miller and Rollnick define motivational interviewing as a "client-centered, directive method for enhancing intrinsic motivation to change by exploring and resolving ambivalence " (Chapter 3). They further describe motivational interviewing as "a way of being with people" and a set of clinical methods that can be taught and learned. Motivational interviewing involves the application of four basic principles:

- Expressing empathy
- Developing discrepancy
- Rolling with resistance
- Supporting self-efficacy

Clinically, approaches related to motivational interviewing can be employed in a variety of ways. These interventions can be the primary treatment or a prelude to another type of treatment in an effort to enhance the client's responsiveness to that treatment. These approaches can also be adapted to combine or integrate with other treatment components or even with entire treatments.

In the research literature, the most widely used approach related to motivational interviewing is one in which the client (usually alcohol- or drug-addicted) is given feedback based on individual results from standardized assessment measures, often the Drinker's Check-Up (DCU; Miller, Sovereign, & Krege, 1988) or a modification of it. The feedback is delivered in a motivational interviewing "style," and discussion of the problem may extend to one or more sessions that continue to embody the fundamental spirit and methods of motivational interviewing. We consider this feedback-based approach— employed in many of the studies reviewed here, including the well-known Project MATCH (1997b)—to constitute an "adaptation" of motivational interviewing (AMI) because it is defined by the presence of the feedback component and not solely by the use of motivational interviewing per se.[1] More broadly, we also apply the term "AMI" to interventions that incorporate additional nonmotivational interviewing techniques while retaining motivational interviewing principles as the core of treatment, as well as to interventions that have been specifically adapted for use by nonspecialists (Rollnick, Heather, & Bell, 1992). It is interesting to note that virtually *all* of the published empirical studies in this area (and therefore in this review) deal with the efficacy of AMIs, with no studies addressing the efficacy of motivational interviewing in relatively pure form.

WHAT HAVE PREVIOUS REVIEWS OF THE MOTIVATIONAL INTERVIEWING LITERATURE FOUND?

Two previous reviews have been published. Noonan and Moyers (1997) reviewed the 11 clinical trials of AMIs available at that time—nine with problem drinkers and two with drug abusers. The authors concluded that nine of these studies supported the efficacy of AMIs for a variety of addictive behaviors.

More recently, Dunn, DeRoo, and Rivara (2001) performed a systematic review of 29 randomized trials of brief interventions claiming to use the principles and techniques of motivational interviewing (or what we have called AMIs) to change behavior in four domains: substance abuse, smoking, HIV risk reduction, and diet and exercise. Data on methodological features were tabled, as were calculations of effect sizes and their 95% confidence intervals.[2] Seventeen studies in substance abuse, two in smoking, four in HIV risk reduction, and six in the area of diet and exercise were reviewed. Overall, 60% of the studies had at least one significant effect size for the AMI under investigation. The strongest evidence for efficacy was found in the substance abuse domain, where AMIs appeared to work well for problem drinkers and improved the rate of entry into and retention in intensive substance abuse treatment. AMI effects did not appear to diminish over time, and the effect sizes for AMIs as preludes to treatment were roughly equivalent to those for AMIs as stand-alone interventions.

WHAT DID WE INCLUDE IN OUR REVIEW?

For this review, we searched through the reference sections of both prior reviews and the motivational interviewing website (*www.motivationalinterview.org*). We also conducted a database search (PSYCINFO) using "motivational interviewing" as a key phrase, and, finally, we sent out an electronic message to all members of the Motivational Interviewing Network of Trainers (MINT) asking for any published or in-press articles relevant to our purposes.

This chapter follows the general guidelines currently employed in reviews of the efficacy of various psychotherapies (see Kazdin, 1992). For this reason, studies had to satisfy the following criteria in order to be included in this review:

- The intervention under study consisted primarily of implementing the motivational interviewing principles just discussed rather than principles of some other approach (such as cognitive-behavioral therapy).
- The intervention was delivered on an individual (one-on-one) and face-to-face basis.[3]
- The efficacy of the individual, face-to-face AMI component could rea-

sonably be imputed from the study design (i.e., without being confounded with self-help, group, or other formats).

- The study design met our criteria for a controlled clinical trial.

In our definition, a controlled clinical trial must use the following: random assignment to groups or an alternate way of equating compared groups
of clients before treatment (e.g., sequential assignment), at least one comparison group, a clear description of the sample, adequate measurement targeting
pertinent problem areas, and the collection of follow-up data. Although the
controlled clinical trial has recently come under some criticism (e.g., Borkovec
& Castonguay, 1998), it remains the gold standard for evaluating treatment
outcome (Miller, Andrews, Wilbourne, & Bennett, 1998).

WHAT KINDS OF CONTROLLED CLINICAL TRIALS
HAVE BEEN CONDUCTED WITH AMIs?

There were a total of 26 studies that met our inclusion criteria.[4] The basic
characteristics of each study, grouped by clinical problem area, are shown in
Tables 16.1a–16.1c. The studies vary widely in terms of settings, sample characteristics, intervention formats, uses of the AMI (e.g., as a prelude to further
services or as a stand-alone treatment), comparison groups employed, intervention quality control, measurement scope, and length of follow-up.

HOW GOOD WERE THESE STUDIES?:
A QUANTITATIVE PERSPECTIVE ON METHODOLOGY

Prior to embarking on a more qualitative look at AMI clinical trials, we will
provide a quantitative evaluation of the methodology and outcome of these
trials, using a system developed by Miller and colleagues (1995). Two independent raters judged the methodological quality of each study on 12 specific
dimensions, with some dimensions (e.g., follow-up rate and length) counting
for more than 1 point, resulting in a maximum possible Methodological Quality Score (MQS) of 17.

Outcome Logic Scores (OLS) reflecting the strength of support for treatment efficacy were also determined for each study. Study outcomes were rated
as providing positive evidence (+ 1; treatment superior to any alternate treatment without a control group, or equal to a more extensive treatment without
a control group) or strong positive evidence (+ 2; treatment superior to no-
treatment or placebo control), negative evidence (−1; mixed or insignificant
results among comparable treatments) or strong negative evidence (−2; treatment worse than alternatives or equal to no-treatment control) for the AMI
intervention under investigation. MQS and OLS were then multiplied for each
study, which yielded a weighted score for each study reflecting its contribution

TABLE 16.1a. Basic Characteristics of Controlled Clinical Trials of AMIs for Alcohol Problems

Study	Setting	Sample characteristics			Intervention type (no. of sessions)	Use of the AMI	Comparison group(s)	Therapist(s) training	Intervention quality control	Measurement type/target	Follow-up interval (% completion)
		Size	Gender (M/F)	Severity							
1*	Psych hospital	28	21/7	AD	AS (1) + MIFB (1) + RT	P	RT	MI	None*	BEH/drinking	3 mo (89%)
2*	VA outpatient SAC	32	30/2	MA	AS (1) + MIFB (1) + SO	P	AP + SO	MI	AUD + COD	BEH/drinking	3 mo (81%) 6 mo (72%)
3	College campus	60	26/34	CB	MIFB (1)	S	No treatment	MI	SUP	BEH/drinking + BEH/ARP + PRO/perceived norms and expectancies	6 wk (98%)
4	College campus	348	160/188	CH	MIFB (1) At 1 yr: MF + possible (10%) MIFB (1)	S	No treatment	AMI	OBS + SUP + MAN	BEH/drinking + BEH/ARP	6 mo 12 mo 2 yr (88%) 3 yr (>80%) 4 yr (83%)
5	Trauma center	762	625/137	SM (83%)	MIFB (1) + SL	S	No treatment	MI	None	BEH/drinking + BEH/ARP	6 mo (74%) 12 mo (53%) 3 yr (on ARP)
6*	SAC	42	30/12	SC	1: AS (2 hr DCU) + MIFB (1) 2: Same + RL	S	6 wk WL then same treatment as I	MI	None*	BEH/drinking	6 wk (93%) 18 mo (76%)
7*	SAC	42	24/18	SC	AS (2 hr DCU) + MIFB (1)	S	1: AS + CFB 2: 6 wk WL then same treatment as I	MI	AUD + COD + OBS + SUP	BEH/drinking + PRO/therapist style	6 wk (100%) 12 mo (83%)

(continued)

221

TABLE 16.1a. (*continued*)

Study	Setting	Size	Gender (M/F)	Severity	Intervention type (no. of sessions)	Use of the AMI	Comparison group(s)	Therapist(s) training	Intervention quality control	Measurement type/target	Follow-up interval (% completion)
			Sample characteristics								
8	Hospital ER	94	60/34	ARE	MIFB (1) + IP + RL	S	5 min talk + IP + RL	MI	RS + VID + SUP	BEH/drinking + BEH/ARP + RC	6 mo (89%)
9*	Prenatal clinic	42	0/42	Varied	MIFB (1)	S	IL	MI	None*	BEH/drinking + RC^l	2 mo (81%)
10*	General hospital	174	174/0	HD	MIFB (1)	S	1: SBC 2: No treatment	MI	AUD + MAN^{SBC}	BEH/drinking + ATI/RC	6 mo (70%)
11a*	5 outpatient SACs	952	688/264	AD or AA	MET (4)	S	1: CBT 2: TSF	MET or CBT or TSF	VID + COD + MAN + SUP	BEH/drinking + ARP + PRO/ therapist style + ATI/RC and others	3 mo 6 mo 9 mo 12 mo 15 mo (90%) 3 yr (85%)
11b*	5 outpatient SACs	774	619/155	AD or AA + IT	MET (4)	S/FU	1: CBT 2: TSF	MET or CBT or TSF	VID + COD + MAN + SUP	BEH/drinking + ARP + PRO/ therapist style + ATI/RC and others	3 mo 6 mo 9 mo 12 mo 15 mo (90%)

TABLE 16.1b. Basic Characteristics of Controlled Clinical Trials of AMIs for Smoking, Drug Addiction, HIV Risk Behavior, and Psychiatric Treatment Adherence

Study	Setting	Sample characteristics			Intervention type (no. of sessions)	Use of the AMI	Comparison group(s)	Therapist(s) training	Intervention quality control	Measurement type/target	Follow-up interval (% completion)
		Size	Gender (M/F)	Severity							
12	Hospital	40	17/23	Teen smokers	MIFB (1) + IP	S	BA + IP	MI	None	BEH/smoking + RC	3 mo (95%)
13*	GMP	536	163/373	Adult smokers	MC (1)	S	BA	MI	MAN*	BEH/smoking + ATI/RC	6 mo (78%)
14	EAP sites	89	73/16	DD	MIFB(1)	Possible P	CFB (1)	MI or CFB	MAN + SUP + RS	BEH/substance use + BEH/work performance + RC	3 mo (87%) 9 mo (71%)
15	Hospital	23	15/8	DC	MIFB (1) + Partial RT	P	SI (1) + Partial RT	MI	None	BEH/substance use + BEH/treatment participation	12 weeks (26%)
16	SAC	192	136/56	IDU	MID (5)	P	RR (5)	MI or RR	AUD + COD + RS	BEH/treatment entry	3 mo
17	SAC	122	79/43	HU	MIF (2) + MT	P	ED (2) + MT	MI	MAN	BEH/opiate use + BEH/ORP + RC	3 mo (75%) 6 mo (60%)
18	SAC	291	224/67	MU	MIFB (2)	S	1: RPSG (14) 2: No treat	MI	SUP + CR	BEH/marijuana use + dependence BEH/MRP	1 mo (88%) 4 mo (82%) 7 mo (81%) 13 mo (87%) 16 mo (89%)
19	SAC	95	44/51	IDU	MIHIV (1) + SH + SO	Adjunct to SO	1: MIHIV (1) + RP (5) + SO 2: BA + IP + SO	MI	MAN + AUD + SUP	BEH/HIV risk behaviors	6 mo (84%)
20	SAC	200	159/41	IDU	MIHIV (1) + RPB	S	No treatment	MI	MAN + SUP	BEH/HIV-risk behaviors	3 mo (60%) 6 mo (44%)
21	Hospital	121	77/44	PSY	MIU (2) + SP	Adjunct to SP	SP	MI	SUP	BEH/treatment adherence	First aftercare appointment

223

TABLE 16.1c. Basic Characteristics of Controlled Clinical Trials of AMIs for Diet, Exercise, and Health Behaviors

| Study | Sample characteristics | | | | Intervention type (no. of sessions) | Use of the AMI | Comparison group(s) | Therapist(s) training | Intervention quality control | Measurement type/target | Follow-up interval (% completion) |
	Setting	Size	Gender (M/F)	Severity							
22	Hospital dietary clinic	121	~60/61	HL	MIM (3)	S	SD (3)	Not reported	MAN + AUD + COD	BEH/diet + PHY/weight + PHY/blood lipids + RC	3 mo (80%)
23	GMP	166	~86/80	HBP	1: HMI (6) + IP + SO 2: LMI (1) + PMI + BM + IP + SO	Adjunct to SO	SO	BM but no MI training reported	None	PHY/weight + PHY/BP + PHY/dietary salt and Fat + BEH/alcohol and smoking + BEH/exercise	18 wk (80%)
24	GMP	523	217/306	Varied adult patients	1: HMI (6) + BF + IP + RL 2: LMI (1) + BF + IP + RL	Adjunct to BF	BF + IP + RL	MI	None	BEH/physical activity score	12 wk (81%) 1 yr (85%)
25	Outpatient clinic	22	0/22	Older obese NIDDM	MISF (3) + GBT	Adjunct to GBT	GBT	MI	None	BEH/treatment adherence + PHY/glucose control	4 mo (73%)
26	Hospital eating disorders clinic	125	0/125	BN	Adapted MET (4)	Possible P	Adapted CBT (4)	MET and CBT	MAN + SUP	BEH/binging + BEH/purging + RC	4 wk (54%)

Notes for Tables 16.1a–16.1c. See references at end of chapter for the list of studies by number.

Studies 11a and 11b are the two different samples of Project MATCH (outpatient and aftercare, respectively). Studies marked with an asterisk (*) involve one of the founders of motivational interviewing (Miller or Rollnick) as an investigator.

Setting: EAP, employee assistance programs; ER, emergency room; GMP, general medical practice; SAC, substance abuse clinic; VA, Veterans Administration

Sample characteristics/Severity: AA, alcohol abuse according to DSM-III-R (DSM, *Diagnostic and Statistical Manual of Mental Disorders*); AD, alcohol dependence according to DSM-III-R; ARE, in emergency room following an alcohol-related event; BN, women with bulimia nervosa according to DSM-IV; CB, college students reporting "binge drinking"; CH, college students reporting "heavy drinking"; DC, diagnosis of substance abuse or dependence with a comorbid mood or psychotic disorder; DD, diagnosis of substance abuse or dependence (with no comorbidity) according to DSM-III-R; HBP, hypertensive (high blood pressure) patients; HD, heavy drinkers as operationalized by > 28 standard drinks/week; HL, patients with hyperlipidemia (total serum cholesterol > 5.2 mmol/liter); HU, heroin users with no polydrug use; IDU, injecting drug users; IT, inpatient treatment of at least 7 days' duration for alcohol-related problems; MA, Michigan Alcoholism Screening Test (MAST; Selzer, 1971) score ≥ 10 ("clinically severe"); MU, marijuana users with no polydrug use; NIDDM, non-insulin-dependent diabetes mellitus patients; PSY, psychiatric inpatients, most (75%) with a mood or psychotic disorder (according to DSM-IV) and a comorbid substance disorder; SC, self-concerned drinkers answering a study-recruitment advertisement; SM, Short Michigan Alcoholism Screening Test (SMAST; Selzer et al., 1975) score of 3–8 ("intermediate").

Intervention type: AS, Drinker's Check-Up (DCU; Miller et al., 1988) or similar assessment device that constitutes part of the intervention (i.e., beyond mere baseline assessment common to all groups); BM, behavior modification techniques; HMI, "high" AMI involving six 45-minute sessions; LMI, "low" AMI involving one 45-minute session; MC, motivational consulting, a brief AMI developed for the study; MET, motivational enhancement therapy, a manualized, four-session AMI (Miller et al., 1992); MF, mailed feedback; MID, AMI for injecting drug users, five 30-minute sessions with no specific feedback component; MIF, AMI for heroin users, a 1-hour session plus a 15-minute follow-up 1 week later (Saunders et al., 1991); MIFB, feedback delivered in a motivational interviewing style; MIHIV, AMI for HIV risk reduction (Baker & Dixon, 1991); MIM, AMI for medical settings (Rollnick et al., 1992); MISF, AMI with some feedback component; MIU, AMI with feedback on URICA (McConnaughy et al., 1989) results; PMI, AMI over the telephone, five 15-minute sessions; RPB, relapse prevention booklet; SH, self-help booklet; SL, summary letter (handwritten) sent 1 month after the intervention; BF, GBT, IP, MT, RL, RT, SO, and SP, see Comparison group for definitions.

Use of the AMI: Adjunct, AMI used as a supplement to other clinical services; FU, AMI used as a follow-up to residential care; P, AMI used as a prelude or preparation for further treatment; S, AMI used as a stand-alone treatment; BF, GBT, SO, and SP, see Comparison group for definitions.

Comparison group: AP, attention-placebo interview, which included some feedback; BA, Brief advice (~5 minutes) to quit smoking or to reduce HIV risk behaviors; BF, brief feedback with normative comparison (regarding exercise levels); CBT, cognitive-behavioral skills therapy (12 sessions); CFB, feedback delivered in a confrontative style; ED, education on opiate-related information, a 1-hour session plus a 15-minute follow-up; GBT, group behavior therapy, a 16-week weight-control program; I, intervention group; IL, informational letter regarding risks of drinking during pregnancy; IP, informational pamphlets/bibliotherapy; MT, methadone clinic, standard treatment; RL, resource list (e.g., treatment agencies, leisure centers); RP, relapse prevention, individual sessions (Marlatt & Gordon, 1985); RPSG, relapse prevention support groups (Stephens et al., 1994); RR, risk reduction, an intervention focusing on a hierarchy of safer injecting practices; RT, residential treatment for alcohol addiction; SBC, brief skills-based counseling; SD, standard dietary intervention; SI, standard preadmission interview and hospital program description; SO, standard outpatient treatment; SP, standard inpatient psychiatric treatment (lasting an average of 14 days); TSF, twelve-step facilitation therapy (12 sessions); WL, waiting list; AS and MIHIV, see Intervention type for definitions.

Therapist(s) training: AMI, adaptation of motivational interviewing; MI, motivational interviewing; BM and MET, see Intervention type for definitions; CBT, RR, and TSF, see Comparison group for definitions.

Intervention quality control: AUD, sessions audiotaped for quality control; COD, session content coded by independent raters; CR, client rating of sessions; MAN, manualized intervention; OBS, therapist(s) observed by peers/supervisors; RS, rating of sessions performed routinely; SUP, ongoing supervision provided to therapist(s); VID, sessions videotaped for quality control.

Measurement type/target: ARP, alcohol-related problems; ATI, client attribute measures; BEH, behavioral measures; BP, blood pressure; I, intervention group; MRP, marijuana-related problems; ORP, opiate-related problems; PHY, physiological measures; PRO, process measures; RC, readiness-for-change measures.

225

to outcome according to its methodological quality. We then summed the cross-product points from all of the studies to derive the Cumulative Evidence Score (CES) for the efficacy of AMIs in each domain, as shown in Tables 16.2a–16.2c. For comparative purposes, Table 16.2d presents a summary of the evidence for the efficacy of several specific treatments for alcohol problems (taken from Miller et al., 1998) alongside the evidence for AMIs in this same domain (from Table 16.2a).

Thus, the cumulative evidence from controlled clinical trials provides strong support for the efficacy of AMIs in treating alcohol problems (CES = +222), with 11 of 12 samples showing positive results. In other problem areas, however, the evidence is less conclusive. Of 10 AMI studies in the domain of smoking, drug addiction, HIV risk behaviors, and psychiatric treatment adherence, five yielded positive outcomes (OLS), with a total CES of –12. Four of five clinical trials for diet, exercise, and other health behaviors showed support for the potential efficacy of AMIs in this realm (CES = + 62).

When AMIs are compared to other common treatments for alcohol problems (Table 16.2d), the results are extremely favorable: AMIs have the highest cumulative evidence total among these different treatment approaches (e.g., CES = +222 for AMIs versus +120 for social skills training and +22 for cognitive therapy). The weight of evidence from controlled clinical trials, corrected for methodological quality, therefore provides good support for the efficacy of AMIs in the treatment of alcohol problems.

DO AMIs WORK?: A QUALITATIVE OUTCOME REVIEW

Although we have just summarized a more quantitative approach to evaluating the efficacy of AMI clinical trials, it is also valuable to consider these studies from a qualitative perspective. In this way, common themes can be highlighted and the most notable studies can be explored in depth in order to give the reader a palpable sense of the current state of clinical research related to motivational interviewing.

AMIs for Alcohol Problems

Nearly half of the studies in this review (11 of 26) have been conducted in the domain of alcohol problems. Two of these (Bien et al., 1993; Brown & Miller, 1993) used an AMI as a prelude to further clinical treatment, while the other nine studies used an AMI as a stand-alone treatment.

AMIs as Treatment Preludes

Brown and Miller (1993) investigated the efficacy of an AMI as preparation for entering residential treatment for alcoholism. The AMI group received an additional (post-baseline) assessment session, followed by a second session in

TABLE 16.2a. Summary of Evidence for the Efficacy of
AMIs for Alcohol Problems

Study	MQS	OLS	CES
1*	10	+2	+20
2*	13	+2	+26
3	9	+2	+18
4	13	+2	+26
5	12	+2	+24
6*	8	−2	−16
7*	14	+2	+28
8	13	+2	+26
9*	9	+2	+18
10*	9	+2	+18
11a*	17	+1	+17
11b*	17	+1	+17
Total CES			+222

TABLE 16.2b. Summary of Evidence for the Efficacy of
AMIs for Smoking, Drug Addiction, HIV Risk Behavior,
and Psychiatric Treatment Adherence

Study	MQS	OLS	CES
12	10	−2	−20
13*	10	+1	+10
14	9	−1	−9
15	6	+1	+6
16	10	−1	−10
17	9	+1	+9
18	14	+2	+28
19	12	−2	−24
20	10	−2	−20
21	9	+2	+18
Total CES			−12

which each person received feedback, in an empathic style, on his or her assessment results. Measurement included pretreatment and postdischarge questionnaires (e.g., the Alcohol Use Inventory [AUI]; Horn, Wanberg, & Foster, 1990; the Brief Drinker Profile [BDP] and the Follow-up Drinker Profile [FDP]; Miller & Marlatt, 1987). As in many of the studies reviewed here, alcohol consumption was converted into standard ethanol content (SEC) units, with one unit equivalent to one-half ounce of ethanol (Miller, Heather, & Hall, 1991), while peak weekly blood alcohol concentration (BAC) levels were projected from self-reported consumption by computer program (Markham, Miller, & Archiniega, 1993) as a reflection of intoxication levels.

TABLE 16.2c. Summary of Evidence for the Efficacy of AMIs for Diet, Exercise, and Health Behaviors

Study	MQS	OLS	CES
22	10	−2	−20
23[H]	8	+2	+16
23[L]	8	+2	+16
24[H]	11	+1	+11
24[L]	11	+1	+11
25	10	+2	+20
26	8	+1	+8
Total CES[†]			+62

TABLE 16.2d. Summary of Evidence for the Efficacy of Specific Treatment Methods for Alcohol Problems

Modality	Average MQS	No. of studies with positive OLS	No. of studies with negative OLS	Total CES
AMIs	11.33	11	1	+222
Social skills training[A]	10.94	11	6	+120
Community reinforcement approach[A]	13.25	4	0	+80
GABA agonist medication[A]	12.00	3	0	+72
Cognitive Therapy[A]	10.26	3	4	+22
Self-help manual[A]	12.00	2	3	+1
Placebo medication[A]	13.00	1	2	−27

Notes for Tables 16.2a–16.2d. See references at end of the chapter for the list of studies by number. Studies 11a and 11b are the two different samples of Project MATCH (outpatient and aftercare, respectively). A, adapted from Miller et al. (1998); CES, Cumulative Evidence Score; H, "high" AMI intervention group in the study; L, "low" AMI intervention group in the study; MQS, Methodological Quality Score; OLS, Outcome Logic Score. Studies marked with an asterisk (*) involve one of the founders of motivational interviewing (Miller or Rollnick) as an investigator. †Two studies in this area (23 and 24) contribute a disproportionate amount of cumulative evidence points to the CES total, since each of these studies employed two distinct AMI groups ("high" and "low"), which are coded separately for treatment effects (OLS).

Three months after discharge, the overall sample showed substantial improvement on both consumption measures. The AMI clients showed significantly more improvement in SEC (but not BAC) relative to the no-treatment controls. Some 57% of the AMI clients versus 29% of the controls were abstinent from drinking 3 months postdischarge.

Bien and colleagues (1993) compared two sessions of an AMI (involving detailed assessment and feedback, as in Brown and Miller, 1993) to an attention-placebo condition in which only brief feedback was provided, along with information about the VA alcohol treatment program. Subsequently, all clients received the standard outpatient treatment (group therapy based on a twelve-step model) available through the Veterans Administration. At 3-month follow-up, the AMI group showed significant reductions on a composite drinking variable relative to the control group, but these differences were no longer significant at 6-month follow-up, probably due to a combination of the AMI group relapsing and the control group catching up.

Both of these studies (Bien et al., 1993; Brown & Miller, 1993) recruited clients in the clinically severe range of alcohol addiction, and both found evidence supporting an AMI as a treatment prelude at 3-month follow-up. Interestingly, the AMI intervention yielded positive outcomes in each study, despite its use as a prelude to a considerably more confrontative treatment approach.

AMIs as Stand-Alone Treatments Compared to No-Treatment Controls

A minimum requirement for demonstrating treatment efficacy is to show that a treatment is more efficacious than the passage of time and reactive effects of measurement. In the area of alcohol problems, six such studies have been published using an AMI as a stand-alone treatment compared to no-treatment controls (Borsari & Carey, 2000; Gentilello et al., 1999; Heather, Rollnick, Bell, & Richmond, 1996; Marlatt et al., 1998; Miller et al., 1988; Miller, Benefield, & Tonigan, 1993). The subject populations have been rather diverse, including high-risk (Marlatt et al., 1998) and binge drinkers (Borsari & Carey, 2000); college students and community samples recruited for drinking feedback (Miller et al., 1988, 1993); patients in a general hospital identified as problem drinkers (Heather et al., 1996); and patients who were hospitalized through the emergency room for alcohol-related accidents (Gentilello et al., 1999).

Five of these studies (all except Miller et al., 1988) demonstrated clear differences between AMIs and no-treatment controls on drinking consumption at short-term (6 weeks) and even longer-term (3 years) follow-ups. Furthermore, while Miller and colleagues (1988) did not report any significant differences *between* the AMI and no-treatment groups at 6-week follow-up, those receiving the AMI did show significant *within-group* reductions in alcohol consumption (SEC) and peak intoxication levels (BAC) through 18 months of follow-up. With some exceptions, these results support the efficacy of AMIs as stand-alone treatments for alcohol problems. We will highlight two of these studies that are particularly noteworthy below.

To evaluate the efficacy of an AMI to reduce the harmful consequences of heavy drinking among college students, Marlatt and colleagues (1998) recruited 506 high-risk college freshmen who were randomly assigned to either a brief AMI or a no-treatment control. The brief AMI intervention, developed by the authors for the college population, involved a single session of drinking-related feedback in a motivational interviewing style, as well as education about alcohol and its effects. After 1 year, those participants whose drinking was considered to be high-risk were given a second AMI feedback session, either by telephone or face-to-face.

Standardized measures of drinking rates, alcohol dependence, and alcohol-related problems were taken, including ratings by collaterals (i.e., significant others in the client's life). While both treatment and no-treatment groups showed improvements at 2-year follow-up, the treatment clients showed significantly greater improvement on both drinking rates and harmful consequences that was maintained at 4-year follow-up (Baer, Kivlahan, Blume, McKnight, & Marlatt, 2001).

Gentilello and colleagues (1999) studied the effects of an AMI on 762 trauma center patients who screened positive for problematic alcohol consumption, using serum measures and the Short Michigan Alcoholism Screening Test (SMAST; Selzer, Vinokur, & Van Rooijen, 1975). The intervention consisted of a single, half-hour feedback session delivered in a motivational interviewing style, in addition to a handwritten letter mailed 1 month later that summarized the session. The study employed two main outcome measures: alcohol consumption and trauma recurrence after hospital discharge.

After 6 months, alcohol intake was significantly reduced in both groups, with no significant between-group differences. At the 12-month follow-up point, the AMI group showed significantly lower weekly alcohol intake than the no-treatment controls. The high attrition (largely due to loss to follow-up) for alcohol consumption assessment (almost 50% at 12-month follow-up) must be borne in mind, however, when interpreting these results.

Trauma recidivism was assessed using a statewide database of emergency department records to detect a return of study patients to the hospital with a new injury. After up to 3 years of follow-up, there was a 48% reduction in hospital admissions for new injuries in the AMI group compared to controls, although this result failed to reach statistical significance.

This study, the first to examine the use of a brief AMI in a trauma center, points to the benefits that AMIs may have in the potentially teachable window after injury. Alcohol consumption was significantly reduced in the AMI group, and, perhaps most importantly, the AMI treatment showed potential to have a lasting (3-year) effect on a socially significant outcome variable—trauma recidivism. While the recidivism measure was crude in the sense that an in-state hospital readmission does not necessarily imply an alcohol-related injury, the measure was nevertheless objective and ecologically valid, which suggests that the inclusion of a single AMI session in trauma centers may have a major effect on the long-term health and future injury risk of such patients.

AMIs as Stand-Alone Treatments Compared to Alternative Treatments

In five of the clinical trials involving AMIs for alcohol problems, the AMI was used as a stand-alone treatment and compared to some other type of treatment. The apparent credibility of these alternative interventions was highly varied. In two studies, the alternatives were weak, consisting either of a 5-minute informational interview with pamphlets and a resource list of alcohol-related services given to participants (Monti, Colby, Barnett, Spirito, &

Rohsenow, 1999), or a brief informational letter describing the risks of drinking during pregnancy (Handmaker, Miller, & Manicke, 1999). In three other studies (Heather et al., 1996; Miller et al., 1993; Project MATCH Research Group, 1997b), the alternative treatments were at least equal in length to the AMI interventions tested. One of these studies (Miller et al., 1993) employed a confrontative feedback session of the same duration as the AMI, while another study (Heather et al., 1996) compared one session of an AMI to one session of a skills-based counseling approach. The strongest comparison of an AMI to alternative treatments was in Project MATCH (1997b), in which four sessions of motivational enhancement therapy (MET; Miller, Zweben, DiClemente, & Rychtarik, 1992) were compared to two empirically supported, 12-session treatments—cognitive-behavioral skills therapy (CBT; Kadden et al., 1992) and twelve-step facilitation therapy (TSF; Nowinski, Baker, & Carroll, 1992).

Not surprisingly, the two studies that compared an AMI to briefer and seemingly less credible alternatives yielded some positive results for the AMI. Monti and colleagues (1999) found that, relative to the comparison treatment, a single 35- to 40-minute session of an AMI delivered in the emergency room after an alcohol-related event significantly reduced several key alcohol-related problems, such as drinking and driving, moving violations, and alcohol-related injuries in the 6 months following the initial emergency room visit. However, this same study did not find any significant group differences in actual alcohol use outcomes at 6-month follow-up. Handmaker and colleagues (1999) studied pregnant drinkers (mild to heavy) and determined that, among women with the highest intoxication levels, an AMI significantly lowered BAC at 2-month follow-up relative to an informational letter, but SEC and total days abstinent were not significantly different between the groups. Overall, then, there appears to be empirical support for the efficacy of AMIs as stand-alone treatments when compared to either no-treatment controls (as in the previous section) or to weak alternatives.

When AMIs have been compared to more viable alternative treatments, however, the AMIs have fared equally well but not better. A study by Miller and colleagues (1993) failed to detect any significant differences between the two intervention groups under investigation—feedback delivered in either a motivational interviewing or a confrontative style—at any follow-up point. Heather and colleagues (1996) also found no significant differences in outcome between participants on general hospital wards who received an AMI and those who instead received a similar quantity of skills-based counseling. Project MATCH (1997b), the largest psychotherapy outcome study conducted to date, found no significant differences between the three treatments tested.

Due to its magnitude, scope, and powerful design, Project MATCH (1997b) will be described in more detail here. The project actually consisted of two separate samples, one involving 952 clients in five outpatient substance abuse clinics, and the other involving 774 clients receiving aftercare treatment following an episode of inpatient or intensive day hospital treatment (i.e., as a follow-up to residential care). The overall objective of each study was to determine whether various subgroups of alcohol-dependent clients would respond differently to three manual-guided, individual treatments.

The AMI in this study was motivational enhancement therapy (MET; Miller et al., 1992), which involved four sessions offered at weeks 1, 2, 6, and 12. The first two sessions consisted of a Drinker's Check-Up (DCU; Miller et al., 1988) combining the clinical style of motivational interviewing with structured personal feedback of the client's assessment results, leading to an individualized change plan. The third and fourth sessions served as check-in visits to review progress, renew motivation for change, and revise the change plan as necessary. Cognitive-behavioral skills therapy (CBT; Kadden et al., 1992), based on social learning theory, views drinking as a problem behavior that is related to other major difficulties in the client's life; it emphasizes building skills to increase the ability to cope with situations that are likely to precipitate relapse. Twelve-step facilitation therapy (TSF; Nowinski et al., 1992) is grounded in the Alcoholics Anonymous concept of alcoholism as a spiritual and medical disease, and it attempts to promote abstinence by fostering acceptance of this disease in concert with a willingness to work through the traditional 12 steps to recovery.

Ten client characteristics were selected as primary matching variables, including motivational readiness to change (measured by URICA; DiClemente & Hughes, 1990) and social support for drinking versus abstinence (measured by the Important People and Activities Instrument; Longabaugh, Wirtz, & Clifford, 1995), as well as secondary matching variables such as readiness to change (measured by the Stages of Change Readiness and Treatment Eagerness Scale [SOCRATES]; Miller, 1992) and anger (measured by the Anger Scale; Spielberger, 1988).

The two primary outcome measures, percentage of days abstinent (PDA) and average number of drinks per drinking day (DDD), were derived from Form 90 (Miller, 1996a), an interview-based assessment device that uses both time-line follow-back methodology (Sobell & Sobell, 1992) and drinking pattern estimation procedures from the Comprehensive Drinker Profile (Miller & Marlatt, 1984). Collateral informants and laboratory tests were employed to monitor changes in client alcohol consumption and to corroborate the self-reported drinking measures. Attrition was low in both samples studied, with data for 85% of clients collected at all follow-up points.

Treatment integrity was clearly safeguarded in this study: All therapists were carefully trained, treatment sessions were monitored by videotape, and therapist behaviors were evaluated by independent raters who were unaware of treatment assignment. In this way, the authors were able to determine that treatment adherence and discriminability among treatments were high, exposure to non-study treatments was minimal, and treatments were comparable with respect to nonspecific dimensions such as working alliance and therapist skill.

At follow-ups conducted from 3 months to 3 years after the first therapy session, participants in all treatment groups showed significant improvements on all drinking measures, with no consistent differences between the groups. There was weak support for the hypothesis that treatment efficacy would be enhanced by matching clients with certain attributes to particular treatment modalities. These matching results from Project MATCH are discussed in further detail later in this chapter.

Project MATCH employed a comprehensive set of outcome measures to assess depression, drinking consequences, percentage of days of paid work, and other life variables that may be affected by alcohol consumption. All of these measures showed improvement in both samples (outpatient and aftercare), with no significant differences between treatment groups. At 15-month follow-up, 43% of clients in the aftercare sample showed substantial improvement (i.e., a reduction in both drinking and related problems), while 52% of the outpatient sample attained this criterion. In both samples, about 35% to 40% of clients did not show any noticeable improvement. In the outpatient sample, for which MET, CBT, and TSF were the only treatments provided, 30% of the clients were abstinent from alcohol at the 3-year follow-up point, while those who did drink were nevertheless abstinent two-thirds of the time in the 90 days before the 3-year interview.

Project MATCH did not have a no-treatment control group, since its primary intention was to investigate treatment matching rather than to test comparative efficacy. Although this limits conclusions about how well the treatments worked on an absolute basis, it remains noteworthy that AMI produced positive outcomes on drinking and related variables with a clinically severe population. Furthermore, AMI performed as well as CBT and TSF, two empirically supported and substantially longer treatment approaches.

AMIs for Alcohol Problems: Discussion

There is cause for optimism regarding the value of AMIs in the treatment of alcohol problems. In general, AMIs have yielded noticeable effects in this domain with relatively small interventions (often no more than a session or two). Furthermore, the positive results of the AMI interventions are sometimes seen as soon 6 weeks posttreatment (e.g., Borsari & Carey, 2000; Miller et al., 1993) and are detectable in follow-ups of up to 4 years (Marlatt et al., 1998).

Moreover, most of these studies have been methodologically rigorous. Almost all of the studies (except Brown & Miller, 1993, and Heather et al., 1996) used true randomization as a means of equating groups of clients before treatment. The dependent measures were focused and precise, targeting pertinent areas of outcome (i.e., alcohol consumption) directly, while some studies also employed secondary outcome measures of auxiliary drinking behaviors and drinking-related consequences. In all of these studies except for Monti and colleagues (1999), Borsari and Carey (2000), and Gentilello and colleagues (1999), the main dependent variables were collateralized so that self-report drinking data could be corroborated, with collateral and self-report measures generally showing high correlations (e.g., correlations exceeding .90 in Brown & Miller, 1993). Furthermore, the majority of alcohol consumption measures used in the studies were derived from self-report questionnaires that have shown good reliability and validity in previous research (e.g., Form 90, Tonigan et al., 1997; AUI, Skinner & Allen, 1983), as well as consistency with laboratory-derived, biological consumption markers (e.g., O'Farrell & Maisto, 1987; Project MATCH, 1997b). Finally, with but one exception (Gentilello et al., 1999), there has been little subject attrition.

In addition to being a sound design aspect, the measurement of collaterals constitutes a key element of these AMI studies: If important others are noticing the client's change in alcohol consumption, then this is likely to be a meaningful change. Moreover, clinical significance is bolstered by the frequent findings that reduction in consumption is associated with other key behavior changes like decreased hospital visits for alcohol-related trauma (Gentilello et al., 1999; Monti et al., 1999), reduced moving violations (Monti et al., 1999), less absence from work (Project MATCH, 1997b), and improved social functioning (Marlatt et al., 1998). These results show promise for AMIs as an intervention with broad-based effects that can precipitate widespread life changes beyond the target problem (Miller, Hedrick, & Taylor, 1983).

Taken together, these studies provide evidence for the clinical utility of AMIs with problem drinkers in a variety of settings—hospitals (Brown & Miller, 1993; Gentilello et al., 1999; Heather et al., 1996; Monti et al., 1999), outpatient clinics (Handmaker et al., 1999; Miller et al., 1993; Project MATCH, 1997b), and even college campuses (Borsari & Carey, 2000; Marlatt et al., 1998)—as well as with both men and women. While selection criteria have varied across studies, most have employed participants who were having serious life problems relating to their alcohol use.

One major shortcoming in most of these studies bears further scrutiny. While the dependent variables are clearly specified in almost all studies, the independent variables—the AMI treatments under investigation—are often vague and imprecise. Treatment fidelity, or how fairly and faithfully a treatment is represented (Kazdin, 1992), is difficult to ascertain because of the paucity of adequate treatment manuals for the AMIs. With the exception of Project MATCH (1997b) and Marlatt and colleagues (1998), the vast majority of studies simply referred to the first edition of this book (Miller & Rollnick, 1991) as the AMI intervention under study. However, as the authors of this book point out, learning motivational interviewing is not merely a matter of reading *about* it (see Chapter 13 in this volume).

Furthermore, treatment integrity, or whether the therapeutic procedures were carried out as intended (Kazdin, 1992), was rarely assessed in these studies. In most cases, training procedures were not carefully described, while integrity checks to measure the implementation of treatment—including videotaping, ongoing supervision, and coding of actual therapist behaviors—were entirely absent from several studies (Brown & Miller, 1993; Gentilello et al., 1999; Handmaker et al., 1999; Miller et al., 1988). Finally, the issue of treatment credibility (whether therapists and clients found the intervention believable) was alluded to only occasionally (e.g., Bien et al., 1993) and was never systematically addressed in any study. Thus, while all of the studies included in this review appeared to have ample treatment fidelity (i.e., the four basic elements of motivational interviewing) in theory, it is impossible to ascertain whether these principles were in fact translated into treatment integrity in clinical practice.

AMIs for Cigarette Smoking

To date, only two controlled clinical trials of AMIs for smoking have been published. Colby and colleagues (1998) compared 5 minutes of advice to quit smoking to a 30-minute AMI for adolescent smokers. Although the results at 3-month follow-up favored the AMI on all measures, none of the comparisons were significant.

Butler and colleagues (1999) studied adult smokers drawn from general medical practices.[5] Similar to Colby and colleagues (1998), the comparison group received brief authoritarian style advice to quit smoking. While both interventions (AMI and advice) were precisely described and manualized (Rollnick et al., 1992), no integrity checks were performed to ensure that the treatment was in fact delivered according to the manual. At 6-months follow-up, the AMI group showed significantly greater improvements than the advice group in four of the eight outcome variables, including decreased smoking in the previous 24 hours, increased delay in time to first cigarette of the day, increased attempts to quit lasting a week or more during the follow-up period, and movement to a more advanced stage of change. However, there were no significant differences between groups on measures that would more powerfully affect the clients' health, such as abstinence rates in the previous month, reduction in the number of cigarettes smoked, and overall quit attempts. On the whole, only 4% of the participants in the study actually quit smoking.

Due to the paucity of studies on AMIs for smoking and the relatively small effects obtained therein, empirical support for the efficacy of AMIs in this area is lacking at the present time and awaits further study.

AMIs for Other Drugs of Abuse

Five studies have been published on the efficacy of AMIs for other drugs of abuse (Booth, Kwiatkowski, Iguchi, Pinto, & John, 1998; Martino, Carroll, O'Malley, & Rounsaville, 2000; Saunders, Wilkinson, & Philips, 1995; Schneider, Casey, & Kohn, 2000; Stephens, Roffman, & Curtin, 2000). Four of these studies (all but Stephens et al., 2000) investigated the utility of an AMI as a prelude to further treatment. Key dependent variables in these four studies included treatment participation (Martino et al., 2000), treatment entry (Booth et al., 1998; Schneider et al., 2000), or intention to seek treatment (Saunders et al., 1995). All four studies used comparison treatments of the same length as the AMI being tested. Two of these alternative treatments appeared to be quite viable (Booth et al., 1998; Schneider et al., 2000), whereas the other two did not (Martino et al., 2000; Saunders et al., 1995). Two of these studies (Saunders et al., 1995; Schneider et al., 2000) employed a specific treatment manual, while two (Booth et al., 1998; Schneider et al., 2000) included extensive intervention quality control such as ongoing treatment integrity checks.

The two studies that compared AMIs to viable alternative treatments (Booth et al., 1998; Schneider et al., 2000) showed quite positive outcomes for the AMI, although there were no significant between-group differences in either study. Schneider et al. (2000) gave substance abusers feedback about their drug use that was delivered in either a motivational interviewing (AMI) or a confrontative style (CI). More than half of the clients subsequently sought additional treatment. In addition, both groups showed significant and equivalent improvements on all substance use measures, with 21% of AMI and 19% of CI clients abstinent after 9 months, as well as significant reductions in the adverse effects of alcohol or drugs on work performance.

Booth and colleagues (1998) studied the effects of an AMI on street-recruited, multiple-injecting drug users. The AMI consisted of five 30-minute counseling sessions focused on the resolution of ambivalence, increasing discrepancy between goals and present drug use, a pro-con drug worksheet, and a specific suggestion of treatment entry as one of a menu of viable options.[6] The comparison group received a similar duration of risk reduction (RR), an intervention that emphasized a hierarchy of safer injecting practices. The main dependent variable was whether clients entered treatment, which was operationally defined as completing the intake procedure for the substance abuse clinic involved in the study. After 3 months, a substantial percentage of clients in both groups entered treatment, but there was no significant difference between conditions: 40% of the AMI and 43% of the RR clients entered treatment.

Two problems with this study must be considered. First, because this study included intervention quality checks (e.g., 40% of sessions were audiotaped and content-coded by independent raters), the authors were able to discover that the AMI was not being properly delivered.[7] Second, treatment entry, the main outcome measure in this study, was not adequately assessed: It consisted only of ascertaining whether a participant filled out an intake form at a single substance abuse clinic, without taking into account actual follow-through or applications to other treatment clinics.

Both studies that compared AMIs to less credible alternative treatments (Martino et al., 2000; Saunders et al., 1995) produced some positive results for the AMIs. Martino and colleagues (2000) gave a single session of an AMI to dually-diagnosed clients who were seeking admission to a partial hospital treatment plan, while control participants received a standard preadmission interview of similar duration. Twelve weeks after discharge from the hospital program, the AMI group was superior to the controls on several measures (less tardiness and early departures throughout the hospital treatment program), but not on measures that reflected actual drug use.

Saunders and colleagues (1995) recruited heroin-dependent drug users who were attending a methadone clinic and provided them with either an AMI or education. Both interventions consisted of one session with a brief follow-up or review session 1 week later. The AMI was adapted by the authors as described in the first edition of this book (Saunders et al., 1991) and included a one-page "decision matrix" regarding the consequences of opiate use.[8] The control condition was an education-based interview in which clients were given drug-related information and referrals in each session. At 6-month follow-up, only two outcome variables attained between-group significance: Compared to controls, the AMI group showed both a decrease in opiate-related problems and greater treatment compliance.

AMI as a Stand-Alone Treatment

Only one study investigated an AMI as a stand-alone treatment for substance abuse (Stephens et al., 2000). In this study, adult marijuana users were assigned either to a delayed treatment control group or to one of the following treatment conditions: two individual sessions of an AMI (which also included cognitive-behavioral strategies) or 14 cognitive-behavioral group therapy sessions based on the relapse prevention model (Stephens, Roffman, & Simpson, 1994). While there were no significant differences between the two intervention groups at any follow-up, both groups showed significantly reduced marijuana use and dependence, fewer marijuana-related problems, and increased abstinence relative to controls (37% versus only 9% for controls). Further, participants in the AMI group were using marijuana less than half as many days at the 16-month follow-up point as they were before treatment. Overall, this well-designed study suggests that a brief course of an AMI may be more efficacious than no treatment and equally efficacious as extended group therapy for a marijuana-dependent population.

In summary, then, there is evidence for the efficacy of AMIs as a prelude to further treatment for drug-addicted populations. In this context, AMIs have been shown to be as efficacious as credible alternatives (Booth et al., 1998; Schneider et al., 2000) and superior to less viable comparison groups (Martino et al., 2000; Saunders et al., 1995). As a stand-alone intervention for marijuana users, one study showed that a relatively brief AMI is as efficacious as more extensive group therapy and significantly more efficacious than no treatment (Stephens et al., 2000).

AMIs for Psychiatric Treatment Adherence in Dually Diagnosed Patients

Only two published studies have addressed the question of whether AMIs are efficacious for dually diagnosed patients—those with concomitant psychiatric and substance use disorders. Martino and colleagues (2000), also discussed in the preceding section, provided some support for the use of an AMI as a preparatory treatment to improve hospital program adherence among psychiatrically ill substance abusers.

Swanson, Pantalon, and Cohen (1999) examined the effects of an AMI for dually diagnosed inpatients, all of whom received the usual hospital treatment that averaged 14 days. One group received an AMI as an adjunct to these clinical services, while the remaining group served as a control. The AMI included a 15-minute session of feedback and discussion on stage of change scores (as assessed by URICA; DiClemente & Hughes, 1990) at the beginning of hospitalization. A second AMI session, lasting an hour, was provided a few days before discharge in order to highlight the patient-stated advantages of change and treatment adherence.

Before discharge from the hospital, all patients were given a referral to an outpatient psychiatric clinic. A significantly greater percentage of the AMI patients than the control patients (47% versus 21%) attended their first aftercare appointment. Taken together with the results of Martino and colleagues (2000), these findings suggest that the addition of an AMI to an inpatient treatment program may have beneficial effects on treatment adherence for dually diagnosed patients.

AMIs for HIV Risk Behaviors

Only two studies have been published on AMIs for HIV risk reduction, both by the same clinical research team. Baker, Heather, Wodak, Dixon, and Holt (1993) tested an AMI as an adjunct to standard treatment with injecting drug users enrolled in a methadone program. The AMI provided a single session of personal risk feedback, along with a motivational interviewing style discussion of high HIV risk behaviors. The comparison treatment included a single session of an AMI, followed by five sessions of relapse prevention (RP; based on Marlatt & Gordon, 1985) that focused on the acquisition of different skills aimed at helping prevent relapse to injecting and unsafe sex. A control group received only brief advice about HIV risk behaviors and an educational pamphlet, while all groups continued to receive the standard methadone program care.

At 6-month follow-up, there were no significant differences among the three groups on HIV risk behaviors. The group receiving both the AMI and RP, however, did show a significant reduction relative to the other two groups for needle-sharing behaviors in the heaviest risk-taking month. This study included several commendable design features, such as the use of collaterals and objective devices (e.g., urinalysis) to corroborate some of the self-report measures, and sound quality control procedures (manuals, supervision, and audiotaping) of the interventions. However, conclusions from this study must remain tentative because the three groups differed significantly on two key pretreatment measures.

Baker, Kochan, Dixon, Heather, and Wodak (1994) recruited 200 injecting drug users who were not currently involved in any form of treatment for drug dependence. The intervention group received a one-session AMI, along with a relapse prevention booklet of cognitive-behavioral coping strategies. There were no significant differences in outcome between this treatment group and a no-treatment control group, while both groups showed improvements at 6-month follow-up. To date, there is no convincing evidence for the efficacy of AMIs in reducing HIV risk behaviors.

AMIs for Diet, Exercise, and Other Lifestyle Changes

Four studies have been published on the use of AMIs for changes in diet, exercise, or other lifestyle habits. One of these (Mhurchu, Margetts. & Speller, 1998) investigated an AMI as a stand-alone intervention, while three (Harland et al., 1999; Smith, Heckemeyer, Kratt, & Mason, 1997; Woollard et al., 1995) tested an AMI as an adjunct to other treatments (usual medical care, brief feedback, or group therapy). Three studies (Mhurchu et al., 1998; Smith et al., 1997; Woollard et al., 1995) recruited adults with medical problems—hyperlipidemia, hypertension, and diabetes, respectively—in an effort to promote lifestyle changes that could slow the effects of the disease.

Only one of these studies (Mhurchu et al., 1998) used a treatment manual (Rollnick et al., 1992) and took steps to ensure therapist adherence to an AMI model, although the study failed to specify the motivational interviewing training obtained by the dietician who conducted the intervention. The other three studies (Harland et al., 1999; Smith et al., 1997; Woollard et al., 1995) lacked any type of intervention quality control beyond the initial therapist training that was reported in two of them (Harland et al., 1999; Smith et al., 1997).

Mhurchu and colleagues (1998) studied patients with hyperlipidemia. A dietician met with clients for three sessions, providing either an AMI or a standard dietary intervention (advice). At 3-month follow-up, both groups showed significant reductions on a variety of outcome measures—dietary habits, fat intake, and body/mass index (BMI)—but there were no significant differences between the two groups. Furthermore, neither intervention led to significant reductions in serum cholesterol, the main target of the study, although this could be due to the uncertain link between dietary advice and cholesterol levels rather than a failure of the intervention itself.

Harland and colleagues (1999) recruited middle-aged adults from a general medical practice to evaluate the efficacy of an AMI for promoting physical activity. In addition to a no-treatment control, the study also employed two separate AMI groups—one consisting of six sessions and the other of a single session—that aimed to increase exercising without prescribing specific activities. At the 12-week follow-up, both AMI groups showed significant and equivalent improvements compared to the control group, but these gains were not sustained through 1 year of follow-up. Several problems with this study may limit its conclusions, such as the use of self-report measurement with no collateral verification, lack of intervention quality control, and participants in the longer AMI group only appearing for half of their scheduled sessions.

Two other studies provided support for the efficacy of AMIs for people with medical problems (Smith et al., 1997; Woollard et al., 1995). Woollard and colleagues (1995) assigned hypertensive patients under medical care to receive either six sessions of an AMI or a single session with five follow-up telephone contacts. Both AMI groups also received some behavior modification (BM) during their sessions, while a control group received the usual medical care without any AMI or BM. At the 18-week follow-up, both intervention groups did equally well and better than the control group. Relative to controls, the six-session AMI group showed significant reductions in both weight and blood pressure, whereas those in the briefer AMI group significantly decreased their alcohol and salt intake. However, two other behavioral targets—physical activity and smoking—were not significantly altered in any group. This study suffers from a number of limitations, including the absence of integrity checks and treatment manuals, no pure AMI group (only AMI plus BM), and inadequate reporting of AMI training. Nevertheless, the effects reported are clinically significant for an important medical target.

Smith and colleagues (1997) produced positive results for an AMI with older, obese women treated for diabetes. All patients were assigned to a standard, 16-week behavioral weight-control program, while one group also received three sessions of the AMI (which included individualized feedback on glycemic control, cardiovascular risk factor status, and behavioral performance) as an adjunct to the program. Those who received the AMI did significantly better than those who did not, as indicated by increased attendance at group therapy, increased food diary completion, more frequent blood glucose recording, and better glycemic control. These results suggest that augmenting a standard behavioral treatment program with an AMI for obese, diabetic women may significantly enhance treatment adherence and control of the disease.

The evidence for AMIs in the area of diet, exercise, and other lifestyle behaviors is mixed. While two studies (Harland et al., 1999; Mhurchu et al., 1998) found either no or short-lived advantages of AMIs over alternative treatments for changing diet or exercise levels, two other studies (Smith et al., 1997; Woollard et al., 1995) found AMIs to be efficacious as an adjunct to usual medical care or group therapy for improving control of medical illness. The possibility that AMIs can help alter the course of potentially life-threatening physical ailments is clearly noteworthy and merits further study.

AMIs for Eating Disorders

Only one controlled clinical trial has investigated the efficacy of AMIs for eating disorders. In the first phase of their ongoing study, Treasure and colleagues (1999) recruited women with bulimia nervosa and assigned them to four sessions of either an AMI or cognitive-behavioral therapy. Both interventions were manualized and conducted by trained therapists under close supervision, although no specific integrity checks were implemented.

At 4-week follow-up, both groups showed significant but equivalent improvements in self-reported bulimic symptoms, including substantial changes in binge eating and vomiting. While this study is limited by the short follow-up period and high attrition (46%), it also represents a promising start to incorporating AMIs into the treatment of eating disorders, especially given the fact that more than half of the women achieved a clinically significant improvement in just 4 weeks of treatment.

Conclusions Regarding the Efficacy of Motivational Interviewing and AMIs

• *There are no studies evaluating the efficacy of "pure" motivational interviewing, as defined by Miller and Rollnick (1991; this volume). Virtually all of the studies in this review evaluate adaptations of motivational interviewing (what we have called "AMIs") that consist of either problem feedback delivered in a motivational interviewing style or other significant modifications.* For the studies evaluating feedback-based AMIs, we have no clear data examining whether it is the feedback, the motivational interviewing style, or the combination that is necessary for positive outcome. Miller and colleagues (1993) explicitly attempted to tease apart these two components by comparing a feedback intervention delivered in a supportive (motivational interviewing) style with one delivered in a confrontative manner. While short-term follow-up data and post hoc analyses favored the motivational interviewing style, the long-term results showed no significant differences between the two feedback styles.

• *In the areas of alcohol problems and drug addiction, relatively brief AMIs (one to four sessions) have yielded moderate to large effects and good maintenance over time.* This conclusion is supported by quantitative analysis (Burke, Arkowitz, & Menchola, 2001; Dunn et al., 2001), methodological ratings (Table 16.2d), and the qualitative review. As yet there are no data on lengthier AMI interventions, leaving open the question of whether there is a "dose effect." It remains to be determined whether lengthier or more intensive interventions will lead to even better outcomes.

• *In general, AMIs are more efficacious than no treatment, and they are not significantly different from credible alternative treatments.* While not all of the studies have employed comparison treatments that were credible and matched to the AMIs in terms of length, those that have done so (e.g., Booth et al., 1998; Stephens et al., 2000) have found equivalent degrees of change in the AMIs and alternative treatments. Further, some studies have demonstrated that relatively brief AMIs perform as well as longer AMIs and more extensive alternative treatments (Harland et al., 1999; Project MATCH, 1997b).

• *AMIs are efficacious, both as stand-alone treatments and as preludes to other treatments.* In psychotherapy and most of medicine, stand-alone treatments are the rule rather than the exception. To our knowledge, it is rare that a treatment can be efficacious both as a stand-alone treatment and as a prelude or adjunct treatment that enhances the efficacy of a variety of other treatments. Yet this is exactly what some of the research on AMIs suggests, even when the treatments with which it is paired are based on models and techniques quite different from those of the AMIs (Bien et al., 1993; Brown & Miller, 1993).

• *While the majority of outcome studies are in the areas of alcohol problems and drug addiction, there are also studies that support the efficacy of AMIs for people with hypertension, diabetes, dual diagnoses, and eating disorders.* Mixed support has been found for AMIs in the domain of cigarette smoking, increasing physical activity, and enhancing dietary adherence in patients with hyperlipidemia. No support has been found for AMIs in the reduction of HIV risk behaviors.

• *Many of the outcomes of AMIs, especially for alcohol problems, not only have been statistically significant but also appear to be clinically significant.* Although none of the studies performed statistical evaluations of clinical significance (Jacobson, Roberts, Berns, & McGlinchey, 1999), there is good reason to believe that AMIs have had substantial clinical effects. For example, drug and alcohol abstinence rates at follow-up have often been considerable (e.g., 37% in Stephens et al., 2000; 57% in Brown & Miller, 1993). In addition, when one examines those measures that most clearly relate to the clients' lives (e.g., the degree of reduction in substance intake, decreases in substance-related problems, ratings by collaterals), it is often the case that the treatment has had a real effect on the problem behavior (e.g., Project MATCH, 1997b; Saunders et al., 1995).

• *Most of the studies on AMIs are quite strong in external validity.* External validity is the degree to which the results of a study can be generalized or extended to settings, populations, or problems other than those in the particular experimental arrangement (Kazdin, 1992). In many cases, participants were recruited directly from real-life settings (i.e., hospitals and medical practices), and even when newspaper advertisements were used in recruitment, the severity of client problems in these studies generally resembles that of people who might seek treatment outside of a research project. Further, most of the studies have not employed extensive exclusionary criteria for participants, so that the subject populations parallel fairly closely those found in actual clinical practice. Moreover, the physical settings in which treatment takes place in these studies are often the very same clinics that offer these services on a nonresearch clinical basis.

• *The internal validity of AMI studies has been quite variable and often weak.* Internal validity is the ability of the research design to rule out alternative explanations of the results. It deals with such issues as the nature and adequacy of control groups, adequacy of the specification of the independent variable (i.e., replicability), integrity of the treatment, adequacy of measurement of the dependent variables, and the reduction or elimination of possible sources of bias. We will consider each of these separately below.

Nature and adequacy of the control groups. As noted earlier in this section, studies comparing AMIs to alternative treatments sometimes did not adequately match the credibility or lengths of the treatments (e.g., 1 hour of an AMI vs. 5 minutes of advice to change the problem behavior). In fact, none of the studies assessed participants' expectations or perceptions of how effective they thought the AMI was in comparison to the alternative treatment(s). If one treatment can generate more positive expectancies for change, then differences in expectancies rather than differences in the efficacy of the procedures can potentially account for any obtained results.

Adequacy of the specification of the independent variable. The majority of studies were quite weak in this respect, thereby jeopardizing any strong conclusions. In many of the studies, neither the credentials of the treatment providers nor the specific training procedures were adequately described. Further, there was little consistency across studies regarding the nature of the AMI interventions tested (except for the common use of problem feedback), resulting in a puzzling heterogeneity of the AMI interventions under study.

Integrity of treatment. Very few studies included a careful evaluation of treatment integrity—that is, whether the treatment providers were actually administering the AMI as directed and whether this could be detected from their interaction with the client. Further, training procedures were rarely standardized (e.g., guided by a manual).

Adequacy of measurement of the dependent variables. The vast majority of studies have included reliable, well-validated, and standardized self-report instruments for the assessment of outcome. In addition, outcome has been measured in several other modalities, including physiological (e.g., urinalysis) and behavioral (e.g., hospital readmissions) realms, as well as ratings by collaterals. Such multimodal measurement constitutes a real strength of most of the AMI studies.

Reduction or elimination of possible sources of bias. Most of the studies left open the possibility of experimenter bias. Often, the alternative treatments were conducted by research staff who knew that the hypotheses predicted the superiority of the AMI, and it is possible that these researcher-therapists also had their own biases in favor of the AMI over the alternatives. It is widely known in the psychotherapy literature that such "therapist allegiances" (Luborsky et al., 1999) may bias results unfairly in favor of one intervention over another.

Despite these problems in internal validity, we have confidence that AMIs are efficacious on two grounds. First is converging evidence: The number of positive outcomes for AMIs from different studies, each of which may contain one or more problems, points inevitably to a consistent and robust effect. Second, there are three exemplary studies that have eliminated almost all problems in internal validity (Miller et al., 1993; Project MATCH, 1997b; Stephens et al., 2000). These three studies provide good support for the efficacy of AMIs in the domain of alcohol problems and drug addiction.

How and Why Do AMIs Work?

Although a substantial amount of thought, practice, and research has already been devoted to motivational interviewing, we are still far from understanding the precise links between processes and outcomes (Miller, 1996b). While Miller and Rollnick (Chapter 1, this volume) speculate about possible therapeutic mechanisms, pointing to the effects of faith and hope, counselor effects (e.g., empathy), and change talk, there is a dearth of evidence regarding how and why interventions related to motivational interviewing might work.

An immediate task for research in this area is to dismantle feedback-based AMIs into their main components—problem feedback and motivational interviewing—to determine their relative contributions to outcome. As discussed in this chapter, we do not yet know whether feedback, motivational interviewing, or the combination is essential to produce a therapeutic effect. In fact, there is some recent empirical evidence to suggest that the feedback component may be more critical than the motivational interviewing component for college student drinkers (Juárez, 2001). Furthermore, the results of two studies suggest that problem feedback may be efficacious whether it is delivered in a motivational interviewing or a confrontative style (Miller et al., 1993; Schneider et al., 2000).

However, using observational coding of therapist behaviors, Miller and colleagues (1993) determined that the two feedback conditions—motivational interviewing and confrontative style—were not substantially different from one another in actual practice. As a result, post hoc correlations were computed between in-session therapist and client behaviors and therapeutic outcomes. Therapist "confrontative" behaviors were directly correlated with client resistant behaviors in the session, while therapist "supportive" (motivational interviewing style) behaviors were correlated with positive change-oriented behaviors from clients. Further, a significant positive correlation was obtained between a single therapist behavior ("confront," consisting of challenging, disagreeing, head-on disputes, incredulity, sarcasm, etc.) and drinking frequency at 1-year follow-up.

There is support for the existence of counselor effects with AMIs. Project MATCH (1998c) found that therapist differences accounted for 6% to 7% of the outcome variance, even after controlling for client severity and site effects. Moreover, exploratory analyses of specific therapist attributes on the Personal Preference Schedule (Edwards, 1953) revealed that better outcomes were significantly associated with higher therapist need for nurturance and lower need for aggression.

The positive effects of AMIs as preludes or adjuncts to further clinical services may be at least partially mediated by increased treatment participation. For example, Brown and Miller (1993) found that clients who received the pretreatment AMI intervention were rated as more involved in subsequent treatment than were the control clients. While several other studies provided support for the ability of AMIs to improve future or concurrent treatment participation (Booth et al., 1998; Martino et al., 2000; Smith et al., 1997; Swanson et al., 1999), none of them (including Brown & Miller, 1993) employed specific mediation analyses in this respect.

There is little direct evidence thus far to suggest that AMIs actually work by enhancing motivation or readiness for change. While AMI clients generally showed an increase in readiness for change after treatment (Handmaker et al., 1999; Mhurchu et al., 1998; Treasure et al., 1999), the AMI interventions— with one exception (Butler et al., 1999)—did not appear to differentially increase readiness for change in comparison to alternative interventions or controls (Colby et al., 1998; Mhurchu et al., 1998; Saunders et al., 1995; Schneider et al., 2000; Treasure et al., 1999). Furthermore, none of these studies performed statistical analyses to determine whether this motivational shift actually mediated client outcome.

Therefore, research suggests that AMIs may be mediated by counselor effects (such as an empathic therapeutic style), by providing feedback on assessment results, or by enhancing future treatment participation. Despite these promising beginnings, we still know precious little about *how* motivational interviewing works.

For Whom Do AMIs Work?

The possibility that some treatments work better for some people and some problems is one that has been widely explored in psychotherapy (Shoham & Rohrbaugh, 1995) and has received attention in the motivational interviewing literature as well. Several clinical trials of AMIs that have looked for such interactions have largely failed to find them (Marlatt et al., 1998; Monti et al., 1999; Project MATCH, 1997a, 1997b, 1998c). In Project MATCH, most of the matching variables did not predict outcome of particular treatments as hypothesized (e.g., stage of change, readiness to change, self-efficacy, or antisocial personality), although two significant matching effects were identified that predicted outcome at the 3-year follow-up period: TSF was more efficacious than AMI for clients whose social networks were highly supportive of drinking, while the opposite was true for clients whose social support networks were low in support for their drinking. This effect reached significance on only one of the alcohol use measures and did not predict success at 1-year follow-up. The most stable and robust interaction effect found in Project MATCH, significant at both 1- and 3-year follow-ups, was that AMI outperformed CBT and TSF on both primary drinking outcome measures for clients high on anger, whereas the converse held true for low-anger clients.

Finally, while two studies provided no support for stage of change as a moderator of AMI treatments (Monti et al., 1999; Project MATCH, 1997a, 1997b, 1998c), two other studies found that those who are least ready to change may derive particular advantage from an AMI over brief advice (Butler et al., 1999) or skills-based counseling (Heather et al., 1996).

THE FUTURE OF MOTIVATIONAL INTERVIEWING RESEARCH: WHERE DO WE GO FROM HERE?

As our review indicates, there has been a real imbalance between internal and external validity in motivational interviewing research thus far. It appears that researchers have been more interested in evaluating the usefulness of AMIs with different populations than in constructing rigorous designs to rule out alternative explanations. In our opinion, the most immediate research need is for studies high on internal validity. Future research could address this by attending to:

- Adequate sample size permitting an appropriate level of statistical power.
- Appropriate control groups that represent clear alternative explanations and are equivalent to the AMIs tested in all other respects (e.g., credibility and length of treatment).
- Careful assessment of treatment fidelity and integrity (see provisional description of skills in Chapter 18).
- Clear description of the motivational interviewing or AMI procedures under study.
- Greater uniformity and comparability of AMIs across studies.

There is another important question that has eluded any direct answer in virtually all of the research that we have reviewed: What is the efficacy of *motivational interviewing* (as opposed to AMIs)? As we have repeatedly noted, there have been no empirical tests of a "pure" form of motivational interviewing, as defined by Miller and Rollnick (1991; this volume). The AMI interventions reviewed here have all involved a motivational interviewing "style" but have also included other elements, such as educational materials, cognitive-behavioral strategies, and, most commonly, problem feedback. We need to know to what extent the positive results of AMIs are due to feedback, motivational interviewing, or the combination. Dismantling studies of this type are necessary to ascertain the active ingredients in AMIs.

There is a considerable amount of theory and research (e.g., Greenberg, Elliott, & Lietaer, 1994; Rogers, 1951) to suggest that motivational interviewing may be a valuable approach, not just for addictions but for numerous other psychological disorders such as anxiety and mood disorders. Motivational interviewing may be seen as an intriguing integration of the principles and strategies of Rogers's (1951) client-centered therapy with more active cognitive-behavioral strategies presented in a way that enhances self-attribution for change. The promise of motivational interviewing is partially supported by the AMI research reviewed in this chapter, but we can only know the extent to which this promise can be fulfilled when we study the process and outcome of motivational interviewing for a wider variety of clinical problems.

SUMMARY

Our review has focused on adaptations of motivational interviewing (AMIs), defined by the presence of feedback or other additional elements—thus far, there have been no studies of "pure" motivational interviewing. The AMI interventions in the studies reviewed here have been relatively brief interventions of between one and six sessions that have been used both as a prelude or adjunct to other treatments and as a stand-alone treatment. The research supports the efficacy of AMIs for alcohol problems and drug addiction, as well as for people with diabetes, hypertension, dual diagnoses, and bulimia. Mixed support has been found for AMIs in the domain of cigarette smoking, increasing physical activity, and enhancing dietary adherence in patients with hyperlipidemia. No support has been found for AMIs in the reduction of HIV risk behaviors (e.g., needle sharing) in the two studies conducted to date.

In general, AMIs have proven superior to no-treatment control groups and less credible alternative treatments, and equal to viable comparison treatments. AMIs have often done as well as other viable treatments that were two or three times longer. AMIs have been quite varied across different studies, making general conclusions about treatment efficacy difficult. More uniformity in the AMI interventions studied would be helpful. In general, research has been strong on external validity but relatively weak on internal validity. The field needs more well-controlled and rigorous trials of AMIs, in addition to studies that attempt to dismantle AMIs in order to evaluate the relative contributions of motivational interviewing and problem feedback. Finally, we need research on "pure" motivational interviewing interventions, as well as process research that elucidates underlying mechanisms so that we can understand more about *how*, *why*, and *for whom* motivational interviewing may work.

NOTES

1. This issue of terminology is discussed further in Chapter 18.
2. See Dunn, De Roo, and Rivara (2001) and Burke, Arkowitz, and Menchola (2001).
3. Group AMI interventions are reviewed separately in Chapter 25.
4. Other chapters in this volume may cover outcome studies related to motivational

interviewing that did not meet our criteria for inclusion here. Thus, it is possible that these other chapters will draw somewhat different conclusions.

5. This intervention did not include any feedback on previous substance-related assessments. However, it did omit the skilled use of reflective listening, which is crucial to the expression of therapeutic empathy. For that reason, we still consider this procedure to be an AMI rather than pure motivational interviewing per se.

6. This intervention employed a combination of motivational interviewing strategies and "role-induction techniques," so we still consider it an AMI rather than pure motivational interviewing per se.

7. According to Chapter 20, this treatment, as planned, may not have been faithful to the principles of motivational interviewing.

8. This intervention was based on an approach to motivational interviewing that "has departed from that espoused by Miller and Rollnick" (Saunders, Wilkinson, & Allsop, 1991), and thus we still consider it an AMI rather than pure motivational interviewing per se.

CONTROLLED CLINICAL TRIALS OF AMIs

1. Brown, J. M., & Miller, W. R. (1993). Impact of motivational interviewing on participation and outcome in residential alcoholism treatment. *Psychology of Addictive Behaviors, 7*, 211–218.

2. Bien, T. H., Miller, W. R., & Boroughs, J. M. (1993). Motivational interviewing with alcohol outpatients. *Behavioural and Cognitive Psychotherapy, 23*, 347–356.

3. Borsari, B., & Carey, K. B. (2000). Effects of a brief motivational intervention with college student drinkers. *Journal of Consulting and Clinical Psychology, 68*(4), 728–733.

4. Marlatt, G. A., Baer, J. S., Kivlahan, D. R., Dimeff, L. A., Larimer, M. E., Quigley, L. A., Somers, J. M., & Williams, E. (1998). Screening and brief intervention for high-risk college student drinkers: Results from a 2–year follow-up assessment. *Journal of Consulting and Clinical Psychology, 66*, 604–615.
   and
   Baer, J. S., Kivlahan, D. R., Blume, A. W., McKnight, P., & Marlatt, G. A. (2001). Brief intervention for heavy drinking college students: Four-year follow-up and natural history. *American Journal of Public Health, 91*(8), 1310–1316.

5. Gentilello, L. M., Rivara, F. P., Donovan, D. M., Jurkovich, G. J., Daranciang, E., Dunn, C. W., Villaveces, A., Copass, M., & Ries, R. (1999). Alcohol interventions in a trauma center as a means of reducing the risk of injury recurrence. *Annals of Surgery, 230*(4), 473–483.

6. Miller, W. R., Sovereign, R. G., & Krege, B. (1988). Motivational interviewing with problem drinkers: II. The Drinker's Check-Up as a preventive intervention. *Behavioural Psychotherapy, 16*, 251–268.

7. Miller, W. R., Benefield, R. G., & Tonigan, J. S. (1993). Enhancing motivation for change in problem drinking: A controlled comparison of two therapist styles. *Journal of Consulting and Clinical Psychology, 61*, 455–461.

8. Monti, P. M., Colby, S. M., Barnett, N. P., Spirito, A., & Rohsenow, D. J. (1999).

Brief intervention for harm reduction with alcohol-positive older adolescents in a hospital emergency department. *Journal of Consulting and Clinical Psychology,* 67(6), 989–994.

9. Handmaker, N. S., Miller, W. R., & Manicke, M. (1999). Findings of a pilot study of motivational interviewing with pregnant drinkers. *Journal of Studies on Alcohol,* 60, 285–287.

10. Heather, N., Rollnick, S., Bell, A., & Richmond, R. (1996). Effects of brief counseling among heavy drinkers identified on general hospital wards. *Drug and Alcohol Review,* 15, 29–38.

11. Project MATCH Research Group. (1997a). Matching alcoholism treatments to client heterogeneity: Project MATCH posttreatment drinking outcomes. *Journal of Studies on Alcohol,* 58, 7–29.
    and
    Project MATCH Research Group. (1998a). Matching alcoholism treatments to client heterogeneity: Project MATCH three-year drinking outcomes. *Alcoholism: Clinical and Experimental Research,* 23(60), 1300–1311.

12. Colby, S. M., Monti, P. M., Barnett, N. P., Rohsenow, D. J., Weissman, K., Spirito, A., Woolard, R. H., & Lewander, W. J. (1998). Brief motivational interviewing in a hospital setting for adolescent smoking: A preliminary study. *Journal of Consulting and Clinical Psychology,* 66(3), 574–578.

13. Butler, C. C., Rollnick, S., Cohen, D., Russel, I., Bachmann, M., & Stott, N. (1999). Motivational consulting versus brief advice for smokers in general practice: A randomised trial. *British Journal of General Practice,* 49, 611–616.

14. Schneider, R. J., Casey, J., & Kohn, R. (2000). Motivational versus confrontational interviewing: A comparison of substance abuse assessment practices at employee assistance programs. *Journal of Behavioral Health Services and Research,* 27(1), 60–74.

15. Martino, S., Carroll, K. M., O'Malley, S. S., & Rounsaville, B. J. (2000). Motivational interviewing with psychiatrically ill substance abusing patients. *American Journal on Addictions,* 9, 88–91.

16. Booth, R. E., Kwiatkowski, C., Iguchi, M. Y., Pinto, F., & John, D. (1998). Facilitating treatment entry among out-of-treatment injection drug users. *Public Health Reports,* 113(Suppl. 1), 116–128.

17. Saunders, B., Wilkinson, C., & Phillips, M. (1995). The impact of a brief motivational intervention with opiate users attending a methadone programme. *Addiction,* 90, 415–424.

18. Stephens, R. S., Roffman, R. A., & Curtin, L. (2000). Comparison of extended versus brief treatments for marijuana use. *Journal of Consulting and Clinical Psychology,* 68(5), 898–908.

19. Baker, A., Heather, N., Wodak, A., Dixon, J., & Holt, P. (1993). Evaluation of a cognitive-behavioural intervention for HIV prevention among injecting drug users. *AIDS,* 7, 247–256.

20. Baker, A., Kochan, N., Dixon, J., Heather, N., & Wodak, A. (1994). Controlled evaluation of a brief intervention for HIV prevention among injecting drug users not in treatment. *AIDS Care,* 6(5), 559–570.

21. Swanson, A. J., Pantalon, M. V., & Cohen, K. R. (1999). Motivational interviewing and treatment adherence among dually-diagnosed patients. *Journal of Nervous and Mental Disease,* 187(10), 630–635.

22. Mhurchu, C. N., Margetts, B. M., & Speller, V. (1998). Randomized clinical trial comparing the effectiveness of two dietary interventions for patients with hyperlipidaemia. *Clinical Science, 95*(4), 479–487.

23. Woollard, J., Beilin, L., Lord, T., Puddey, I., MacAdam, D., & Rouse, I. (1995). A controlled trial of nurse counseling on lifestyle change for hypertensives treated in general practice: Preliminary results. *Clinical and Experimental Pharmacology and Physiology, 23,* 466–468.

24. Harland, J., White, M., Drinkwater, C., Chinn, D., Farr, L., & Howel, D. (1999). The Newcastle exercise project: A randomized controlled trial of methods to promote physical activity in primary care. *British Medical Journal, 319,* 828–831.

25. Smith, D. E., Heckemeyer, C. M., Kratt, P. P., & Mason, D. A. (1997). Motivational interviewing to improve adherence to a behavioral weight-control program for older obese women with NIDDM: A pilot study. *Diabetes Care, 20*(1), 53–54.

26. Treasure, J. L., Katzman, M., Schmidt, U., Troop, N., Todd, G., & de Silva, P. (1999). Engagement and outcome in the treatment of bulimia nervosa: First phase of a sequential design comparing motivation enhancement therapy and cognitive behavioural therapy. *Behaviour Research and Therapy, 37,* 405–418.

CHAPTER 17

Motivational Interviewing in Medical and Public Health Settings

KEN RESNICOW, COLLEEN DIIORIO, JOHANNA E. SOET,
BELINDA BORRELLI, DENISE ERNST, JACKI HECHT, *and*
ANGELICA K. THEVOS

Whereas much of the initial applied and empirical work in motivational interviewing has centered on addictive behaviors, most notably alcohol use, in recent years, there has been considerable interest on the part of public health (PH) and medical professionals in utilizing motivational interviewing to address other health behaviors and conditions, such as smoking, diet, physical activity, diabetes control, pain management, screening, sexual behavior, and medical adherence (Berg-Smith et al., 1999; Colby et al., 1998; Emmons & Rollnick, 2001; Ershoff et al., 1999; Miller, 1996b; Rakowski et al., 1992; Resnicow, Jackson, Wang, Dudley, & Baranowski, 2001; Smith, Heckemeyer, Kratt, & Mason, 1997; Stott, Rollnick, & Pill, 1995; Taplin et al., 2000; Velasquez et al., 2000).

This chapter will examine medical and public health applications of motivational interviewing. We begin by providing an overview of some conceptual and pragmatic nuances that are associated with the use of motivational interviewing in these settings and, in particular, application to chronic diseases and nonaddictive behaviors. Then we explore issues related to training PH and medical personnel in its use. We next describe the application of motivational interviewing to specific behaviors and health conditions and conclude with a summary and discussion of future research directions.

CONCEPTUAL ISSUES: APPLICATION OF MOTIVATIONAL INTERVIEWING TO NONADDICTIVE AND CHRONIC DISEASE BEHAVIORS

Given its roots in addiction counseling, it is important to examine how motivational interviewing may function differently in theory and practice when applied to nonaddictive behaviors and chronic diseases. For example, an essential element of motivational interviewing is working through ambivalence about change (Miller & Rollnick, 1991; Resnicow, DiIorio, et al., 2001; Rollnick, Butler, & Stott, 1997), and this technique appears to be particularly effective among individuals who are initially at low readiness to change (Butler et al., 1999; Heather, Rollnick, Bell, & Richmond, 1996; Resnicow, Jackson, et al., 2001). It can be posited that the nature and magnitude of ambivalence, as well as the reasons for change, differ in kind (not only in degree) between addictive and nonaddictive behaviors. Modifying behaviors such as fruit and vegetable intake or physical activity may not entail the intensity of resistance or convey the depth of psychologic and interpersonal meaning as does ending alcohol or heroin use. For nonaddictive behaviors, less time (though not necessarily less skill) may be needed to resolve client ambivalence, and such encounters may involve a more behavioral than cognitive focus. Moreover, if the nature and magnitude of ambivalence is substantively different for nonaddictive behaviors, and if resolving ambivalence is a major reason that motivational interviewing is effective, then perhaps motivational interviewing will be less effective in the PH and medical setting. Conversely, there may be considerable ambivalence, resistance, and denial about health behaviors such as medical adherence, obtaining screening and diagnostic tests, increasing exercise, and others, and motivational interviewing may be equally effective in these settings (Prochaska et al., 1994).

Another difference may lie in the fact that for many addictive behaviors—for example, cigarette use—the behavior change process often entails a discrete "quit day." Although target goals and timing are important for changing behaviors such as eating and physical activity, the pattern of change is often quite different. The concepts of abstinence and relapse are perhaps less tangible for some health-promoting behaviors.

Finally, in addiction counseling, the client often has been referred to or has sought treatment for their condition, whereas in the medical and PH settings, clients may have sought care for another condition or concern, and the practitioner may raise issues such as smoking, diet, or exercise (see Chapter 18, in this volume). Given that the client may not have initiated the discussion of the topic, perhaps there will be less interest or willingness to address such behaviors within this context. Conversely, some patients may specifically schedule a periodic checkup with their physician, with the explicit expectation that their diet, physical activity, substance use, screening history, or other health behaviors will be addressed. Whether practitioner-initiated motivational interviewing intervention functions differently than those that are client-initiated has not been empirically determined.

PRAGMATIC ISSUES: DURATION, FREQUENCY, AND MODALITY OF CONTACT

Perhaps the most limiting factor in using motivational interviewing in PH and medical settings is time. Whereas full-blown motivational interviewing for addiction counseling may involve multiple sessions of considerable duration, in medical settings (particularly primary care), patient encounters typically range from 10 to 15 minutes (Emmons & Rollnick, 2001; Goldstein et al., 1998). Moreover, medical practitioners may have only a single contact with a patient for a particular health behavior. For example, in a public hospital walk-in clinic or emergency room, a physician may be able to broach the topic of behavior change—for example, quitting smoking. However, this physician may never see that patient again. Similarly, in some managed care systems, patients are not always linked to specific practitioners (Goldstein et al., 1998). Even when there is continuity of care, difficulty obtaining reimbursement for behavioral counseling further limits practitioners' ability and motivation to deliver intensive motivational interviewing.

Numerous implications arise from these constraints. First, there is a need to adapt motivational interviewing into a briefer format that is suitable to limited client contact. This briefer format (referred to elsewhere as "brief negotiation") is referred to in this text as an adaptation of motivational interviewing (AMI; Rollnick & Miller, 1995). Rollnick and others have developed motivational interviewing–based techniques tailored to brief encounters. One example is the 0–10 importance/confidence (i.e., readiness ruler) strategy described elsewhere in this text, which allows physicians and other health care practitioners to assess motivation and facilitate client or patient movement along the change continuum (Butler et al., 1999; Rollnick et al., 1997; Rollnick, Mason, & Butler, 1999). A useful feature of these techniques is their algorithmic nature, which fits well with the general medical framework for decision making.

Brief adaptations of motivational interviewing (see also Chapter 18) are distinguished from full-blown motivational interviewing in several ways. First, when there is limited client contact, either in terms of duration or frequency, it is generally not feasible to employ the full range of motivational interviewing techniques nor is it possible to build the depth of rapport that may be needed to maximize therapeutic effect. For example, in medical settings, physicians may not have sufficient time to fully explore client ambivalence or to engage in extensive reflective listening. In some cases, the goal of brief interventions may simply to be engage the client to accept a referral or to think about making future changes.

The method of delivering motivational interviewing may be different in medical and PH settings, where they may be part of multicomponent interventions that include education materials, as well as non–motivational interviewing individual and group interactions (Glasgow, Whitlock, Eakin, & Lichtstein, 2000; Resnicow, Coleman-Wallace, et al., 2000; Resnicow, Jackson, et al., 2001). In addition, motivational interviewing is often delivered via telephone (Berg-Smith et al., 1999; Glasgow et al., 2000; Ludman, Curry, Meyer, & Taplin, 1999; Resnicow, Coleman-Wallace, et al., 2000; Resnicow et al., in press; Resnicow, Jackson, et al., 2001; Sims, Smith, Duffy, & Hilton, 1998; Taplin et al., 2000; Woollard et al., 1995). When motivational interviewing interventions are conducted by telephone, both counselors and clients operate with limited nonverbal cues and depth of rapport, and, therefore, the effect of treatment may be compromised (Soet & Basch, 1997). The efficacy and cost–benefit ratio of telephone versus in-person intervention merits further study.

PROFESSIONAL DEVELOPMENT AND TRAINING ISSUES

In the addiction field, motivational interviewing interventions have typically been delivered by individuals with training in psychology or counseling. Training such professionals in use of motivational interviewing often represents only a moderate refinement of skills. Although within PH and medical settings psychologists and social workers (Ludman et al., 1999; Resnicow et al., in press; Smith et al., 1997; Velasquez et al., 2000) have been used to deliver motivational interviewing, more commonly nurses (Doherty, Hall, James, Roberts, & Simpson, 2000; Velasquez et al., 2000; Woollard et al., 1995), physicians (Doherty et al., 2000; Rollnick et al., 1997); dietitians (Berg-Smith et al., 1999; Mhurchu, Margetts, & Speller, 1998; Resnicow, Coleman-Wallace, et al., 2000; Resnicow, Jackson, et al., 2001), or health educators (Harland et al., 1999) have been employed. For these professions, learning motivational interviewing may represent a total retooling of their orientation. (Emmons & Rollnick, 2001; Rollnick, 1996). Physicians, nurses, and dietitians have traditionally been trained to provide expert (often unsolicited) advice about the benefits of health behavior change (Goldstein et al., 1998). These disciplines are heavily based on instructional methods and sharing of information (Glanz, 1979; Rollnick, 1996). Nurses and dietitians sometimes go beyond providing advice by educating patients, in a prescriptive way, about steps they can take to change health behavior. A challenge for many healthcare practitioners is adopting the more facilitative and collaborative spirit of motivational interviewing in place of the more prescriptive, practitioner-centered, and directive techniques that are traditionally employed in medical settings. This represents a formidable barrier to training PH and medical practitioners.

An illustration of the contrast between motivational interviewing and the traditional patient education or medical model can be captured in how information is presented. In the traditional paradigm, the health practitioner often provides information about the risks of continuing a behavior or the benefits of change with the intent of persuasion. This may include statements (perhaps more accurately, appeals) such as "This is very important for your health because . . ., " "This behavior poses great risk," "It is essential that you change because. . . . " Implicit in such statements is an evaluative interpretation. In contrast, within motivational interviewing, information is presented in a more neutral manner, and the client is asked to do the work of interpretation. A practitioner may state to a client who does not exercise that "There are some scientific studies that have found that people who walk 2 miles or more per week have half the risk of heart disease compared to those who walk less than 1 mile. What do you make of that?" Or, rather than stating that "It is important for you to quit smoking because . . ., " practitioners might be trained to state that "It is a medical fact that smoking can increase a person's chances of having another heart attack, and I have seen this happen to several of my patients. But what is important to me is what you think about this." Thus, many health care practitioners need to be trained to avoid persuasion with "predigested" health messages and instead allow the client to process the information, find their own personal relevance, evaluate their own risks and rewards, and convince themselves to change rather than be convinced by the practitioner (see Chapter 18; Rollnick et al., 1999).

Another challenge facing PH and medical practitioners is the amount of time available for training in motivational interviewing (Emmons & Rollnick, 2001; Stott et al., 1995; Velasquez et al., 2000). Limited time for training and follow-up supervision can make it difficult for some health care providers to "buy into" the philosophy and thus experience the effectiveness of this approach, as well as to "let go" of the reflex to provide information (Pill, Rees, Stott, & Rollnick, 1999). For example, Stott and colleagues (1995) trained practitioners to deliver adaptations of motivational interviewing to address diabetic care using a "client-centered" approach whereby the number of training sessions and strategies for training were negotiated with the practitioners. While the majority of practices chose two to three training sessions lasting 1– 1.5 hours each, few opted for additional training. Practitioners were willing to observe role-play demonstrations, yet few were willing to practice these skills. Velasquez and colleagues (2000) trained several groups of PH nurses, all of whom participated in the role plays and experiential aspects of the training. While these nurses reported high levels of satisfaction with the motivational strategies, many nurses found it difficult to actually implement this style of intervention with their clients because of competing patient care needs, limited time, and lack of confidence. Finally, on-going supervision in these settings may not be very intensive or rigorous (Borrelli et al., 1998; Pill et al., 1999; Velasquez et al., 2000).

A key clinical and research question that remains to be determined is the extent to which such professionals, with limited postgraduate training, can be "retro-fitted" to become skilled motivational interviewing counselors. Practitioners not primarily schooled in client-centered counseling may be able to learn the basic techniques of motivational interviewing, but without extensive training they may be unable to achieve the whole that is greater than the sum of its parts. Technical skills are necessary but insufficient to achieve the spirit of motivational interviewing. Whereas such professionals, with a few hours or days of training, may be able to employ some of the core motivational interviewing skills and strategies (e.g., asking open-ended questions, setting agendas, obtaining permission, minimizing unsolicited advice, and basic reflective listening), mastering deeper level reflection, handling resistant statements or clients, and applying motivational interviewing across a range of health behaviors often requires a degree of training, practice, and supervision that is not practical in most health care settings. Chapter 16 looks to the future and discusses some ways of resolving this issue.

While practitioners' acceptance of a motivational style is important, it is also essential to consider patients' perspectives. In studies where nurses incorporated a motivational style of counseling, patients reported being highly satisfied with the intervention (Borrelli et al., 1998; Emmons et al., in press). Similarly, a study of patients' perceptions of the doctor's advice to quit smoking demonstrated that the interventions patients found most acceptable were those that considered the patient's receptivity, conveyed a respectful tone, avoided preaching, and showed caring and support of the individual (Butler, Rollnick, Pill, Maggs-Rapport, & Stott, 1998). The fact that motivational interviewing interventions may result in improved provider–patient relationships and consumer satisfaction is an underdeveloped and potentially powerful selling point to providers and health care agencies.

DIET AND PHYSICAL ACTIVITY CHANGE

Nuances associated with changing diet and physical activity patterns relevant to motivational interviewing include the fact that these behaviors generally involve modification rather than elimination; reshaping rather than abstaining. Whereas there is generally no "quit day," there may be concrete behavioral targets such as eating five servings of fruits and vegetables per day, reaching a daily caloric or fat-intake limit, or exercising a specific number of days or minutes per week. In addition, diet and physical activity change may be elements of multicomponent programs to reduce risk factors such as dyslipidemia, diabetes, high blood pressure, obesity, and recurrence of heart disease. Particularly for secondary prevention, changes in these domains must be long-term, if not for a lifetime: for example, reducing saturated-fat intake for a hyperlipidemic individual. Thus, ambivalence may center around the long-term burden of change. Motivational interviewing for such individuals could focus on helping them come to grips with the chronic nature of their condition, as well as identify ways to reduce what can be perceived as an overwhelming burden. Moreover, although generally not considered addictive behaviors, giving up or reducing the intake of favorite foods or reducing preferred sedentary behaviors are often perceived as unpleasurable or a sacrifice, and such changes can manifest similar to withdrawal. Thus, a key goal for a motivational interviewing counselor may be to help an individual reframe their change in positive terms—for example, what is gained versus what is lost—as well as to conceptualize their change in other than hedonic terms: for example, the effect on or the reduced anxiety about their disease risk rather than focusing on the taste of broccoli.

Five controlled outcome studies[1] and one uncontrolled outcome study using motivational interviewing to modify diet and physical activity behaviors were identified. (Most of the published controlled studies are also reviewed in detail in Chapter 16 and are therefore only briefly addressed here.) In addition, there are numerous ongoing studies in the United States and abroad that will be completed over the next few years. The outcome studies include four secondary prevention trials for patients with diabetes, hyperlipidemia, or hypertension (Berg-Smith et al., 1999; Mhurchu et al., 1998; Smith et al., 1997; Woollard et al., 1995) and two primary prevention trials in well populations (Harland et al., 1999; Resnicow, Coleman-Wallace, et al., 2000; Resnicow, Jackson, et al., 2001) .

The first of the secondary prevention trials was a pilot study conducted by Smith and colleagues (1997). Twenty-two overweight women with non-insulin dependent diabetes mellitus were randomized to receive a standard 16-week group behavioral weight control intervention or the same intervention with the addition of three individual motivational interviewing sessions. Motivational interviewing sessions were delivered by experienced psychologists. The motivational interviewing involved one session before group treatment and two at midtreatment, and it included individualized feedback on glycemic control. At posttest, women in the motivational interviewing group showed significantly better glycemic control than the standard intervention group, and they were more likely to monitor their blood glucose. The motivational interviewing group also showed significantly higher session attendance and they turned in more diet and activity diaries.

Mhurchu and colleagues (1998) randomized 121 patients with hyperlipidemia, which is usually secondary to coronary heart disease. The same dietician met with them for three sessions, either using motivational interviewing–based counseling or a standard dietary intervention. At 3-month follow-up, there were no significant between-group differences for any of the main outcomes.

Woollard and colleagues (1995) randomly assigned 166 hypertensive patients in general medical practices to receive either "high" motivational interviewing, consisting of six 45-minute sessions every fourth week, or "low" motivational interviewing, which comprised a single face-to-face session plus five additional brief telephone sessions. Both groups received their usual GP care, in addition to an educational manual. A control group was also used that consisted only of the usual GP care. At 18-week follow-up, there were no significant differences between the two motivational interviewing groups. However, both motivational interviewing groups had better outcomes than the controls.

Finally, in the Dietary Intervention Study in Children, children initially aged 8 to 10 years, who had elevated LDL cholesterol, received three years of dietary intervention (Berg-Smith et al., 1999). As the cohort moved into adolescence, the investigators elected to add a motivational interviewing intervention to "renew" adherence to the prescribed diet among the original intervention group (there was no control group for this phase). The counselors were primarily masters'-level health educators and dietitians who received 18 hours of training. There was one in-person session and one follow-up session either in person or by telephone. Data from the first 127 youth to complete the two sessions indicated that the proportion of calories from fat and dietary cholesterol (assessed by three 24-hour recalls) was significantly reduced at 3-month follow-up, and overall adherence scores improved. Adolescent satisfaction with the motivational interviewing intervention was high. A unique element of this intervention is the exquisite detail provided by the authors regarding the theoretical basis for the intervention (Berg-Smith et al., 1999).

With regard to primary prevention, Harland and colleagues (1999) recruited 523 general medical practice patients to evaluate the efficacy of motivational interviewing for promoting physical activity. The population was sedentary but otherwise healthy. The study employed four intervention groups. Two groups received a single 40-minute motivational interviewing session, and two groups received six 40-minute motivational interviewing sessions delivered over 12 weeks. Approximately half of the participants in the motivational interviewing groups also received vouchers for free aerobics classes. There was also a control group that received no motivational interviewing. A physical activity score was assessed by an exercise questionnaire that was completed at 12-week and 1-year follow-ups. At the 12-week follow-up, there was a significant improvement in this score in the four intervention groups relative to the controls (38% improved vs. 16%) but no significant differences between the "high" and "low" motivational interviewing groups. At 1-year follow-up, there were no significant differences in physical activity between the intervention groups, either combined or separately, relative to the control group. This was because of a deterioration in effects in the intervention group, as well as a slight improvement among the control group.

Resnicow and colleagues (Resnicow, Coleman-Wallace, et al., 2000; Resnicow, Jackson, et al., 2001) recently completed the Eat for Life (EFL) trial, a multicomponent intervention to increase fruit and vegetable consumption among African American adults, delivered through black churches. Fourteen churches were randomly assigned to three treatment conditions: (1) comparison;

(2) culturally tailored self-help intervention with one telephone cue; and (3) self-help intervention, one cue call and three motivational interviewing counseling calls. Cue calls were intended to increase use of the self-help intervention materials and were not structured as motivational interviewing contacts.

Motivational interviewing counselors, who were either registered dietitians or dietetic interns, participated in three, 2-hour training sessions conducted by the first author (KR) and were observed performing at least two phone counseling encounters before being certified. They received ongoing supervision from doctoral level staff. The primary outcome, assessed at baseline and at 1-year follow-up, was fruit and vegetable intake, assessed by food frequency questionnaires (Resnicow, Odom, et al., 2000). Change in fruit and vegetable intake was significantly greater in the motivational interviewing group than in the comparison and self-help groups. The net difference between the motivational interviewing and comparison group was approximately 1.1 servings of fruits and vegetables per day, whereas the net difference between the motivational interviewing and the self-help group was approximately 1.0 serving. Despite these promising results, however, preliminary analysis of tape-recorded motivational interviewing sessions indicated only moderate fidelity on the part of the dietitians to the spirit and techniques of motivational interviewing.

Resnicow and his colleagues are currently conducting another study based on the Eat for Life trial (Resnicow et al., in press), entitled Healthy Body, Healthy Spirit. This is a randomized effectiveness trial with three experimental conditions. Group 1 receives standard nutrition and physical activity intervention materials; Group 2 receives culturally tailored self-help nutrition and physical activity interventions; Group 3 receives the same intervention as Group 2, plus four telephone calls with motivational interviewing counseling. Unlike the Eat for Life trial, where the motivational interviewing intervention was delivered by dietitians, here the motivational interviewing is being delivered by masters'-level counseling psychologists, who were originally trained in the person-centered model of R. R. Carkhuff (1969; Carkhuff, Anthony, Cannon, Pierce, & Zigon, 1979).

A unique element of the motivational interviewing intervention in the Healthy Body, Healthy Spirit trial is the use of a values clarification strategy, based on the work of Miller and C'de Baca (1994). In the original method, the client was asked to sort a list of approximately 70 values in terms of personal importance and to select around 5 that are most important. The revised protocol uses a modified and shortened set of values or attributes, as shown in Table 17.1. Clients are asked to briefly discuss why the values or goals selected are important to them, and then they explore what connection, if any, they see between their current health behavior and their ability to achieve these goals or live out these values. Alternatively, the counselor may ask how changing their health behavior may be related to these goals or values. Initial results using this strategy appear promising. In the process of linking health behavior to core values, considerable change talk has been elicited.

TABLE 17.1. List of Values, Attributes, and Goals and Rates of Endorsement in the Healthy Body, Healthy Spirit Project

Value, attribute, or goal	Rate of endorsement (%)	Value, attribute, or goal	Rate of endorsement (%)
Good parent	49	Attractive	5
Good spouse/partner	38	Disciplined	16
Good community member	13	Responsible	22
Strong	13	In control	10
On top of things	7	Respected at work	8
Competent	8	Athletic	2
Spiritual	55	Not hypocritical	7
Respected at home	4	Energetic	10
Good Christian	46	Considerate	18
Successful	13	Youthful	3
Independent	16		

Note. $n = 135$. Percentages represent the rate of endorsement by participants in the HBHS project to date of each of the core values.

One difference between the Eat for Life and Healthy Body, Healthy Spirit projects is that in the latter, counselors have referred many clients to project dietitians for additional nutritional follow-up such as information about diabetes and weight control. Thus, although using trained counselors, as opposed to dietitians, to provide the motivational interviewing may yield an intervention of greater fidelity, the fact that these interventionists do not possess a great deal of expertise in nutrition or exercise counseling has necessitated considerable additional follow-up.

In sum, the evidence for the efficacy of motivational interviewing in the area of diet and exercise is mixed, with two studies showing little or no advantage of motivational interviewing over comparison treatments (Harland et al., 1999; Mhurchu et al., 1998), and four showing positive effects (Berg-Smith et al., 1999; Resnicow, Jackson, et al., 2001; Smith et al., 1997; Woollard et al., 1995). Despite the positive effects observed in these four studies, internal validity is threatened by the fact that the motivational interviewing interventions were additive to other interventions (or the Dietary Intervention Study in Children did not have a control group). Client contact was not comparable across conditions, as the comparison groups did not receive any "sham" or alternative counseling. Finally, in two studies, higher-dose motivational interviewing interventions failed to produce greater treatment effects (Harland et al., 1999; Woollard et al., 1995). Together, these findings raise questions about the extent to which treatment effects can be attributed to motivational interviewing as opposed to attention effects or generic elements of counseling that are not unique to motivational interviewing (e.g., empathy). In addition, intervention fidelity generally has not been adequately assessed or controlled for. Thus, negative or weak results may have been the result of poor intervention delivery, as opposed to ineffective intervention per se (see Chapter 16).

Key questions that merit examination in this area include the following: Which professions are most willing and able to effectively deliver motivational interviewing interventions? For example, are dietitians and exercise professionals the best candidates, or are such interventions best delivered by individuals with a background in counseling? Which is more important: specific content knowledge on the part of the practitioner or counseling skill and style?

SMOKING CESSATION

Motivational issues are important not only in the decision to attempt quitting but also in maximizing treatment adherence and in minimizing relapse. Motivational interviewing may therefore have a role across the entire spectrum of smoking control. Although pharmacological treatments and counseling guidelines have been shown to be effective in helping *motivated* smokers quit (U.S. Department of Health and Human Services, 2000), these treatments are less helpful for smokers who are *less motivated* to quit. Those motivated to quit represent only the minority of smokers (Richmond, Bell, Rollnick, & Heather, 1996; Velicer & DiClemente, 1993) and in routine medical care, health care practitioners are more likely to encounter smokers who are unmotivated to quit. Therefore, strategies are needed to help clinicians work with unmotivated and ambivalent smokers.

Standard care usually takes the form of physician advice, which is largely a prescriptive approach. When repeated over time it may be iatrogenic—actually undermining quit attempts and increasing patient resistance and attrition (Butler, Pill, & Stott, 1998). Instead, Butler, Pill, and Stott (1998) suggest that practitioners take into account the smokers' receptivity and convey support in a respectful, nonjudgmental, manner.

There have been several published studies that used adaptations of motivational interviewing for smoking cessation, primarily in clinical settings (Butler et al., 1999; Colby et al., 1998; Ershoff et al., 1999; Glasgow et al., 2000; Lando, 2001; Velasquez et al., 2000). (See Chapter 16 for additional details.)

Borrelli and colleagues (1998) are currently evaluating both short-term and long-term (12 months post-treatment) cessation outcomes in older, homebound medically ill adults. In this study (Project CARES), home health care nurses are randomly selected to provide either an adaptation of motivational interviewing or brief advice to their patients during their routine home care visits. Nurses in the intervention group are trained to deliver the motivational interviewing intervention that includes physiologic feedback about patients' levels of expired carbon monoxide. Physiologic feedback can be a powerful mechanism to highlight discrepancies between personal risk perception and current behavior. Feedback may be particularly salient for older smokers because this group tends to have difficulty connecting their physical symptoms with their smoking. Intervention nurses also enhance optimism about change by talking with patients about the benefits of quitting and emphasizing that it is never too late to quit. Preliminary data indicate that the intervention is acceptable to both patients and to home healthcare nurses (Emmons et al., in press).

Despite the potential role for motivational interviewing in cessation counseling, outcomes from randomized trials thus far have been mixed. Some of the studies with negative results, however, do suffer from methodological problems such as inadequate length of or description of motivational interviewing training, lack of treatment fidelity monitoring procedures (Butler et al., 1999), and low rates of treatment completion (Glasgow et al., 2000). Another reason for the mixed results of motivational interviewing for smoking cessation is the short-term follow-up (Colby et al., 1998). Since the emphasis in motivational interviewing is often on the decisional processes for change, not only change itself, more proximal indicators of future cessation such as stage of change should be assessed. Some remaining research questions are the following: Which components of motivational interviewing are critical for smokers? Is feedback a critical motivational component, and what types of feedback are most effective? What are the important moderating variables? Is motivational interviewing more effective with some smokers than with others?

MEDICATION ADHERENCE

Poor medication adherence is a concern for many, if not most, medications, across virtually all socioeconomic populations. This topic is also addressed in detail in Chapter 20. People who accept their health condition, who are able to incorporate taking medication into their lifestyles, who have more severe health conditions, and who believe their medication reduces symptoms or disease risk—all these have higher levels of adherence than those who deny their illness or attach negative meanings to taking medications (Cramer, Mattson, Prevey, Scheyer, & Ouellette, 1989; Creer & Levstek, 1997; DiIorio, Faherty, & Manteuffel, 1994; Shope, 1988; Singh, Squier, Sivek, & Wagener, 1996; Trostle, 1988; Turner et al., 1998). In addition, people who have health conditions that are intermittent and unpredictable have more problems with adherence. However, beyond these illness and cognitive variables, when asked why they do not take their medication more regularly, people generally note that they simply forgot. The usual remedies for forgetfulness include pill boxes, timers, beepers, calendars, and other planning strategies. Reminder systems are not effective when failure to adhere relates to side effects of the medication, ambivalence about the disease or treatment, fear of harm from treatment, negative meanings attached to medicines, representations of the illness that are inconsistent with medication taking, and stigma.

Moreover, although forgetfulness appears to be a major cause of low adherence, forgetfulness may reflect an underlying ambivalence about the disease or its treatment. Despite the benefits of taking medication, some individuals may want to avoid the associated inconvenience and side effects, and, emotionally, individuals may not want to confront the fact that they have an illness. Motivational interviewing may be effective for individuals whose adherence is related to ambivalence regarding the pros and cons of taking their medications or who have not come to grips with their condition and all that it may imply. Giving such individuals an opportunity to express their concerns may be particularly helpful in resolving their mixed emotions, as well as in overcoming the more pragmatic barriers they may face.

In several studies Kemp and colleagues have tested the use of an intervention based on motivational interviewing to promote medication adherence among people with psychosis (Hayward, Chan, Kemp, & Youle, 1995; Kemp, Hayward, Applewhaite, Everitt, & David, 1996; Kemp, Kirov, Everitt, Hayward, & David, 1998). In a pilot study, they (Hayward et al., 1995) tested a motivational interviewing–based approach to encourage medication adherence among patients who had been prescribed neuroleptic drugs. Twenty-one patients diagnosed with schizophrenia or affective disorders were randomly assigned to compliance therapy or nondirective discussion sessions. A therapist trained in motivational interviewing techniques met with each patient for three 30-minute sessions. Although there were no differences between the treatment and control groups in attitudes toward medication, insight, or compliance, the changes in the treatment group were in the expected direction. In a second study, patients in a psychiatric ward were randomly assigned to receive either compliance therapy based on motivational interviewing principles or supportive counseling (Kemp et al., 1996). Each group received four to six sessions of counseling by a research psychiatrist or clinical psychologist who was trained in techniques of motivational interviewing. Participants who received motivational interviewing showed significantly greater improvements in attitudes to drug treatment, greater insight into their illness, and more compliance with their treatment than did participants in the supportive counseling group at 6-month follow-up. In a subsequent study, participants who received four to six sessions of compliance therapy delivered by a trained therapist demonstrated significantly greater insight, more positive attitudes toward treatment, and greater observer-rated compliance than did participants who receive nonspecific counseling. These changes were retained over an 18-month follow-up period (Kemp et al., 1998).

DiIorio and colleagues (1994) are currently conducting a study using motivational interviewing to promote adherence to antiretroviral medications among people diagnosed with HIV. The project, entitled Get Busy Living, is a randomized trial with one group receiving the usual adherence education and the other receiving usual nurse education plus one in-person motivational interviewing session followed by four telephone counseling sessions over a 3-month period. Nurses received three 4-hour training sessions and were evaluated using a "standardized patient" before they began the intervention. As part of each session, participants are asked to first rate their motivation for taking each HIV medication (up to four), and then they are asked to rate their confidence in taking each. They also complete the values clarification activity described earlier to help link their medical adherence and health to other core values and life goals. Information gained from these assessments is used to reveal discrepancies between motivation and behavior and strategies to foster adherence.

Thus, motivational interviewing appears to have a potentially useful role in helping individuals improve their medical adherence, in particular by exploring their pros and cons and by giving voice to underlying fears and anxiety about their illness. There is insufficient empirical evidence to make firm conclusions regarding when and how motivational interviewing may be best used in this regard; however, current studies will further elucidate many of these key issues.

HIV PREVENTION

Transmission of the human immunodeficiency virus (HIV) is perhaps the number one public health problem in the world today. The most common causes of HIV infections are sharing unsterilized needles among drug users and unprotected sexual intercourse. Absent a cure or vaccine, behavioral approaches remain paramount. The most effective HIV behavioral interventions have been based on cognitive-behavioral theories (Kelly, 1995; NIMH Multisite HIV Prevention Trial, 1998). However, these interventions assume that the participants are in the "action phase" and ready for change. Less attention has been paid to individuals who are not aware of their own risk of infection or who believe that their behaviors do not place them at risk. Motivational interviewing may have a promising role, and several studies have explored its application in this regard.

Carey and colleagues (1997) randomly assigned 102 women considered at risk for HIV infection to a treatment or wait-list control group. The treatment group met in groups of 8 to 13 participants for four 90-minute sessions. The intervention was delivered by two trained therapists; it included elicitation of self-motivational statements, summarizing concerns regarding HIV risk, and feedback about behaviors. Participants in the intervention group, compared to the control participants, demonstrated significant increases in HIV knowledge and risk awareness and intentions to adopt safer sexual practices; they also engaged in fewer acts of unprotected intercourse.

Carey and colleagues (2000) replicated their first study by using a second sample of 102 low-income women. Women in the control group received a four-session health-promotion program. Participants in the treatment group increased their knowledge and their intentions to reduce their risky behaviors. Although there were no differences in the treatment and control groups relative to other outcomes, participants in the intervention who had less than perfect intentions increased their condom use, talked more with their partners about condoms and HIV testing, and were more likely to refuse unprotected sex.

Belcher and colleagues (1998) used motivational interviewing as the basis for a single 2-hour session to promote HIV risk–reduction practices among low-income urban women. They found that the participants' knowledge and self-efficacy did not improve over those of a control group who received a 2-hour session on AIDS education. However, participants in the intervention did report significantly higher rates of condom use at followup. The results of these studies suggest that there is a role for motivational interviewing in HIV prevention. However, further research is necessary to determine if motivational interviewing is more useful as an adjunct to the usual cognitive-behavioral group interventions common in HIV prevention or whether motivational interviewing is more effective as a stand-alone intervention. An important issue for investigation is determining which types of HIV prevention interventions are best delivered by HIV counselors, as opposed to people who may possess a more extensive counseling background.

ISSUES RELATED TO CARDIOVASCULAR AND DIABETES MANAGEMENT

Diabetes and cardiovascular disease (CVD) are chronic illnesses that are best managed when health behaviors become integrated into long-term lifestyle habits. Management of diabetes and CVD requires controlling numerous health behaviors, such as diet, physical activity, smoking, and, in some cases, self-monitoring and medication adherence. The complexity of the behavioral regimen makes it difficult to assess patient adherence, as patients may routinely comply with certain recommendations, yet not with others.

Strategies are needed to motivate patients to consistently follow these complex treatment regimens. As noted earlier, Smith and colleagues (1997) evaluated the result of adding a motivational component to a standard behavioral obesity intervention among women with non-insulin-dependent diabetes mellitus. Those who received the additional motivational sessions had significantly better attendance at the group program, better compliance with filling out food diaries and self-monitoring blood sugars, and better glycemic control.

When working with people who have chronic illnesses, such as diabetes and CVD, it is important to assess patients' readiness to adopt each health behavior individually, rather than viewing adherence as an "all or nothing" phenomenon. Because controlling these conditions often implies multiple and complex behaviors, prioritizing which behaviors to address and when may be particularly important elements of motivational interviewing intervention in these contexts. Patients may also benefit from affirmations and problem-solving skills to help them sustain behaviors they are committed to, along with motivational strategies that help them better understand their risks for disease-related complications.

SCREENING

Obtaining screening services represents a behavioral choice for which there may be considerable ambivalence. Individuals may avoid screening tests because they fear the worst, or they simply may want to avoid the associated pain and discomfort, cost, or time commitment. Motivational interviewing has been used to modify screening behaviors in two studies: one looked at increasing screening rates for mammograms (Ludman et al., 1999; Taplin et al., 2000), and another addressed both mammogram and Pap smears (Lando et al., 2001). Both studies were conducted in large health maintenance organizations among women who had not received needed services within the HEDIS 3.0 guidelines. Initial contact was made by mail with a follow-up phone call at 2 and 6 months. Both studies had semistructured protocols, and checklists were completed at each encounter. In one study, two types of phone calls were compared: a brief reminder/scheduling call and a 5- to 10-minute motivational interviewing call designed to identify concerns and address barriers. The interventions were conducted by counselors at the masters' level with training in psychology. Ongoing supervision, including some tape review, was done by the initial trainer. Both phone interventions were equally effective in increasing screening rates for women who had not received a mammogram within the 2-year window. However, the motivational interviewing call was less cost-effective because of training and supervision costs (Fishman, Taplin, Meyer, & Barlow, 2000). The second study compared an enriched usual care (which included generic reminder calls and letters for many women) with an outreach mail and phone motivational interviewing contact and an inreach (an attempt to intercept women at scheduled clinic visits) contact, which also entailed motivational interviewing (shown to not add any additional effect due to low clinic visit rates among women needing screening). For the outreach and combined groups, the responses—primarily on barriers, beliefs, and readiness to obtain screening—were used to tailor a letter encouraging the women to schedule the screening. These women were aged 50 to 69 and met the HEDIS 3.0 criteria for needing both mammograms and Pap smears. The interventions were conducted by noncounselor research specialists. Ongoing intervention meetings were used to discuss issues and concerns with the intervention. At 14 months, women who received the outreach motivational interviewing had significantly higher rates of screening for both tests, compared to the usual care in all subgroups except for women over age 65. Taken together, these studies indicate that motivational interviewing is a promising strategy to increase the use of screening tests, at least among women with poor screening histories.

INTERNATIONAL APPLICATIONS: PREVENTING INFECTION

The studies already discussed here were conducted in developed and industrialized countries. There are serious health problems in developing countries, however—for example, diarrheal diseases, malaria, and malnutrition—that affect vast numbers of economically disadvantaged individuals. Motivational interviewing has potential application in these areas.

Thevos and colleagues have conducted several studies in African peri-urban communities where local health promoter volunteers were trained in motivational interviewing (Thevos, Kaona, Siajunza, & Quick, 2000; Thevos, Quick, & Yanduli, 2000). Their studies have focused principally on decreasing diarrheal diseases through safe water treatment and storage behaviors at the household level. The first trial was 8 weeks in length and measured disinfectant residuals in stored household water in 166 (out of 185 that began the study) randomly selected households. Either standard health education alone or an adaptation of motivational interviewing was delivered in four weekly household visits. Health counselors received 5 hours of training in motivational interviewing over three sessions. The results showed a high adherence rate to disinfectant use in both groups across the 8 weeks of assessment (range 71.1% to 94.7%), that was not statistically different. Possible explanations for the null findings include the provision of free disinfectant to both groups and inadequate statistical power (Thevos, Quick, & Yanduli, 2000). Another mitigating factor was insufficient training of the health promoters. Originally, 10 to 12 hours of training were planned; however, because of scheduling difficulties and illness, only 5 hours were actually delivered.

The second study, conducted in a different community, included 332 households in two geographically separate areas. Five local health promoters were assigned to deliver either standard health education alone or motivational interviewing. In each condition, health promoters made at least four household visits to discuss safe water. They received 8 hours of training in motivational interviewing plus field supervision. At the 8-month follow-up, there was a statistically significant 71% higher sales of water disinfectant in the motivational interviewing group (Thevos, Quick, & Yanduli, 2000). In a follow-up study in the same community that was conducted 16 months after the intervention, significantly higher rates (twofold) of detectable disinfectant in household water persisted in the motivational interviewing group (Thevos et al., 2001).

A third study coincided with a social marketing campaign to promote household water disinfection practices (Thevos, Kaona, et al., 2000; Thevos et al., 2001). Local health promoter volunteers received either the health education training associated with the campaign or the same training, supplemented with motivational interviewing. Eighteen health promoters received four full days of training in motivational interviewing, plus ongoing supervision. A total of 198 households from two different geographic areas within one community were included in the study. All households in the entire community received the social marketing campaign. At the 3-month follow-up, a statistically significant sixteenfold increase in the use of water disinfectant was observed in the motivational interviewing area over the area receiving health education and social marketing alone (Thevos, Kaona, et al., 2000).

In all these studies, the quality of delivering the motivational interviewing intervention was assessed. The health promoters completed self-rating scales and were independently rated by trainers in the field. These data indicated stable, high ratings on essential elements of motivational interviewing, such as expressing empathy and avoiding argumentation. The use of other quality-assurance techniques, such as tape recording, was not feasible in these settings (Thevos et al., 2001).

Together these studies suggest that, with adequate training, interventions using motivational interviewing have the potential to ameliorate some public health problems that confront developing nations. However, successful adaptation of motivational interviewing for these settings requires creativity and flexibility, along with an appreciation of cultural differences.

SUMMARY AND FUTURE DIRECTIONS

Health care and public health settings represent potentially important channels for delivering motivational interviewing, as health care providers can exploit "teachable moments," in which patients may be more receptive to modifying their behaviors. While the literature in this area is still emerging, available evidence suggests motivational interviewing holds considerable promise as a behavior change approach for PH and medical settings. It should be noted that there are at least 15 current U.S. National Institutes of Health–funded studies where motivational interviewing is being tested as a primary or adjunct intervention for health behavior change, with varying types of counselors and delivery modalities, and the results of these trials will considerably inform the direction of practice, policy, and research (Resnicow, DiIorio, et al., 2001)

A key issue that must be addressed in future studies relates to internal validity (see Chapter 18), in particular, the use of appropriate controls for the motivational interviewing intervention and rigorous assessment of treatment fidelity. Few studies to date adequately describe methods used for training and "certifying" providers (Glasgow et al., 2000; Smith et al., 1997), and the extent to which fidelity to motivational interviewing was attained is often unclear. Failure to account for quality and quantity of treatment delivery could result in Type III error—that is, erroneously concluding an intervention failed when, in fact, it wasn't delivered with adequate dose or fidelity (Basch, Sliepcevich, Gold, Duncan, & Kolbe, 1985). Research is currently being conducted to elucidate the active ingredients of motivational interviewing and to determine the optimal dose of motivational interviewing needed for effective behavior change. Determining the internal validity of motivational interviewing interventions can be achieved by comparing motivational interviewing head to head to other counseling methods, holding constant the attention effects, dose, and delivery modality. Additionally, by coding motivational interviewing encounters with such systems as the Motivational Interviewing Skill Code; Miller & Mount, 2001), dose–response analyses can be performed. It can be hypothesized that individuals who received counseling that was of higher fidelity should have better outcomes than those who received less-skilled motivational interviewing counseling. Studies that measure dose and fidelity of motivational interviewing interventions will help to illuminate its essential elements, as well as the optimal dose.

Ultimately, the essential question may not be whether motivational interviewing works in PH and medical settings, but how well, in what populations, for which conditions and behaviors, and at what cost. Other issues are which professions are able to deliver motivational interviewing with sufficient fidelity, and how much training is needed to raise competence to adequate levels. How will different health care delivery systems (e.g., public vs. private hospitals; health maintenance organizations vs. preferred provider plans) be willing and able to incorporate motivational interviewing into clinical practice, and how will practitioners be reimbursed for training and delivery of motivational interviewing? What is the efficacy and cost-effectiveness of telephone versus in-person delivery of motivational interviewing? Other important research issues include the effectiveness of motivational interviewing across different sociodemographic populations, as well as its cost effectiveness relative to other methods for changing health behaviors.

ACKNOWLEDGMENT

Development of this chapter was supported by National Cancer Institute Grant No. CA-69668 and National Heart, Lung, Blood Institute Grant No. HL64959 to Ken Resnicow and by Grant No. HL62165 to Belinda Borrelli.

NOTE

1. In considering which studies to include in this chapter, we relied almost entirely on authors' self-descriptions of their interventions. Thus, any intervention that was described as motivational interviewing, or informed by motivational interviewing, was considered to be such. In most cases, there was little published information to determine the extent to which interventions adhered to motivational interviewing principles or the extent to which such interventions were delivered with fidelity. Therefore, it is likely that the studies included here are highly variable with regard to their fidelity to motivational interviewing (see Chapter 16 for further discussion of this issue).

CHAPTER 18

Variations on a Theme

Motivational Interviewing and Its Adaptations

STEPHEN ROLLNICK, JEFF ALLISON, STEPHANIE BALLASIOTES,
TOM BARTH, CHRISTOPHER C. BUTLER, GARY S. ROSE, *and*
DAVID B. ROSENGREN

Soon after an initial effort was made to adapt motivational interviewing for brief interviews (Rollnick, Heather, & Bell, 1992) it seemed as if more method development was needed. Colleagues were addressing a range of problems in settings that were quite different to the specialist addiction counseling world in which motivational interviewing was born (see Chapter 17). Time pressures were often greater; there was less time for training practitioners who might not have a background in counseling; and the recipients might not even want help in the first place!

Between them, Chapters 16 and 17 clarify questions about effectiveness and about why and how these adaptations were developed. This rising interest in the flexibility of motivational interviewing undoubtedly presents a challenge to practitioners and trainers who are committed to implementing high-quality interventions. For example, one of us (Rollnick) received a call from a senior researcher who seriously wondered whether a 2-hour classroom introduction to the stages of change model would be an adequate training in motivational interviewing, not to mention a call about applying the technique to obese household pets!

How far can motivational interviewing be adapted before its goals, skills, and spirit are diluted beyond recognition? If a method is not actually motivational interviewing, then what is it? If one ventures away from home territory, what other models and methods might inform our understanding and thereby enrich clinical practice? The aim of this chapter is not to summarize or review the adaptations of motivational interviewing that have been described elsewhere, but to formulate some answers to these questions. To this end, the present team of authors—experienced clinicians and trainers from a range of backgrounds—set out to clarify and improve the usage of terms and to develop consensus about the content of motivational interviewing and its relatives. The outcome is a provisional framework for understanding approaches to behavior change, in which three forms of intervention—brief advice, behavior change counseling, and motivational interviewing—are compared and contrasted. The implications of this framework for practitioners, trainers, and researchers are then discussed.

BLAMING, LABELING, AND THE RIGHTING REFLEX

If motivational interviewing emerged as a reaction to blaming, labeling, and the righting reflex in the addictions field, it could find a comfortable home in a host of other contexts where behavior change is a regular topic of conversation. This much will be recognized by people who work in criminal justice, psychiatric, chronic disease, and primary care settings, to mention just a few. Despite the creative construction of methods like the patient- or client-centered approach, telling people what to do about behavior change is still often embedded in language, role definitions, routine procedures, training courses, and even, it could be argued, in the design and layout of rooms and clinics.

The righting reflex is usually expressed in the form of a strong persuasive effort in which the practitioner takes center stage in making the case for the other to change behavior. While this may be useful in some circumstances and with some recipients, our assumption is that *in consultations about behavior change* this might be self-defeating, so that a key task is to facilitate self-directed change as much as possible.

WHAT'S IN A NAME?

Almost from the outset, adaptations of motivational interviewing have appeared in the literature. One only need look as far as the chapter by Saunders, Wilkinson, and Allsop (1991) in the first edition of this volume to find a new name and a different perspective. Since then, the development of these adaptations have been fast and furious, taking on names such as brief motivational interviewing, brief negotiation, motivational enhancement therapy, motivational consulting, motivational intervention, and motivationally informed intervention, to name just a few. These terms are also sometimes confused with names given to methods that are not connected to motivational interviewing, like FRAMES, brief intervention, and brief therapy. Sometimes the term "motivational intervention" is given to a method that bears little or no relation to motivational interviewing, but through the use of the term "motivation," it somehow gains a kind of spurious respectability. After all, a horsewhip might be called a motivationally informed intervention, but it clearly lies outside the confines of this review! Even in this book, we find our colleagues in Chapter 16 obliged to use the phrase "adaptations of motivational interviewing." Given this state of affairs, a number of questions arise: Why did this naming occur? What attitude and skills are needed when talking about behavior change? What are the similarities and differences between various methods?

Protecting Motivational Interviewing

One reason for the variety of names used is a reluctance to use the term "motivational interviewing" itself, because it might dilute the parent method beyond recognition (Rollnick & Miller, 1995). For example, an adaptation with a strong technical orientation might place too little emphasis on empathic listening to bear much resemblance to motivational interviewing. Scrutiny of these adaptations reveal that they vary quite widely in their reliance on different principles and key elements of motivational interviewing. Caution about calling them motivational interviewing would thus seem to be justified. Understanding the skills involved would appear to be essential.

Are They Different Methods?

It is one thing to avoid the dilution of motivational interviewing, quite another to give every adaptation a new name. On the one hand, those who developed each method probably sincerely felt that their method was different to some degree from others. The dimensions along which they vary include the length of the intended consultation; the setting (emergency room, through hospital inpatient and outpatient departments to primary health care settings); the identified problem; whether or not the recipient is help-seeking; practitioner background, training, skill level; and so on. On the other hand, when one listens to practitioners talking about these methods, their similarities are often more striking than their differences: They all seem to be delivered in a nonconfrontational style, with a common goal—to elicit motivation to change and to encourage the person to take responsibility for decision making.

The proliferation of different methods runs against the trend in the world of specialist therapies, where it is generally very difficult to demonstrate specific effects of well-defined treatments (Mattson, 1998), and there is a discernable movement toward producing generic, transtheoretical models and methods. It is difficult to argue that these methods all have a content and treatment effect that allows us to distinguish one from the other. Two of us (Butler et al., 1999; Rollnick et al., 1992) viewed our own contribution of two names with such reservation that in a subsequent book (Rollnick, Mason, & Butler, 1999) we gave the method no name at all! There is a strong possibility that proliferation of names will lead to confusion.

What Happens Inside?

How might one make a decision about what method to practice, teach, or evaluate? Our initial thought was to produce a taxonomy of different methods, with guidelines about what to use where and when. Unfortunately, the absence of a clear definition and a statement of the skills involved rendered this aspiration unrealistic. We therefore decided to put these methods to one side and to start with the more general question of what attitude and skills could be used for what purpose in consultations about behavior change. What emerged was a provisional descriptive framework in which three forms of intervention can be identified.

BRIEF ADVICE, BEHAVIOR CHANGE COUNSELING, AND MOTIVATIONAL INTERVIEWING

To help the potentially bewildered practitioner, researcher, trainer, and academic reviewer, as well as the more experienced motivational interviewing practitioner and researcher, we have suggested a provisional framework (Box 18.1), which identifies three kinds of intervention: brief advice, behavior change counseling, and motivational interviewing. They are differentiated by the intervention context and goals, as well as the practitioner's style and skills. These factors may operate independently but tend to co-vary. Box 18.1 is merely a framework for bringing them together in a coherent manner. However, as it stands, all three methods focus on the task of talking about behavior change. We use the terms "practitioner" and "recipient" or "client" to denote the two individuals involved in these interactions. As ungainly as these terms may be, they are broad enough to encompass the range of circumstances within which these interventions occur.

Some Practical Examples

Here are a few examples of useful exchanges between practitioners and recipients, taken from the everyday practice and training experience of the authors; which of these scenarios, we asked ourselves, involved motivational interviewing? If they were not motivational interviewing, what skills and methods were being used?

BOX 18.1. Three Kinds of Behavior Change Interventions

	Brief advice	Behavior change counseling	Motivational interviewing
Context			
Session time	5–15 minutes	5–30 minutes	30–60 minutes
Setting	Mostly opportunistic	Opportunistic or help-seeking	Mostly help-seeking
Goals		BA goals, plus:	BA and BCC goals, plus:
	Demonstrate respect Communicate risk Provide information	Establish rapport Identify client goals Exchange information Choose strategies based on client readiness	Develop relationship Resolve ambivalence Develop discrepancy
	Initiate thinking about change in problem behavior	Build motivation for change	Elicit commitment to change
Style			
Practitioner–recipient	Active expert–passive recipient	Counselor–active participant	Leading partner–partner
Confrontational or challenging style	Sometimes	Seldom	Never
Empathic style	Sometimes	Usually	Always
Information	Provided	Exchanged	Exchanged to develop discrepancy
Skills[a]			
Ask open-ended questions		**	**	***
Affirmations		**	**	***
Summaries		*	***	***
Ask permission		**	***	***
Encourage recipient choice and responsibility in decision making		**	***	***
Provide advice		***	**	*
Reflective listening statements		*	**	***
Directive use of reflective listening		*	*	***
Variation in depth of reflections		*	**	***
Elicit change talk		*	**	***
Roll with resistance		*	***	***
Help client articulate deeply held values		*	*	***

[a]Skills range from nonessential to essential using a 3-point scale (one, two, or three asterisks).

Example 1: Brief Advice

> A social worker conducts a routine visit to a vulnerable young mother with whom he has a good relationship. He asks about her concerns, and she says that her boyfriend has been smacking the child, not particularly hard, but that she is unhappy about this. The social worker suspects that drugs are being used by this couple. He apologizes for having so little time to talk things through and asks her permission to be frank about his views and concerns. He tells the mother that because the child's safety is paramount, the smacking is a cause for serious concern. He also mentions that if she is using drugs, this could harm her and her child's development. The mother becomes tearful; she readily agrees to contact the social worker if she needs help and to receive him again in 2 days' time. He acknowledges the courage she has shown in trying to solve her problems and encourages her to take stock of her situation and make choices in her own best interests and those of her child.

In this meeting, traffic was almost all one way and consisted mainly of an outline of risks of certain behaviors. Nevertheless, under the circumstances, it was carried out in a clear and compassionate manner.

Example 2: Behavior Change Counseling

> A junior doctor seized the moment and conducted a 6- to 7-minute interview about smoking at the bedside of a man who had recently had a heart attack. Afterward, the man said that he had been made to think very seriously about giving up smoking and that he was surprised that the young doctor had not given him a lecture; she seemed to listen and to want to understand. When asked what she had done in this consultation, the doctor replied, "I didn't push; I listened and let him tell me about why he might quit." She said she had remembered two things from a series of brief behavior change workshops: letting people tell you why and how they might change, and not jumping ahead of readiness to change.

This clinician clearly had an interest in communication, some ability to listen, and an awareness of the patient-centered model. Was she using motivational interviewing? Our guess is that, according to the framework (see Box 18.1), this was probably an example of behavior change counseling. Without listening to or looking at a recording of her interview, it is difficult to be sure; but there is little reason to believe she was using motivational interviewing. The influences on her practice came from undergraduate communication skills training in patient-centered consulting and workshops on behavior change.

Example 3: Motivational Interviewing

> A probation officer is about to drive a client on a supervision order to visit his young daughter who is living with the client's ex-wife. Before set-

ting out, they discuss the offender's feelings of frustration and loss at no longer living with his wife and daughter and how much he misses them. The probation officer steers the conversation to the course of events that led to the breakdown of the marriage—due to the client's drug use and dealing—and the client says how very much he would like to reestablish the marriage. The probation officer elicits from the client a clear intention to achieve abstinence to demonstrate his love and commitment to his family. The client's goals and values become clearer, as his own understanding of his future options comes into sharper focus.

This is a good example of motivational interviewing. Helping the person resolve the contrast between personal values and the behavior problem is another characteristic of motivational interviewing (develop discrepancy). It is likely that a lot of the directing and steering was done by using reflective listening and selective reinforcement.

Example 4: Not Really a Behavior Change Consultation

A home visitor, described by colleagues as a "born listener," has had little professional training. She did attend 2-day training in motivational interviewing. She goes to an overcrowded flat in a poor township where a pregnant mother is overwhelmed by a host of problems, including alcohol dependence, depression, and physical conflict with her boyfriend. She says that she has no hope for either herself or her child, and she wishes that the pregnancy could have been aborted. The home visitor stays for an hour and arranges more appointments. The home visitor said that she did a lot of listening and also talked a little bit about what could improve the baby's health; the mother seemed brighter when she left and had expressed some concern about alcohol damaging the fetus.

This example raises the distinction between using listening skills in the form of generic counseling (probably used here) and more focused talk about behavior change (little evidence here). Motivational interviewing and behavior change counseling involve more than listening empathically. There is a clear focus on behavior change.

Three Kinds of Intervention

The descriptive guide in Box 18.1 reflects expert judgment and consensus. As a work in progress, its ongoing development will continue to be informed by clinical research and practice. The category labels represent best clinical practice; there is no attempt to assert relative value of the skills and strategies. Although most skills listed may be employed in any of three categories, we differentiate the relative emphasis, occurrence, and necessity of each to brief advice, behavior change counseling, and motivational interviewing; excluded are elements or characteristics that we consider equivalent across all categories. The interventions might be used in more than one meeting with the patient. The focus is on the skills necessary to the intervention, not the skills of the practitioners. We do not assume that brief advice or behavior change counseling is employed by a less-skilled practitioner.

Brief Advice

This cluster of skills is fairly easy to characterize, so well engrained is it in everyday conversation in health, social care, and other settings. In this context, however, we look to characterize advice giving in a way that maximizes its potential for effectiveness, as it is delivered in a sensitive manner.

The context of brief advice helps explain its character. Brief advice is typically short in duration and focused on a specific problem area (e.g., diabetes), although more than one behavior may be addressed within that domain (e.g., diet, exercise, and so on). Brief advice often occurs within an opportunistic setting. That is, the recipient may not be directly seeking assistance for the behavior or situation to which the brief advice is directed. Instead, the practitioner takes advantage of a circumstance where brief advice may prove helpful. This opportunity may spontaneously arise or be a component of the planned intervention. For example, a client visits his or her physician about joint pain, and a discussion about weight loss ensues.

The style of brief advice suggests an inequality of roles between the practitioner and recipient. The practitioner has taken on an expert role, and the client is the recipient of this expertise. Although this may imply a somewhat more passive participant stance, this does not have to be the case. Good practice standards in this circumstance are designed to diminish this inequality and passivity, thus increasing the likelihood of change. Of considerable importance here is the demonstration of respect in the manner in which the participant is addressed, privacy is ensured, and permission is requested before offering advice.

Denise Ernst (personal communication, March 2000) identifies three situations in which brief advice is appropriate: (1) the recipient asks for information; (2) the practitioner has information that might be helpful to a participant; or (3) the practitioner feels ethically compelled to provide advice. In the first two situations, brief advice is usually prefaced by a request for permission. In the last circumstance, the practitioner may or may not ask permission to proceed. In all instances, however, we might expect the practitioner to elicit participant response to the advice and its pertinence to current life circumstances. Participant responsibility and choice are also emphasized.

The skills here include identifying an appropriate circumstance for brief advice, raising the subject in a respectful manner that does not elicit unnecessary resistance, and then presenting information, often about risk, to the recipient. Open questions might occasionally be asked to assess the recipient's reactions. Listening skills are usually limited to brief summaries and perhaps surface-level reflections. Other skills, including the use of deeper reflections, receive little emphasis in this approach. Stage of change or readiness to change may occasionally inform the advice given, but does not play a central role in this intervention.

The overall goal of brief advice, as with all three interventions, is to facilitate behavior change. In brief advice, the specific tasks of the practitioner are to communicate risk, provide information, and initiate a behavior change sequence.

Behavior Change Counseling

Behavior change counseling is derived from the patient-centered method (Stewart et al., 1995), with some principles and skills linked to the more specific subject of health behavior change (Rollnick et al., 1999) and motivational interviewing. The context for behavior change counseling is often broader than for brief advice, including more problem areas and behaviors, but is not typically the systemic change that may be included in a motivational interviewing encounter. Systemic change involves the client deciding that a major shift in identity or behavior patterns, or both, is required. For example, a client addicted to alcohol not only stops drinking but also takes on the identity of a nonuser, with its accompanying behavior shifts in several categories.

Although it can be very brief in nature, behavior change counseling also extends to longer time frames. Still, the overall brevity remains a defining factor. Behavior change counseling may also be opportunistic, but more often it is a planned element of the encounter. For example, a person with diabetes meeting with a dietician may discuss diet, exercise, and meal planning but could also discuss identity issues related to having diabetes. Awareness of stages of change and client readiness drives the content and process of the session. The practitioner does not look to actively develop discrepancy, this being a guiding principle of motivational interviewing, where, for example, the discrepancy between personal values and a potentially destructive behavior is actively explored.

The roles of the practitioner and recipient are more egalitarian than in the brief advice session. The practitioner using behavior change counseling operates as an adviser to a client who is an active and engaged participant. The encounter is more collaborative than typically observed with brief advice, and greater attention is placed on building rapport. However, this does not necessarily require the same intensity of relationship building that is essential to the good practice of motivational interviewing. Behavior change counseling often has a task-oriented flavor. This form of counseling, therefore, does not derive its content only from motivational interviewing but from the patient- or client-centered method that is so commonly taught and practiced in healthcare and social care settings (see, e.g., Rollnick et al., 1999). The "spirit" of this activity is one of shared decision making.

The difference between behavior change counseling and motivational interviewing skill clusters narrows. They employ many overlapping skills, although in a somewhat different manner. In behavior change counseling, open questions and reflective listening statements are used to understand the client's views and feelings about the why, how, and when of behavior change (lifestyle habits, medication use, etc.). However, the reflective listening used may be less directive. That is, the practitioner follows the client in listening rather than directing the process. The focus is less on eliciting change talk and more on understanding the person. The practitioner avoids engendering resistance and negotiates an agenda that is sensitive to the readiness of the person.

The practitioner's tasks include those described in brief advice while adding specific elements that are designed to identify the client's goals (rather than those of the practitioner), select strategies based on the goals and the client's readiness, and then work purposively to build motivation for change. Information is exchanged rather than provided (see Rollnick et al., 1999); to achieve this, open questions and reflective listening are used to elicit the client's knowledge and information needs and to elicit his or her personal interpretation of the information provided.

Motivational Interviewing

The third kind of intervention, for which we have reserved the term "motivational interviewing," clearly includes high-quality listening as described under behavior change counseling, but it also requires the strategic use of specific psychotherapeutic methods to diminish resistance, resolve ambivalence, develop discrepancy, and trigger behavior change. With behavior change counseling, for example, the practitioner asks open questions to encourage the client to talk and then offers reflective listening statements to convey an understanding of what the client says. With motivational interviewing, the practitioner asks *particular* open questions that are intended to elicit certain kinds of speech (change talk) and *selectively* reflects the elements of client speech that enhance motivation for change, promote the resolution of ambivalence, and reinforce behavior change. The practitioner may invite (not impose) new perspectives and resolutions that are compatible with the client's value system. When responding to resistance, the practitioner using motivational interviewing chooses responses that are intended to diminish and defuse resistance and redirects the client to change talk. The principle difference between behavior change counseling and motivational interviewing, then, is the practitioner's conscious and strategic use of his or her own responses to elicit and reinforce certain kinds of speech from the client, while reducing other types of client responses.

Because of its emphasis on listening, as well as the broader goals included in this approach, motivational interviewing tends to happen less in brief opportunistic settings than it does in help-seeking settings. It can also be used where the client is obliged to attend counseling—for example, in criminal justice settings. The practitioner often has a background in counseling, although this is not a requirement. The practitioner works in a collaborative manner with the client, with a primary emphasis on building the relationship. The "spirit" of this activity can be likened to that of a dance, where the practitioner leads a delicately balanced collaborative effort.

COMMON ELEMENTS: THE SPIRIT OF BEHAVIOR CHANGE ENCOUNTERS

Conversations about behavior present a fairly unique challenge: the aspirations about change of practitioner and recipient don't necessarily fall on peaceable common ground (see Rollnick et al., 1999). One can sometimes almost touch the tension in the atmosphere. Feelings of disengagement, optimism, hope, and fear of impending conflict can swing back and forth, sometimes expressed, often not. Each of the three methods described in Box 18.1 is an attempt to steer a constructive path through this kind of conversation, to avoid the righting reflex, and to encourage, as one of us (Allison) often puts it, dancing rather than wrestling. The danger with a list like that in Box 18.1 is that is does not adequately capture the less tangible tone of the consultation. All of these methods require the capacity to be flexible, to tolerate uncertainty, to allow silence to generate thoughtfulness but not unnecessary anxiety, and—particularly with behavior change counseling and motivational interviewing—the ability to refrain from providing solutions or arguments for change.

SOME IMPLICATIONS

Practice

These three methods for talking about behavior change are not separate entities, as Box 18.1 clearly illustrates. They overlap in some senses, and they contain some distinct characteristics, much like three different styles of regional cooking might vary. How does one choose what method to use? We have suggested that this is largely determined by context: the time one has available, and whether or not the client is actively seeking help about a behavior change issue. Another possibility we gave serious thought to is that the more intensive methods are better suited to client problems that are more intractable. While this rings true for us as practitioners, we hesitate at this stage to go beyond describing methods into the world of client–treatment matching, knowing how difficult it has been for research on specialist therapy to match client problems to different treatments (Mattson, 1998).

Care should be taken to avoid oversimplifying the question of *skillfulness* in using these methods. An understandable temptation is to view the more complex method, motivational interviewing, as more skillful. However, the conceptually simpler method, brief advice, can be far from easy to use well. Anyone who has been in a situation like that encountered by the social worker in the first example here knows that to use brief advice in such a situation requires considerable skill. Indeed, many seasoned practitioners have been heard to observe, after a career embracing many thousands of consultations, that experience has taught them to simplify the communication skills they use, for example, by using shorter questions and empathic listening statements, and by avoiding overambitious goals for the consultation. This is what an experienced cook will often say: the art is in knowing what to leave out rather than what to put in. Brief advice, done well, can have an artful quality that matches the sophistication of motivational interviewing. Time and resources are often critical considerations. Brief advice can represent effective use of limited resources. It can also reflect a considered ethical judgment not to go into more personal matters with a client who has consulted for some other reason. Choice about what method to use involves weighing up what kind of skills are required for what situation.

When looking at Box 18.1 practitioners will inevitably move from the question of what method to use to a comparison of their own skills with those listed. Through self-guided learning, supervision, and training it should be possible to identify gaps in their skills portfolio. After considering the framework, a practitioner might say, "I want to be practicing motivational interviewing, but after examining this framework, I realize reflective listening skills should be more central to my practice. But let me remind myself. What exactly is reflective listening? What are the skills? How do I learn these skills, and how do I practice them?"

Learning and Training

This topic has been addressed in Chapters 13 and 14, and is also identified as a serious challenge in public health applications in Chapter 17. Relevant here are the implications of the framework presented in this chapter. Essentially, we hope that it will help learners find out where they are in the spectrum of behavior change interventions and to decide what skills they will need for their practice to be congruent with a given method. Trainers and facilitators should be able to establish jointly agreed learning objectives with practitioners. As training progresses, the framework allows all concerned to assess progress and consider the extent to which practitioners need to add new skills to their repertoire.

The list of skills in Box 18.1 are by no means comprehensive or the last word on this subject. Facilitators might well ask practitioners how valid are the skills from their perspective? What should be left out, and what needs to be put in? Do the categories in Box 18.1 have face validity? What empirical support exists for these categories?

Among the more specific implications for learning that emerge from the framework are that it will take more effort to achieve competency in motivational interviewing; that in learning brief advice and behavior change counseling, one often needs to encourage practitioners to "not do" things, to "unlearn" old habits that are usually connected to telling people why or how they might change, or to using a confrontational interviewing style; that some practitioners, because of their background, work circumstances, and learning preferences might not wish to or may not be well suited to doing certain kinds of interventions; and that undergraduate or prequalification training might focus initially on brief advice and some of the key elements of behavior change counseling.

Research

In pursuing the aim of this chapter, to clarify the inner working of behavior change efforts, one implication for research is strikingly clear—evaluating a complex intervention is no simple matter. Writers and reviewers of grant proposals might find the framework in this chapter useful for locating and understanding the method to be evaluated. Studies will benefit from developmental work which precedes the end-stage question of the effectiveness of a given method (see Chapters 16 and 17). This might include addressing the following questions:

- What does existing practice look like, and what skills are used by practitioners?
- How might a chosen method fit into this context? What skill combination and method best suits this setting? What are the reactions of clients?
- How well have practitioners acquired competence in training? What training methods were used? Were practitioners able to transfer skills into real consultations?
- Was the delivery of the method adequately monitored with reliable and valid measurement tools?

This list is by no means comprehensive, neglecting, for example, the assessment of outcome. However, it demonstrates that unless attention is paid to what practitioners *actually do* in training and in real consultations, the conclusions of a study will inevitably be tinged with reservations and uncertainty, a theme that is clearly running through the review in Chapter 16.

BRIEF ADAPTATIONS REVISITED

In light of the framework in Box 18.1, one might conclude that, by default, many of the adaptations reviewed in Chapters 16, 17, and 20–24 are examples of behavior change counseling or even brief advice. We are obliged to speculate about this, because it is not clear exactly what skills were used by the practitioners involved. For example, the first study of an adaptation (Rollnick et al., 1992) used a reasonably well-documented method that was called, perhaps ambitiously, brief motivational interviewing. However, the refined use of reflective listening was not built into the method, and its delivery was not properly monitored. The fact that recipients changed—that they might have engaged in change talk under difficult circumstances in a busy hospital ward environment—does not mean that motivational interviewing was used by the practitioners involved. The framework presented here should enable those developing adaptations of motivational interviewing to avoid inaccuracies of this kind.

CONCLUSIONS

A look back over the last 10 years at the field of motivational interviewing and its relatives might give the impression of practitioners, trainers, and researchers learning as they go along! There is a lot of truth to this assertion. Inductive processes have undoubtedly played a major role in the development of methods, informed by clinical encounters, training experiences, and the challenges thrown up by trying to evaluate efficacy and effectiveness. This has led to some confusion about what method to learn, practice, and evaluate, and it has also generated creativity. The aim of this chapter has been to encourage this activity to move forward on a surer skills-based footing, freer from a potentially misleading array of names of methods. Three methods, that vary in complexity, have been proposed as a possible way forward.

There has undoubtedly been a yearning for the quick fix in some quarters, where the search for a really brief method is associated with a desire to have something that can be applied *to* or *on* people; in truth, a high-quality exchange about behavior change is a demonstration of skillfulness that is not equivalent to following a recipe. The technical fix, therefore, might exist, but it will not be based on motivational interviewing, behavior change counseling, or the patient-centered method.

ACKNOWLEDGMENTS

Stephen Rollnick coordinated the writing of this chapter. The remaining authors all contributed equally, and are therefore listed in alphabetical order. We are sincerely grateful to our colleagues in the international Motivational Interviewing Network of Trainers who also contributed to this effort in its early stages—Hal Arkowitz, Chris Dunn, William Miller, and Ken Resnicow.

CHAPTER 19

The Role of Values in Motivational Interviewing

CHRISTOPHER C. WAGNER *and* FRANCISCO P. SANCHEZ

If you bring forth what is within you, what you bring forth may
save you.
                                                    —GOSPEL OF THOMAS

People change their behavior and lifestyle for many reasons. Some change because their current lifestyle no longer brings them sufficient pleasure. Some
change because external forces constrain them. Still others change because
their lifestyle no longer fits their identity. In each of these situations the person's values are elements of the change process.

This chapter focuses on using clients' values as a means to increase motivation to move toward a more satisfying lifestyle (issues related to counselor
values are addressed in Chapter 12). Focusing on values helps the person appreciate those things in life that are more vital to the person than drug use or
other problematic behaviors (Miller, 1998). Focusing on values can help clients define the kind of life they want to lead and the kind of person they want
to be, thus fortifying their determination to make adaptive changes.

VALUES AND BEHAVIOR

What Are Values?

For an overview of values, we turn to two authors whose work is directly applicable to motivational interviewing. Carl Rogers (1964), whose person-centered therapy provides conceptual underpinnings for motivational interviewing, proposed definitions for two types of values. He defined "operative values" as "the tendency for any living beings to show preference, in their actions, for one kind of object or objective rather than another" (p. 14). "Conceived values" were defined as "preference(s) of the individual for a symbolized object" (p. 14). The preferences in the first term are behavioral and in the second they are conceptual. Milton Rokeach (1973, 1979) believed that one function of values is to motivate, and he conceptualized values as either modes of conduct (instrumental values, such as obedience, helpfulness, and loving) or end states of existence (terminal values, such as wisdom, social recognition, and pleasure). Instrumental values motivate because they represent the idealized modes of behavior that are necessary to reach desired end states. Terminal values are motivating because they represent the desired end states.

In this chapter we draw from these definitions to conceptualize values as either *behavioral ideals* or *preferences for experiences*. As behavioral ideals, values function as judgments about what is good and not good with corresponding prescriptions for behaving consistent with the beliefs. When a person expresses that an important value is "to love one another," that person is indicating that it is "bad" to intentionally harm or perhaps even ignore others. As preferences for experiences, values guide individuals toward seeking situations in which they may experience excitement, relaxation, novelty, competition, comfort, belongingness, or security. While the person may have beliefs corresponding to these activities (e.g., "Being active keeps me healthy . . . "), often it is the experience that is at the center of the value (e.g., " . . . But more important, running just feels good").

The Structure of Values

Abraham Maslow's (1970) motivational pyramid, traditionally described as one of "needs," proposes a hierarchical structure of values. In Maslow's scheme, biological needs are prepotent—people generally value (and will seek) sustenance of the body, protection from pain or danger, and facilitation of pleasure in preference to activities that do not serve this end. When biological needs are largely satisfied, social needs (values) are pursued: acceptance by others; a sense of belongingness; receipt of attention, approval, and praise. Once secure in the social realm, psychological values—those regarding achievement, knowledge, and understanding—are often pursued. Finally, people tend to pursue even "higher" values of beauty, self-actualization, creation, and transcendence of identity barriers.

One implication of Maslow's structure is that when a person is forced to choose between a behavior that only fulfills a lower-order need and one that only fulfills a higher-order need, it is natural to choose the former. Thus, when drug use or another problematic behavior helps a person escape pain or gain pleasure, then it is natural for the person to continue that behavior, despite social rejection. When the problem behavior meets both biological and social needs, such as belonging to a peer group, it is natural for the person to continue the behavior even when it interferes with the pursuit of higher-order strivings toward achievement or self-actualization. To choose a behavior that meets these higher-level needs over the problem behavior that meets lower-order needs requires either confidence that the new behavior will continue to meet the lower-order needs or a transcendence of the natural order of motivations. From this point of view, behavior that conforms to higher-level values may be the exception, not the rule.

Schwartz and Bilsky (1987) proposed another structural model by classifying values into three types: biological, interactional, and social institutional. Using the Rokeach value survey (1973), they validated seven value domains that lead toward individualistic or collectivistic goals: enjoyment, achievement, self-direction (individualistic), maturity, security (mixed), conformity, and prosocial (collectivistic). They proposed another domain, social power, but there were no markers in the Rokeach lists to investigate it. This study suggested the presence of bipolar value dimensions of individualistic vs. collectivistic goals: self-direction vs. conformity, and achievement vs. prosocial values. They also reported some support for a dimension of enjoyment vs. prosocial values. These findings do not mean that a person cannot simultaneously hold opposing sets of values; in fact, there is some evidence that people have different value structures for different life roles (work vs. social; Brown & Crace, 1996).

Consistency between Values and Behavior

It is tempting to believe that behavior is generally consistent with values. A person who values fairness doesn't cheat; a person who values honesty doesn't lie. The evidence for the influence of other factors on behavior is strong, however. For example, immediately after declaring that "caring for others" is the basis of their religious faith, seminary students on their way to lecture on the Good Samaritan parable step over men slumped in doorways, moaning for help, simply because the students were told they are late for their presentation (Darley & Batson, 1973). Concerned bystanders ignore calls for help from victims of accidents, stabbings, and other emergency situations, apparently inhibited by the presence of other nonintervening onlookers (Darley & Latane, 1968; Latane & Darley, 1968). Even when reduced to "twitching, stuttering wreck(s)," individuals continue to deliver apparently painful shocks to innocent volunteers simply because the experimenter tells them that they "have no choice" (Milgram, 1963, p. 377). These studies do not negate the fact that people often behave in congruence with their expressed values, although they do call into question the strength of these values when the situational pull is in an opposite direction.

Although the influence of situations on behavior is undeniable, it is not absolute. Instead, behavior is the result of an interaction between the situational pull and personal tendencies. Individuals select the situations in which they participate, interpret the meaning of situational attributes, and make behavioral choices. Motivation to behave in a values-congruent manner appears to be enhanced when a person identifies higher personal values as salient to the situation, has strong attitudes about the situation based on personal experience (Schuman & Johnson, 1976), and has well-defined, challenging behavioral goals (Locke & Latham, 1990). A positive outcome expectancy or sense of self-efficacy further enhances the values-behavior consistency (Bandura, 1986; Feather, 1992), as does a positive mood state (Feather, 1992).

However, several factors appear to lessen the congruence between values and behavior. Lack of recognition of the relevance of values to specific behavioral choices appears to lessen congruence (Kristiansen, 1985), as does a lack of recognition of the negative consequences of the behavior upon oneself or others (Schwartz, 1974). When individuals deny personal responsibility for behaving in a values-congruent manner or for the resulting consequences (attributing responsibility instead to the situation itself or to other persons involved), value-behavior congruence is also diminished (Schwartz & Howard, 1980). In addition, values–behavior congruence appears to decrease when positive role models express rejection of relevant values or when negative role models endorse those values (Schwartz & Ames, 1977).

These and other findings suggest possibilities for facilitating increased consistency between values and behavior in counseling. The counselor might encourage the client to adopt the role of a self-investigator (Hermans, 1987) and to carefully contemplate the relationship between personal values and behavior (Conroy, 1979; Kristiansen, 1985; Wojciszke, 1987), considering past personal experiences and reliable external information (Fazio & Zanna, 1981; Schuman & Johnson, 1976). The counselor could help the client define goals, appreciate the value choices offered by various situations and the consequences of making certain choices, and increase hope, confidence, and a positive attitude. Through discussion, the client may come to experience his or her value system as increasingly stable and clear (Schwartz & Howard, 1980), yet not inflexible (Rogers, 1961). Over time, the client may take increasing responsibility for making values-congruent behavior choices (Schwartz & Howard, 1980), as well as for the consequences of those choices (Schwartz, 1974).

These findings provide some guidance for counselors who are encouraging clients to move in a values-congruent direction, although there appears to be an important caveat: one needs to be seen by clients as a "positive referent" or risk fostering opposition to the information or suggestions provided (Schwartz & Ames, 1977).

Values and Problematic Behavior

We focus on three viewpoints found in the literature regarding the relationship between values and problematic behavior: problematic behavior may be primarily self-oriented (good for the individual, but harmful to others), short-sighted (good for the individual now, bad for the individual later), or inefficient (satisfies some needs or values, but prevents satisfaction of others). To help explain these points and for subsequent discussion, we present the case example of Tina.

> Tina is a 33-year-old woman who presents for substance abuse treatment at an inner-city agency, following an arrest for possession of cocaine. She appears unhealthy and exhausted. She reports smoking cocaine over extended weekends, smoking a pack of cigarettes per day and drinking beer and wine while using cocaine. She lives in public housing with her mother. She is currently unemployed, and her only source of income is money she makes through "running" drugs between dealers and buyers. She has two daughters, ages 8 and 11, whom she regularly leaves with her mother while she goes on her binges. She previously spent considerable time with her daughters, helping them with homework, playing games with them, and shopping, but this has decreased substantially over the past year.

People who display problematic behavior are sometimes perceived as "lacking in values." They may be seen as selfish, choosing personal pleasure over other values promoted by society such as caring for one's family or being involved in community affairs (Peele, 1990). One example of such thinking is the moral model of addiction, which considers problematic drug use to be an immoral and unrestrained pursuit of self-centered values. In our example, Tina's cocaine consumption could be considered representative of self-oriented values as she has neglected her daughters while using cocaine.

"Short-sighted" behaviors are those that reap short-term rewards while ignoring long-term negative consequences. Substance use and other problematic behaviors often lead to immediate rewards of increased pleasure or relaxation, as well as other short-term rewards such as excitement or a sense of belonging to a peer group. It is typically over the long term that these behaviors are unsatisfying. For example, it is healthy to desire to be part of a peer group that shares experiences and viewpoints, but when the common denominator among group members is use of substances, one may find one's needs for belonging are met only temporarily; the social bonds may dissolve as the substances disappear. In our case example, Tina's problematic behaviors are short-sighted; they provide pleasure and excitement now, but over the long term they may lead to a dissatisfied sense of self, a feeling that life has been wasted, and legal consequences that prevent her from obtaining a satisfying job or lifestyle.

"Inefficient" behaviors fulfill certain needs at the expenses of others. Intensive substance use may fulfill values of relaxation and pleasure, as well as belongingness, while simultaneously reducing achievement and self-esteem. Tina's cocaine use produces pleasure and she finds the surrounding lifestyle exciting, yet these needs are fulfilled at the expense of other values she holds about parenting, achievement, and self-esteem.

While these focus areas can help in analyzing clients' problem behaviors, it is best to avoid strong initial assumptions about what values drive those behaviors. Our preconceptions about which values are most important may blind us to a thorough understanding of clients' own value system. Counselors can reduce the influence of their own biases by exploring these notions with clients, asking clients to identify potentially self-oriented, short-sighted, or inefficient behaviors for consideration. Discussion of problematic behaviors in the context of the values they serve may decrease resistance because it is the clients themselves who identify the behaviors and any conflicts or undesired consequences with the values held. Once these relations are identified, clients may determine that they do not need to change their values per se but must simply find different ways to fulfill their preferences for experiences. Although the counselor can inform the client of ways that others have achieved this, no one but the client can discover which other behaviors meet needs and conform to personal ideals. Creativity is helpful in this venture, as the behaviors that "work" may be social, vocational, educational, recreational, artistic, or spiritual in nature. For Tina, who values both excitement and autonomy, the goal may not be to change those values but perhaps to find less problematic ways of achieving them, whether that be through dancing, career building, or perhaps even kick boxing!

VALUES AND PSYCHOTHERAPY

Theoretical Perspectives

One foundation for considering the role of values in motivational interviewing is humanistic theory. Among its basic tenets are assertions that people are motivated by the desire for growth and self-direction (Rogers, 1964) and are continually striving for the actualization of their potential (Maslow, 1967). Rogers proposed that as children and adolescents experience reward or rejection for various behaviors, they learn to value or devalue those aspects of self that underlie the various behaviors. As certain behaviors are consistently (or intensely) met with rejection or punishment, individuals tend to "close off" or disown those "parts" of their self. Individuals receiving considerable rejection, or "negative regard," become more likely to lack recognition of personal problems, lack desire to change, lack awareness of internal feelings and values, avoid close relationships, and be unwilling to communicate with others about their inner experiences. Rogers's client-centered therapy involved providing an interpersonal atmosphere in which clients would increasingly become aware and accepting of their experiences and values, the disowned aspects of self, and a sense of self-direction. Rogers (1961) reported that clients often would increasingly value self-direction, flexibility of behavior and sense of self, acceptance of their internal complexity and contradictory feelings, an openness to internal experiences that were previously ignored or rejected, acceptance of others, and self-trust. In addition, clients were observed to increasingly reject facades and compulsions to live by others' standards, expectations, or rewards.

Mowrer's (1945) work on integrative learning suggests that learning can be interrupted by the time delay between contradictory short- and longer-term results of a given action, setting up a "vicious circle" or nonintegrative strategy. For example, Tina's use of cocaine provides excitement. Finding ways to afford and obtain the drug feeds her desires for adventure and achievement. Running drugs provides interpersonal reinforcement, as both the dealers and the buyers enjoy seeing her and reinforce her for helping. Using cocaine is a reward for successfully completing her "mission," and its euphoric properties add to her positive feelings. At the end of a several-day run, however, Tina ends up feeling ashamed for neglecting her daughters, feels she has been "used" by the dealers and buyers, and experiences depressed mood, feeling that she once again let herself and her family down and "wasted" several days' time. In this situation, focusing on her values about parenting and achievement may promote insight about the nonintegrative nature of her behavior pattern. This insight may be obscured by the delay between the desirable short-term consequence of enjoyment, excitement, and adventure and the undesirable longer-term consequences of experiencing shame and depressed mood.

Mowrer's (1966) "integrity therapy" helps clients willingly claim appropriate responsibility for actions they find troubling. Mowrer attributed psychological distress to the lack of integrity or correspondence between a person's behavior and moral beliefs; psychological relief begins with acknowledgment of the troubling nature of the behavior. According to Mowrer, "it is the truth we ourselves speak rather than the treatment we receive that heals us" (1966, p. 114). He called the speaking of such truth a "painful but liberating self-disclosure." Once discovering themselves in a genuine way, including the discrepancy between behavior and ideals, individuals liberate themselves from their distress.

Rokeach (1979) proposed that values function as motivational guideposts, stimulating an increase in value-behavior consistency, thus improving self-esteem. Rokeach also believed that although different individuals may hold similar values, differences in the relative importance of each value may account for differences in behavior. His values self-confrontation (VSC) approach involved individuals rank-ordering their value preferences, comparing their ordered list with that of a positive reference group, and discussing the implications of the ordering priority.

Empirical Studies

Although we uncovered relatively few published outcome studies that focused on values-oriented approaches with problematic behaviors, those that we found are instructive. A study of heavy smokers who received treatment at a smoking cessation clinic found posttreatment differences in smoking rates between a group that participated in a values ranking and examination process versus a control group. At the conclusion of the 19-day clinic, the control group was smoking at 28% of its pre-clinic average, while the values group was at 5%; this difference was maintained at 2-month follow-up (Conroy, 1979).

Schwartz and Inbar-Saban (1988) used Rokeach's VSC method with overweight individuals interested in losing weight. They assessed individuals' value priorities, then discussed the congruence of these priorities with the rank-ordered priorities that differentiated between weight-losing (wisdom = 2, happiness = 11) and non-weight-losing (e.g., wisdom = 5, happiness = 5) groups in a pilot study. Individuals undergoing VSC lost more weight over the following 2 months than a nontreatment group or than a discussion-control group, and they continued to lose more weight than the discussion-control group over the following 12 months (during which time the nontreatment group received VSC and subsequently also surpassed the discussion group in weight loss). The VSC method produced values change among participants toward congruence with the positive reference group, and the value change mediated the weight loss, presumably by increasing dissatisfaction about the discrepancy between the individuals' and reference groups' scores.

Although not using an explicitly values-oriented approach, Downey, Rosengren, and Donovan (2000) reported that the perception of discrepancy between substance use and self-standards was a significant motivator of abstinence among individuals who participated in public-sector addiction treatment, including a brief motivational intervention. Their article also reviews the literature on the relationship between addictive behaviors and identity issues, which is a focus closely related to that of this chapter.

VALUES AND MOTIVATIONAL INTERVIEWING

Why Focus on Values?

From a humanistic viewpoint, motivational interviewing involves assisting individuals to define their current and ideal selves, then pursue movement from the current self toward the ideal. Thus, a focus on values may help increase an individual's sense of the importance of change, as well as define the direction of change. The counselor may assist clients to more fully appreciate their current self by eliciting discussion of problematic behaviors in relation to self-oriented, short-sighted, or inefficient value choices. This can assist clients to uncover reasons for continuing to engage in less-than-optimal behaviors, despite resulting negative consequences. When the problematic behaviors can be seen as (misguided) choices to achieve valued ends, individuals may become less defensive about protecting those choices and more open to exploring other means of achieving their values.

A values focus can help a person define his or her "ideal self" by exploring those behavioral ideals to which the person resonates. Sometimes, individuals have forgotten about these values or have rejected them as naive or unachievable. Simply focusing on these ideals can help a person detect current behaviors inconsistent with the ideal. In our case example, Tina's explicit focus on her ideal self as healthy parent and provider may help her appreciate the problems posed by her attempts to live an exciting, fast-paced, glamorous lifestyle. In this way, the person's values guide the direction of change.

A focus on values may stimulate motivation for change. Focusing on discrepancies between ideal life conditions and actual conditions may induce a desire to "recalibrate" daily behaviors to be more congruent with deeply held beliefs. Awakened to a deeper sense of self and values, the person may become increasingly aware that the problematic behaviors meet certain short-term needs but do not lead to fulfillment of more deeply held values or long-term satisfaction. Focusing on ideals can help decrease clients' defensiveness and increase desire for change by shifting the focus away from consideration of "negative" behaviors or lifestyle, toward a focus on a positive, more deeply satisfying lifestyle that can be pursued and enjoyed. Clients may come to perceive that they do not necessarily have to purge valued aspects of their current self; instead, they need to restrain certain tendencies in order to develop a deeper, more aware self and live with a greater sense of purpose (importance) and power (confidence). By doing this, they may also reduce the negative emotions that are often related to the identification of a discrepancy between values and behavior (Avants, Singer, & Margolin, 1993–1994).

Ambivalence about various possibilities can be viewed in part as the experiential result of multiple conflicting values. In our example, Tina's ambivalence can result from a conflict between her short-term values of excitement and a glamorous lifestyle and her longer-term values of good parenting and a lifestyle that permits sustained achievement, despite its "ordinary" nature. While ambivalence may be resolved from concluding that longer-term values take precedence over short-term values, there are other paths to its resolution. Sometimes, it is not so much a conflict between the long- and short-term values themselves but an issue that the strategies for fulfilling short-term values are precisely those strategies that prevent fulfilling the longer-term values. There are ways to gain excitement other than using cocaine and living a fast lifestyle. By seeking with the client the positive motivations behind the problematic behaviors, we can open the door to consideration of alternative behaviors that address short-term needs without unduly interfering with the pursuit of long-term goals.

Similarly, ambivalence can arise from conflicts between individualistic and collectivistic values (e.g., self-direction vs. conformity), or from valuing one behavior or experience that interferes with another valued behavior or experience (e.g., partying late at night with friends makes it difficult for Tina to get up and help the kids off to school). Clarifying the relative importance of these values may help reduce ambivalence.

Highlighting Values in the Practice of Motivational Interviewing

The use of values can be incorporated into the practice of motivational interviewing in many ways. The most obvious way is to "keep an ear open" for clients' values. Many of the underlying principles and practices of motivational interviewing already focus on clients' values or can be easily adapted to do so.

In helping a client to better understand the values guiding everyday behavior, two of the motivational interviewing principles are especially useful. When expressing empathy, counselors can focus on unspoken values behind a client's statements. For example, one day Tina arrives late for her appointment, explaining that the kids have been sick and her mother relies too much on junk food, so Tina made the kids a good breakfast before leaving the apartment. A counselor could interpret this situation in many ways. The counselor may interpret the explanation as unimportant, as a need to vent stress, or perhaps as a test of the therapeutic relationship. Given the client's history of tending to her own needs over her childrens', the counselor may view this behavior as a sign of resistance to treatment or even doubt the veracity of the report itself. Depending on the interpretation, the counselor may explore the perceived resistance, reflect the client's frustration, reassure the client that the counselor won't reject or punish her for arriving late, or simply shrug off the explanation. Using the principle of expressing empathy and focusing on the values of the client, the counselor could respond, "It seems like it's important for you to be a good mother and do the best you can for your kids, even if you have to sacrifice some things for yourself or if other people might not understand." This response expresses the counselor's understanding of the meaning of the client's behaviors and refocuses the conversation on a deeply held value (e.g., caring for her children), its relation to current behavior (feeding the kids nutritious foods in case her mother doesn't), and the importance of the value (it's worth risking the counselor's misunderstanding, disbelief, or annoyance).

Rolling with resistance is typically discussed in terms of the momentary interpersonal behaviors of the client and counselor. The counselor does not oppose resistant behaviors. When a client argues, the counselor explores the client's views, changes topics or does anything other than argue back. When a client withholds his or her opinion, the counselor does not insist the client explain it. In terms of values, the resistant behaviors may indicate some opposition between the client's competing internal values, between the values of the client and counselor, or between the values of the client and society. For example, although she desires a more sustainable lifestyle that builds toward a better future, Tina may perceive available employment opportunities as too menial or unrewarding. Similarly, she may be attached to aspects of her current lifestyle that likely decrease her chances of developing a more sustainable one, such as buying expensive clothes and jewelry. Challenging her on these values may increase resistance. "Rolling with" these issues by explicitly acknowledging her valuing meaningful employment and a sense of social status may help develop an atmosphere in which she is able to consider these value conflicts in a less defensive manner.

Whereas the previous two principles focus on understanding current behavior, the principle of developing discrepancy is intended "to create and amplify . . . a discrepancy between present behavior and . . . broader goals and values" (Chapter 4 in this volume). In the practice of motivational interviewing, the counselor does not dramatically point out the discrepancy (e.g., "So having social status is more important to you than saving money to give your children a better life?"). Instead, the counselor develops the theme of discrepancy bit by bit over an extended conversation or across counseling sessions. One may elicit the development of discrepancy from the client rather than leading with an interpretation regarding apparent conflicts between values and behavior (e.g., "We've talked several times about how important it is to you to 'get somewhere' in life. At the same time, you like buying fashionable clothes, and being looked up to by others and you feel like it's drudgery to go to work every morning. How do these fit together?").

Standard motivational interviewing strategies may be adapted to focus explicitly on clients' values. In early discussions, these strategies may help clients define their current self in light of their values. Using the opening strategies, the counselor may directly ask about clients' values (both ideals and preferences for experiences), reflect statements related to ideals or preferences, summarize described experiences in light of clients' values, and affirm the effort involved in determining clients' ideals and their relation to current lifestyles. Emphasizing personal choice in behavior or lifestyle may prompt exploration and ownership of values (e.g., "It's up to you to decide which kind of life you want to lead—what's important to you?"). Counselors can review a typical day to help clients define their preferences for experiences, as well as gather information for the later consideration of discrepancies between current behavior choices and values. When providing assessment feedback, counselors can determine clients' reactions to the results and explore any dissatisfaction in terms of clients' values.

Double-sided reflections can be expressed as mirroring the ambivalence that results from an underlying values conflict. The exploration of good things/less good things is essentially a values clarification exercise already, and counselors can make an explicit link to client values when summarizing this topic (e.g., "So while you view your current lifestyle as exciting and you like leading a fast life, you also feel like you're not getting anywhere and you think it's not-so-good for your kids, which bothers you because it's important to you to build a career and to be a good mother"). Focusing on values as preferences for experiences can help clients improve their understanding of the functions of their current behavior, as well as help them formulate a clearer sense of the values they are seeking to fulfill through the behavior.

Motivational interviewing strategies may directly assist clients in their attempts to define their core values and ideal self. When looking forward, clients can be asked to consider possible futures that may result from particular choices in relation to deeper values (e.g., "Looking ahead, how do you expect things to be a year from now if you continue to focus on excitement and being 'part of the scene'? How might things be different if you focus that time on your desires to achieve more?"). The decisional balance exercise is a values exercise similar to good things/less good things, except with a focus on future behavior. Once the pros and cons have been identified, counselors may ask clients to consider which of these options best meet clients' ideals while also fulfilling their preferences for experiences. Counselors may reflect that clients have the opportunity to create different lifestyles and to choose in part who they will become in the future through the course of action they choose. Use of the importance ruler is another strategy with an obvious relation to values. Valuing a behavior, choice, or situation means that one considers these things important. When counselors reflect clients' statements regarding what makes a particular choice important (or not), it is a natural time to incorporate a more general discussion of the clients' values.

Values can also play a role in increasing confidence. Increasing awareness of one's ideals leads to making more conscious choices about the extent to which one will strive to live in consonance with those values. Intentionally recalling both ideals and preferences for experiences may be useful to clients in tempting or stressful situations and can help fortify clients against making harmful choices. For Tina, intentionally recalling her ideals of being a good mother and personal achievement through building a career may help her refuse a friend's offer to take her out on the town or share some cocaine with her. Recalling that her desire to participate in these is related to her preferences for exciting experiences may then cue her to actively seek another exciting experience in order to help protect her against relapse.

The role of values may again be highlighted during the change planning process, when clients are asked to state why the chosen plan is important to them. When clients make a commitment to a particular behavior plan (e.g., to quit smoking), it can be useful to reflect that they are at another level making a commitment to a particular identity (e.g., an ex-smoker). Further, it may be useful to review any previous unsuccessful attempts to implement changes and look for values that may have been neglected. For example, Tina quit using drugs and alcohol on several previous occasions, motivated by self-directed anger about neglecting her children's needs, as well as by the desire to improve her lifestyle. Each time, after a period of working full-time, developing more intimate relationships with her children, and using her earnings almost entirely to provide for the family, Tina relapsed. Although her change attempts produced positive short-term results, her zeal for improving things for her daughters and for "making up for lost time" created a situation in which her values regarding excitement and sociability were left unfulfilled and the situation became nonsustainable over time.

Incorporating Other Promising Techniques

Various clinicians and researchers have added values-oriented techniques into their practice. One common approach has been to adapt Rokeach's card sort and values self-confrontation (VSC) approach.

Brown and Peterson (1990) describe using VSC to treat addictive behaviors, having clients rank their top values, then discussing those values in comparison to those of successfully recovering individuals (with high rankings of the terminal values of inner harmony, self-respect, and wisdom and the instrumental values of honesty and forgiveness). Following the discussion, clients recorded daily ratings of their value-behavior consistency for each of their ranked values.

Sanchez (2000) studied the outcome of a values card sort exercise with alcohol abusers in a 1-hour motivational interviewing format, based in part on the work by Miller and C'de Baca (1994). Topics discussed included the meaning of the various values statements, evaluation of current value-behavior consistency, perceived barriers to and opportunities for increasing value-behavior consistency, and personal evaluation of the extent to which the use of alcohol plays a role in achieving or preventing consistency. An attention-control group viewed addiction-related videos in the presence of the interventionist. The values group had better outcomes on measures of drinking behavior and consequences at 3-month and 6-month follow-up. Sanchez reported impressions that the technique increased the ease of practice, as well as client engagement.

De Francesco (2001) reports using the values card sort approach with firefighters, focusing on exercise and dietary behaviors. Firefighters were asked to discuss how their health goals fit with their values. De Francesco describes how this can resolve ambivalence and increase motivation by helping participants more closely tie their behavioral goals to their own specific values (e.g., leading an active lifestyle vs. losing weight). One participant reflected his perception that he may have previously failed at weight loss because he was essentially doing it for the "wrong" reasons, that is, reasons unrelated to his values (i.e., he valued "looking good" more than the health benefits that result from exercise and his focus during previous change attempts had been on improving health).

Other motivational interviewing practitioners have incorporated a focus on values-behavior consistency into their work with persons with HIV (Ryan,

Fisher, Krutch, & Downey, 2001), in motivational counseling groups (Ingersoll, Wagner, and Gharib, 2000), and in efforts toward health promotion (Chapter 17 in this volume).

Rusk and Ervin (1996) outlined a somewhat different values clarification approach named "guided self-change" (no apparent relation to the similarly named approach of Sobell & Sobell [1998]). They described the goal not as curing of illness but "healing of spirit." They proposed several principles that resemble those of motivational interviewing. First, labeling is viewed as counterproductive because it focuses clients on deficits and distracts them from their values. Second, an essential task for clients is "compassionate self-observation," carefully monitoring behavior in light of values without passing judgment or self-criticism. Third, clients are encouraged to take personal responsibility for developing and implementing change plans. Clients are provided with audiotapes of each session and are encouraged to review them privately, in order to facilitate further consideration of the values discussed in session. Between sessions, clients are encouraged to implement real-life experiments that clarify or amplify personal values or increase value–behavior consistency. Perhaps somewhat different from the practice of motivational interviewing, the therapist is viewed as a mentor or guide who offers specific values for clients to consider as ideals: respect, understanding, caring, and fairness. (In the Schwartz–Bilsky [1987] structure, these are most representative of the prosocial, maturity and self-direction domains.)

Simon, Howe, and Kischenbaum (1995) offer several additional promising techniques, such as having clients write words ending in "ing" that tell something about who they are (e.g., loving, hard-working). Discussion of the implications of the self-identity words as reflected in the person's life may focus on the present. However, counselors can listen for underlying values and help clients explore those further. The authors offer other existential techniques, such as having the person write down several answers to the question "Who are you?" then exploring the answers provided in relation to the values implied in the client's answers. Similarly, they suggest having the person imagine a life-threatening experience, then focus on questions such as "What do you have yet to get out of life that is important?" or "What contributions would you like to make in this life that you have not yet completed?"

SUMMARY

Incorporation of a values perspective in the practice of motivational interviewing is supported from both conceptual and practical bases. Focusing on clients' values is consistent with the self-directedness of the person-centered framework underlying motivational interviewing and may help clients view behavior change more as desired movement toward a more fulfilling lifestyle than an undesired loss of familiar and reinforcing habits and ways of being. Initial attempts to explicitly incorporate a values focus have yielded positive preliminary empirical findings as well as positive comments from practitioners and clients. This chapter has suggested several other specific ways in which a focus on values may be explicitly incorporated in order to help clients change.

ACKNOWLEDGMENTS

We thank Jessye Cohen, Karen Ingersoll, and David Rosengren for their thoughtful reviews of an earlier version of this chapter.

CHAPTER 20

Motivational Interviewing and Treatment Adherence

ALLEN ZWEBEN *and* ALLAN ZUCKOFF

> It is not patients who should comply with their doctors' demands, but doctors who should comply with their patients' informed and considered desires.
>
> —S. Holm, cited by Barry Blackwell,
> *Treatment Compliance and the Therapeutic Alliance*

WHAT DO WE MEAN BY "ADHERENCE"?

Terms such as "compliance" and "adherence" have been used interchangeably in the pharmacotherapy and psychosocial treatment literature, to refer to individuals' entering into, attending, and completing treatment, as well as to their performance of treatment activities and tasks. We have chosen not to use the term "compliance" because of its connotation of obedience to authority, and association with such concepts as "resistance" or "denial"; clients labeled "noncompliant" have often been seen as personally deficient in motivation or said to possess character traits that make them prone to failing to engage in and sustain a treatment relationship.

Consistent with the outlook inherent in motivational interviewing, we make no assumptions about the personalities of those who participate inconsistently in treatment or choose not to attend as expected; rather, we start from the belief that these decisions and behaviors are determined in large part by the interactions of treatment seekers with treatment providers and systems (Daley & Zuckoff, 1999; Zweben, Bonner, Chaim, & Santon, 1988). We therefore use the more neutral term "adherence" to describe the extent to which people follow through with agreed-on or prescribed actions, or do what providers expect them to do, where treatment is concerned. This term may designate keeping appointments and maintaining timely attendance, taking medications as prescribed, or completing specific tasks between appointments (e.g., attending support groups, selecting a significant other to participate in sessions, doing reading or writing assignments, engaging in activation tasks for depression or exposures for anxiety disorders, self-monitoring, or taking medication for various medical conditions). Adherence, then, is broadly defined to encompass those factors that may have an impact on how fully a particular treatment is delivered as a result of participant decisions and actions.

WHY IS IT IMPORTANT TO ENGAGE AND MAINTAIN CLIENTS IN TREATMENT?

Those who do not adhere to a therapeutic regime can represent a costly and troublesome problem for treatment providers. When clients attend inconsistently or participate halfheartedly in therapy activities, clinicians can become frustrated and even demoralized. At the same time, individuals who occupy available slots without fully using the treatment offered can reduce access for others who want it; and, because many will eventually need additional services, health care costs overall may be unnecessarily increased (Carroll, 1997). As pressure has been brought to bear on treatment programs to maintain economic viability in the context of the demands of managed care, frequent missed appointments and high rates of dropout have drawn increasing systemic and administrative attention.

More important, mounting evidence of a relationship between treatment adherence and treatment outcome (Brown & Miller, 1993; Corrao et al., 1999; Daley, Salloum, Zuckoff, Kirisci, & Thase, 1998; Fiorentine & Anglin, 1996; Hu et al., 1998; Simpson, Brown, & Joe, 1997; Walker, Minor-Schork, Bloch, & Esinhart, 1996) has made problems of adherence a focus of professional concern. Response to both pharmacological and psychosocial treatment has been shown to depend on producing an adherence effect (Volpicelli, Alterman, Hayasguda, & O'Brien, 1997). Significant relationships have been found among treatment retention and symptomatic improvement, life functioning, and client well-being (Daley et al., 1998; Mattson et al., 1998; Westerberg, 1998). Thus, individuals who adhere to a treatment regime appear to have a better chance of success than do those who do not.

The magnitude of the adherence problem is quite striking and has been well-documented in the mental health, substance abuse, and medical fields over the past 25 years (Baekeland & Lundwall, 1975; Blackwell, 1976; Chen, 1991; Dobscha, Delucchi, & Young, 1999; Garfield, 1994; Hochstadt & Trybula, 1980; Hser, Maglione, Polinsky, & Anglin, 1997; Ito, Donovan, & Hall, 1988; Joyce, 1990; Krulee & Hales, 1988; Matas, Staley, & Griffin, 1992; Onken, Blaine, & Boren, 1997; Owen, Rutherford, Jones, Tennant, & Smallman, 1997; Solomon & Gordon, 1988; Stark, 1992; Wolpe, Gorton, Serota, & Wright, 1993; Wright, 1993). Dropout rates among psychiatric patients are between 31 and 56% prior to the fourth session (Carroll, cited in Mattson et al., 1998); about 30% of alcohol clients drop out between 2 and 5 months of treatment while only 26% remain in treatment past 6 months, and only 58% of scheduled psychotherapy appointments are kept (Carroll, cited in Mattson et al., 1998). Pharmacotherapy studies have reported sample rates of failure to take medications for such conditions as rheumatic fever, diabetes, heart disease, tuberculosis, and even leprosy to be anywhere from 37% to 67% (Wright, 1993). These figures raise serious questions about whether persons in need of help with psychiatric, substance use, or medical problems are adequately receiving that help.

It should be acknowledged that the specific nature of the relationship between treatment adherence and treatment outcomes remains uncertain and requires further investigation. Retention in psychosocial treatment is not always associated with better outcomes (see, e.g., Crits-Cristoph et al., 1999). Furthermore, although adherence predicts better outcomes in many contexts (Westerberg, 1998), it is not always clear that adherence is the source of those improved outcomes. For some clients, staying in treatment longer may spur greater efforts to change; for others, improved attendance may simply reflect the fact that these clients were more "ready" to begin with. To illustrate, in Project MATCH (Project MATCH Research Group, 1998b), a multisite, client–treatment matching study dealing with alcohol problems, pretreatment motivational readiness predicted both treatment adherence *and* treatment outcomes.

Nonetheless, the bulk of the evidence in both pharmacological and psychosocial interventions leads to the conclusions that without adequate levels of treatment attendance, it would be difficult for persons to take maximum advantage of treatment (Mattson et al., 1998); without participants' active cooperation, treatment cannot have its desired impact. Developing more effective approaches to improve adherence is thus arguably a critical challenge confronting providers.

WHAT IS THE EVIDENCE THAT MOTIVATIONAL INTERVIEWING CAN BE USED TO IMPROVE ADHERENCE?

What Research Has Been Done?

Table 20.1 summarizes all the published or presented tests of motivational interviewing of which we are aware that include findings on adherence effects. The adaptations of motivational interviewing (AMIs; see Chapter 16, this vol-

TABLE 20.1. Adherence Effects of Adaptations of Motivational Interviewing

Study	Sample	Interventions	Adherence effects	Caveats
Miller et al. (1988)*	42 problem drinkers, recruited by advertisement; moderate severity	AMI (DCU or DCU + referral vs. wait list control (DCU deferred 6 wk)	*Treatment entry* 14.3% overall at 6 wk, 33.3% overall at 18 mo	Integrity? No control.
Kuchipudi et al. (1990)	114 male acute inpatients admitted to a VA hospital with alcohol-related illness + past medical advice to quit drinking	AMI (3 brief interviews with medical staff, 1 long interview with social worker, 1 group with psychiatric nurse) vs. NIC, added to standard care	*Treatment entry* AMI = NIC (18.4% overall at 10–16 wk)	Intervention as described conflicts with principles of motivational interviewing.
Bien, Miller, & Burroughs (1993)*	32 men entering VA outpatient alcohol treatment; high severity	AMI (DCU) vs. diagnostic control, prior to start of standard treatment	*Treatment entry* AMI = diagnostic control (81.2% overall)	Therapist effects?
Brown & Miller (1993)*	28 alcohol-dependent adults entering private residential treatment	AMI (DCU) vs. NIC, at start of standard treatment	*Task performance* Compliance and goal attainment (therapist rated): AMI > NIC	Integrity? Therapist effects?
Saunders et al. (1995)	122 opiate-dependent adults entering a methadone program	AMI (no feedback) vs. EC: 1 extended session, brief follow-up session at 1 wk	*Retention* Days in treatment: 151 AMI vs. 127 EC Wk in study: 22.3 AMI vs. 17.8 EC Study follow-up contact: AMI > EC (1 wk, 3 and 6 mo)	Integrity? Therapist effects?
Smith et al. (1997)*	22 obese women, age 50+, with NIDDM and able to exercise, recruited to a 16-session group behavioral weight control program by advertisement or letter	AMI (1 session at initiation, 2 at midpoint, with feedback), vs. NIC, added to standard treatment	*Attendance* Sessions: 13.3 AMI vs. 8.9 NIC *Retention* Completion (16 wk): AMI = NIC (77% overall) *Task performance* Food diaries submitted: 15.2 AMI vs. 10.1 NIC Days glucose monitored: 46.0 AMI vs. 32.2 NIC Days exercised: 35.2 AMI vs. 23.7 NIC ($p = .07$) Days recorded calories: 76.8 AMI vs. 55.7 NIC ($p = .07$)	Integrity? Manual? Training? AMI was the only 1:1 contact provided.
Aubrey (1998)*	77 adolescents entering outpatient polysubstance treatment; high severity	AMI (DCU) vs. NIC, at start of standard treatment	*Attendance* Sessions: 17 AMI vs. 6 NIC	Integrity? Therapist effects?
Booth et al. (1998)	192 intravenous drug users; recruited through community outreach; high severity	AMI (MI and RI, no feedback) vs. RR: 5 sessions, 1/2 hr each, + offer of free vs. pay treatment; rapport-building first session in AMI and RR	*Treatment entry* AMI = RR (at 8 week) *Attendance* Intervention sessions: AMI = RR (3.94 overall)	Strategies used in AMI found not to be tailored to subject readiness to change.
Daley et al. (1998)*	23 depressed cocaine dependent psychiatric inpatients, discharged to dual-diagnosis aftercare on antidepressant medication	AMI (MI and DDRC, no feedback) vs. TAU: 5 1:1 and 4 group sessions during first month of aftercare	*Retention* 30 days: 100% AMI vs. 41.7% TAU 90 days: 72.7% AMI vs. 8.3% TAU *Attendance* Intervention sessions (9): 7.2 AMI vs. 2.7 TAU	Integrity? Nonrandomized (consecutive assignment). TAU unspecified.

TABLE 20.1. (*continued*)

Study	Sample	Interventions	Adherence effects	Caveats
Daley & Zuckoff (1998)*	100+ adults with substance and psychiatric diagnoses in a psychiatric hospital, referred to dual-diagnosis aftercare.	AMI (MI and DDRC, 1 session, no feedback) vs. NIC, added to usual discharge planning.	*Treatment entry* 67% AMI vs. 35% NIC	Analysis? Integrity? Nonrandomized (historical control, not described).
Kemp et al. (1998)	74 adults with psychotic diagnoses in a psychiatric hospital on antipsychotic medication; 60% involuntary	AMI (MI and CT, no feedback) vs. NSC: 4–6 sessions + optional boosters, added to routine management and aftercare	*Task performance* Medication compliance (observer-rated): 5.5–5.7 AMI vs. 3.5–4.3 NSC on 7-point scale (postintervention and at 3, 6, 12, and 18 mo)	Integrity?
Mattson et al. (1998)	1,726 alcohol-dependent adults voluntarily seeking aftercare or outpatient treatment at 9 sites	MET (4 sessions) vs. CBT (12 sessions) vs. TSF (12 sessions)	*Retention* Wk in treatment: 8.8 CBT vs. 8.1 TSF (8.3 MET, ns) *Attendance* Sessions: 80% MET vs. 68% CBT vs. 63% TSF	Fewer MET sessions offered; wk in treatment for MET could be 1, 2, 6, 12 only.
Mhurchu et al. (1998)	121 adults with hyperlipidemia referred to a hospital-based dietetic department for diet advice	AMI (MI and advice, with feedback) vs. TAU: 3 interviews over 3 mo	*Task performance* Dietary intake reductions: AMI = TAU (at 3 mo)	Therapist effects? Training? Baseline dietary intake was low.
Berg-Smith et al. (1999)	127 adolescents in the Dietary Intervention Study in Children (DISC) since age 8–10	AMI (initial session with 4–8 week follow-up, 5–30 min each, with feedback), assessed pre/post	*Task performance* Action plan formulation (interviewer report): 94% Action plan implementation (interviewer report): 89%	Analyses? Integrity? No control.
Harland et al. (1999)	523 adults 40–64, not engaging in regular exercise, recruited from a primary medical practice	Brief (1 session) vs. intensive (6 sessions in 12 wk) AMI, with or without vouchers, vs. BA, all with feedback	*Task performance* Activity/vigorous activity/moderate activity: Brief AMI = intensive AMI > BA (at 12 wk) Brief AMI = intensive AMI = BA (at 1 yr)	Integrity? Manual? Therapist effects? Training?
Swanson et al. (1999)	121 adults admitted to psychiatric units of two private hospitals; psychiatric (100%) and substance abuse (77%) diagnoses; voluntary	AMI (brief URICA feedback at admission, 1-hr interview predischarge) vs. NIC, added to standard care; all received URICA and aftercare referral	*Treatment entry* All: 47% AMI vs. 21% NIC Dual diagnosis: 42% AMI vs. 16% NIC Psychotic diagnoses: 47% AMI vs. 21% NIC Affective diagnoses: 50% AMI vs. 20% NIC	Integrity? Manual?
Treasure et al. (1999)	125 women diagnosed with bulimia nervosa at a hospital eating disorders unit	MET vs. CBT: 4 weekly 1:1 sessions, as first phase of sequential treatment, followed by group or individual CBT	*Retention* Intervention completion (4 wk): MET = CBT (66.7% vs. 76.3%, ns)	Integrity? Pretreatment waiting list of up to 3 years.
Connors et al. (2000)*	126 adults diagnosed with alcohol dependence or abuse admitted to a 12-wk outpatient 1:1 and group treatment program	AMI (DCU) vs. RI vs. NIC, prior to start of standard treatment	*Retention* Completion: AMI > NIC, RI = NIC *Attendance* Group: AMI > NIC, RI = NIC 1:1 and group: AMI > NIC, RI = NIC	None.

(*continued*)

TABLE 20.1. (*continued*)

Study	Sample	Interventions	Adherence effects	Caveats
Dench & Bennett (2000)	51 alcohol-dependent adults entering a 6-wk day treatment program	AMI vs. EC (replication of Saunders et al., 1995)	*Retention* Completion (6 wk): AMI = NIC (66.7% overall) *Attendance* Days (completers): AMI = NIC (28.0 vs. 26.0, ns) Days (dropouts): AMI = NIC (17.2 vs. 19.7, ns)	Therapist effects? Training?
Martino et al. (2000)*	23 adults with substance and mood or psychotic diagnoses entering a 12-wk partial hospital program; high severity	AMI (with feedback) vs. SI: 1 session, 45–60 min, at start of standard treatment; both vs. historical NIC	*Attendance* Days: 31 AMI vs. 17 NIC (22 SI, ns) Tardiness index: 0.00 AMI vs. 0.18 SI Early departure index: 0.00 AMI vs. 0.17 SI *Task performance* Days medication compliant (self-report): AMI = SI (89% vs. 86%, ns)	Integrity? Manual? Therapist effects?
Schneider et al. (2000)	89 adults diagnosed with substance abuse or dependence at 14 EAP sites; moderate severity	AMI (DCU) vs. DCU-C; all received neutral initial assessment, personal feedback report in second interview, and written disposition	*Treatment entry* AMI = DCU-C (66% professional, 60% self-help overall at 3 mo) *Task performance* Followed initial treatment plan: AMI = DCU-C (63% vs. 54% at 3 mo, ns)	Source of provider adherence ratings unclear.
Donovan et al. (2001)	654 drug-dependent adults evaluated, referred, and placed on wait list for publicly funded inpatient or outpatient treatment	AMI (SC +DCU, scheduled clinical follow-up, unscheduled support services) vs. SC. All received assessment, resource booklet, weekly study contract	*Treatment entry* AMI = SC (71% overall) *Retention* Completion: AMI = SC (71% overall)	High refusal/exclusion rate
Lincourt et al. (in press)	167 men with substance use diagnoses mandated to treatment, unable to identify treatment goals	Group AMI (6 sessions, with assessment and feedback) vs. NIC, at start of standard treatment	*Retention* Completion: 56% AMI vs. 32% NIC *Attendance* Sessions: AMI = NIC (16.2 vs. 18.2, ns) Missed appointments: 17% AMI vs. 24% NIC	Integrity? Training? Archival study; study condition self-selected.

Note. All adherence effects reported are statistically significant unless otherwise noted. *Published information supplemented by personal communication with study author.

Abbreviations: AMI, adaptation of motivational interviewing; BA, brief advice control; CBT, cognitive-behavioral therapy; CT, cognitive therapy; DCU, Drinker's Check-Up (assessment + 1 feedback interview); DCU-C, DCU with confrontational feedback; DDRC, dual disorders recovery counseling; EC, education control; MET, motivational enhancement therapy (4 sessions, feedback); MI, motivational interviewing; NIC, no-intervention control; NSC, nonspecific counseling control; RI, role induction; RR, risk reduction intervention; SC, Standard Care control; SI, standard interview control; TAU, treatment-as-usual control; TSF, twelve-step facilitation; URICA, University of Rhode Island Change Assessment.

Caveats: Analysis?, no statistical analyses of significance of results; Integrity?, no measures described to ensure that providers adhered to intended intervention; Manual?, no written intervention manual or curriculum described; No control, absence of control condition for adherence outcomes; Therapist effects?, Possibility of therapist effects due to single or unspecified intervention provider(s); Training?, training and supervision of intervention providers not described or inadequately described.

ume) employed in these studies include "check-up" (assessment and feedback) interventions and AMIs without feedback, single- and multiple-session interventions, add-on AMIs and integral treatment modules, and interventions given individually and in groups. These studies also span a range of populations and settings, from alcohol and drug treatment to treatment of psychiatric disorders to medical and behavioral health applications. Table 20.1 describes the nature of the interventions and their measured effects on various aspects of adherence and offers caveats for interpreting individual studies, allowing us to describe our conclusions about the data while leaving readers free to make their own assessments. (We do not include information on outcomes; these are well covered in Chapter 16.) All reported findings are statistically significant unless noted.

What Does the Research Show?

The available studies can best be described as providing preliminary guidance and directions for further investigation where treatment adherence is concerned. With only a few exceptions, most of these studies were designed to assess treatment outcomes, and adherence effects were looked at secondarily (and at times peripherally) rather than systematically. In addition, many of these studies are limited in ways that require caution in interpreting them.

   We have included two unpublished studies and several which do not meet the methodological requirements of the randomized controlled trial (RCT); we have done so because these studies provide data on adherence effects in areas with little or no coverage in available RCTs (adolescents, health behavior change in primary care, dual diagnosis aftercare, group motivational interviewing).

   Though results of these studies must be treated with caution, this is also true of RCTs with other limitations of internal validity (see Chapter 16, this volume). Sample sizes are often small; interventionist training is often either left undescribed or, when described, too limited to ensure that those providing the intervention are competent to do so effectively; measures to ensure that the intervention delivered matches the one intended by the researcher (manuals, tape recording and monitoring of sessions, ongoing supervision) are often absent; interventions are often performed by one person, raising the question whether it is the intervention or the unique qualities of the individual that accounts for the effect; and limited description of interventions often makes it difficult to assess the extent to which the spirit and practice of motivational interviewing are incorporated. In some cases in which descriptions are given, serious questions can be raised, as the interventions either are at odds in important ways with motivational interviewing or reduce motivational interviewing to its strategies while neglecting its spirit and its focus on communicational process (e.g., Booth, Kwiatkowski, Iguchi, Pinto, & John, 1998; Kuchipudi, Hobein, Fleckinger, & Iber, 1990; Mhurchu, Margetts, & Speller, 1998).

Studies that correct for these problems in internal validity are under way, including studies being conducted by at least four of the researchers listed in Table 20.1 (Booth et al., 1998; Daley et al., 1998; Martino, Carroll, O'Malley, & Rounsaville, 2000; Smith, Heckemeyer, Kratt, & Mason, 1997). Randomized controlled designs with adequate power to detect moderate adherence effects, interventions sensitive to adherence-influencing factors such as level of motivational readiness, and routine collection of data on adherence as well as physiological, psychiatric, and substance use outcomes will in time allow us to pass more definitive judgment on the adherence effects of AMIs.

What conclusions can we draw now (however tentatively and preliminarily) where enhancement of adherence is concerned? In the majority of controlled studies (12 of 21), AMIs were found to produce significant adherence effects. The effects of AMIs in five studies were equivalent to those produced by other well-specified or standard interventions with which they were compared (Booth et al., 1998; Mattson et al., 1998; Mhurchu et al., 1998; Schneider, Casey, & Kohn, 2000; Treasure et al., 1999), and in four others add-on AMIs produced no incremental benefit where adherence was concerned (Bien, Miller, & Burroughs, 1993; Dench & Bennett, 2000; Donovan, Rosengren, Downey, Cox, & Sloan, 2001; Kuchipudi et al., 1990). Of the two studies that assessed adherence following an AMI intervention but did not include a comparison group, one appeared promising (Berg-Smith et al., 1999), the other less so (Miller, Sovereign, & Kriege, 1988).

The findings of adherence effects in the preponderance of studies leave us cautiously optimistic about motivational interviewing as an add-on adherence intervention. In several of these studies, across multiple populations, the adherence findings were quite robust; Connors, Walitzer, and Derman (2000) are especially impressive in that a single motivational interviewing session led to significantly greater treatment attendance (and also significantly better drinking outcomes) compared not only to a no-treatment control but also to a role-induction interview, a well-researched and empirically supported treatment preparation intervention (Walizter, Derman, & Connors, 1999).

We can also discern a number of patterns in these studies that provide the beginnings of a more nuanced picture. One is that AMIs seem to be effective in facilitating transition of clients from one level of treatment to another; in Swanson, Pantalon, and Cohen (1999), receiving an AMI more than doubled aftercare entry rates among all subjects as well as specifically among clients with affective disorders, psychotic disorders, and dual (psychiatric and substance use) disorders, whereas in Daley and Zuckoff (1998) the intervention fell just short of doubling aftercare entry. This result also raises a question as to whether intervention effects may be greater for groups of clients in transition, as opposed to nonclients being recruited into treatment (as in Booth et al., 1998; Miller et al., 1988; and Schneider et al., 2000), where AMIs either failed to outperform their alternatives or produced limited effects on treatment entry. Preliminary results of one ongoing study of nonclient recruitment

(Zuckoff, Ryan, & Thoma, 2000) also suggest that the effect under such circumstances may be expected to be smaller.

A second finding is that AMIs may exert their effects on outcomes at least in part by promoting adherence. Brown and Miller (1993), the only investigators to examine this hypothesis explicitly, found that an adherence effect mediated improved residential treatment outcomes among those who received an AMI intervention. Five other studies (Aubrey, 1998; Connors et al., 2000; Daley et al., 1998; Kemp, Kirov, Everitt, Hayward, & David, 1998; Lincourt, Kuettel, & Bombardier, in press; Saunders, Wilkinson, & Phillips, 1995; Smith et al., 1997) found effects on a variety of measures of attendance, treatment commitment, readiness to change, and task completion, as well as on treatment outcomes. These findings suggest that examination of relationships between adherence effects and outcomes is an important direction for future research.

A third pattern can be found in the relative effectiveness of single-session and multiple-session interventions. Six single-session interventions (excluding assessment, putting Drinker's Check-Up interventions in that category) were associated with improved adherence (Aubrey, 1998; Brown & Miller, 1993; Connors et al., 2000; Daley & Zuckoff, 1998; Harland et al., 1999; Martino et al., 2000); in four others, AMIs were either not superior to alternate interventions (Mhurchu et al., 1998; Schneider et al., 2000) or produced small (Miller et al., 1988) or no (Bien, Miller, & Burroughs, 1993) adherence effects. Multiple-session interventions account for nine findings of improved adherence (Berg-Smith et al., 1999; Daley et al., 1998; Harland et al., 1999; Kemp et al., 1998; Lincourt et al., in press; Saunders et al., 1995; Smith et al., 1997; Swanson et al., 1999); in five others, AMIs were not superior to alternate interventions (Booth et al., 1998; Treasure et al., 1999) or produced no incremental benefits in terms of adherence (Dench & Bennett, 2000; Donovan et al., 2001; Kuchipudi et al., 1990). In the one study that compared single- and multiple-session (six offered, mean attended = 3) AMIs (Harland et al., 1999), no significant overall differences were found, but subjects who received the multiple-session AMI plus vouchers for free use of exercise facilities increased their general activity level significantly more than did those in any other condition. When we recognize that in a number of successful interventions "multiple" denoted only a second, brief contact, and that these interventions are otherwise dissimilar in terms of structure and the populations on which they were tested, the added value of at least one follow-up session would appear to be worth the additional effort and expense required.

Fourth, an important question, in light of the limited resources of many treatment programs, is whether a group intervention can be of comparable effectiveness in promoting adherence as those delivered individually (see Chapter 25, this volume). Lincourt and colleagues (in press), in an archival study, found that a six-session AMI group significantly enhanced adherence compared with treatment as usual. Daley and Zuckoff (1998), in a nonrandomized, open-treatment trial, found that offering a single-session AMI in small groups enhanced treatment entry compared with an historical control. These studies suggest that group AMIs may be at least potentially useful in promoting treatment adherence, but a definitive judgment must await more rigorously designed trials.

We have focused thus far on the implications of studies in which AMIs produced improvements in treatment adherence. What can be learned from those studies in which significant differences between AMI and control or comparison conditions were not found? In some cases, the implications of these studies are difficult to interpret. In Project MATCH, for example, clients receiving motivational enhancement therapy (MET) attended a significantly higher proportion of their sessions than did those receiving cognitive-behavioral therapy (CBT) or twelve-step facilitation (TSF) over the course of a 12-week treatment period (Mattson et al., 1998). However, these differences could be accounted for by the differential task demands between the three treatment conditions; MET clients were required to attend only 4 sessions in contrast to 12 for CBT or TSF. In Treasure and colleagues (1999), dropout during the first 4 weeks of treatment was equivalent between MET and CBT conditions; however, the fact that clients in this study had been on a waiting list for up to 3 years prior to receiving treatment limits the generalizability of these results.

One conclusion that can safely be drawn is that, unsurprisingly, adherence interventions are subject to the law of diminishing returns: where measured adherence is already relatively high, there may be little to be gained in trying to boost it further. For example, in Bien, Miller, and Burroughs (1993), the only adherence measure used was subjects' attendance at the first treatment session; with over 81% of subjects overall attending, there may have been little room for the intervention to show an effect. Two other studies of alcohol- and drug-dependent samples in which no incremental effect was shown may also have involved relatively high baseline adherence for the population. In Donovan and colleagues (2001), 71% of all drug-dependent subjects entered treatment after an average wait of 22 days, a proportion that compares very favorably with other, similar samples (Hser et al., 1997; Stark, 1992). In Dench and Bennett (2000), 63% of all subjects completed treatment according to stringent criteria; subjects receiving the control intervention attended an average of 97% of contracted sessions, compared with 98% among AMI subjects; among treatment completers, controls attended 26 of 30 possible treatment days, compared with 28 among AMI subjects. While AMI subjects dropped out after marginally fewer days than controls, they did show significant differences in the direction of readiness to change in all three subscales of the SOCRATES from pre- to postintervention. Finally, in a study of weight control, Mhurchu, Margetts, and Speller (1998) noted that target dietary intake was low among all subjects prior to the interventions; the findings of no difference on adherence outcomes between the AMI and standard dietary advice groups seems clearly related to a ceiling effect, especially in light of the significant further dietary reductions in both conditions.

A second, obvious conclusion is that AMIs are less likely to show adherence effects when they deviate excessively from the core principles of motivational interviewing. For example, Kuchipudi and colleagues (1990) have been cited (Rollnick & Miller, 1995) as an illustration of the problem of drift in the dissemination of innovations (see Chapter 18, this volume). Subjects were given the same message (the need to stop drinking and the importance and effectiveness of treatment) repeatedly by one treatment team member after another in an effort to use the authority of the medical director to directly persuade subjects to enter a treatment program. No reference is made to any motivational interviewing principles or strategies other than a generic "compassionate and concerned" style, and no evidence is presented that subjects were asked for their own thoughts about their behavior or changes that might be beneficial. Because provider training in motivational interviewing is not mentioned—and social workers who provided some of the sessions were said to be "experienced in alcoholism treatment," presumably from a traditional perspective—this should not seem surprising.

What Questions Remain to Be Answered?

As we began by noting, the current state of research regarding the relationship of motivational interviewing-based interventions and treatment adherence can best be described as preliminary. We can identify a number of issues that require clarification via further research.

What Is the Relationship between Adherence Intervention and Treatment Outcome?

Adherence to treatment is important to the extent that it leads to improved treatment outcomes. Though the correlation between adherence and more successful outcomes is well established, little is known about the circumstances and conditions under which adherence interventions result in greater gains in treatment. Specifically, what kinds of clients receiving which kinds of treatments (e.g., medical or psychosocial treatments) might benefit from adherence strategies? For example, in certain medical treatments such as antiretroviral treatment of AIDS, enabling patients to take medications exactly as prescribed is crucial to outcome, while in some psychotherapy models the relationship between adherence and outcome may be much less clear. Clearly, studies that, like Brown and Miller (1993), systematically investigate relationships between interventions, adherence, and measures of outcomes are needed to elucidate these relationships.

Is Motivational Interviewing Specifically Efficacious in Promoting Treatment Adherence Compared with Other Forms of Intervention?

Studies over the past 40 years have shown that treatment adherence may be enhanced by interventions ranging from brief and opportunistic contacts (Carr, 1985; Chafetz, 1961, 1968; Chafetz et al., 1962, 1964; Fiester, Cooley,

& Bausinger, 1979; Hochstadt & Trybula, 1980; Koumans & Muller, 1965; Koumans, Muller, & Miller, 1967; Olfson, Mechanic, Boyer, & Hansell, 1998; Turner & Vernon, 1976), to treatment contracting (Lash, 1998; Lash & Blosser, 1999), to role induction (Zweben & Li, 1981), vicarious therapy pretraining, and experiential pretraining (Walizter et al., 1999). The studies we have reviewed suggest that motivational interviewing adds something meaningful, and that employing it is at least as useful as adding other well-specified treatment preparation interventions . As indicated earlier, these studies tend to focus mainly on treatment outcomes rather than adherence per se. Only Connors and colleagues (2000) provide the first clear evidence that employing a motivational interviewing approach may at least in some situations be preferable not just to no intervention but to other forms of adherence intervention. Clearly, comparative randomized trials, which attend to both adherence and motivational concerns along with the issues of internal validity, are required to definitively answer the question we posed previously.

What Are the "Effective Ingredients" of Motivational Interviewing Used as a Treatment Adherence Intervention?

The issue of how motivational interviewing exerts its effects on outcomes has been raised repeatedly by Miller (e.g., 2000) and others, and this question may be asked with equal urgency in the area of adherence effects. Many candidates for "effective ingredient" can be identified: eliciting of change talk, emphasis on personal choice and control or "autonomy support" (Foote et al., 1999; see also Deci & Ryan, 1985), a specific style of responding to expressed resistance (Miller, Benefield, & Tonigan, 1993), the way in which advice is presented and plans for change are negotiated, and so on. However, current research provides limited assistance in evaluating the importance of these aspects of AMIs in promoting adherence. Dismantling studies, as well as post hoc analyses and qualitative studies examining counseling process, may in time provide a clearer picture.

Among the components for which data are currently available is formal feedback. A majority of the interventions under consideration here incorporate a feedback process, although it should be noted that these interventions vary from DCU-style feedback reports to systematic but less structured feedback processes to feedback on a single measure of readiness to change. Overall, it appears that AMIs incorporating feedback display somewhat more consistency in enhancing adherence than those that do not, but an important question is whether and how different kinds of feedback may elicit differing effects.

One variation is between differing styles in which feedback can be provided. Schneider and colleagues (2000) found that "confrontational" presentation of feedback was as effective in eliciting treatment entry as was feedback done in the style of motivational interviewing. However, Schneider and associates did not investigate the effects of what study therapists actually did, as opposed to what they were assigned to do. Miller and colleagues (1993) had similarly found no statistically significant main effect of motivational versus confrontational styles on reductions in drinking; it was only in the post hoc analysis, in which they linked the actual practice of therapists to client outcomes, that Miller and associates found confrontational therapist behaviors to be significantly related to worse drinking outcomes.

A second variable is the nature of the feedback itself. Preliminary results presented by Zuckoff and colleagues (2000) suggested that providing limited versus extensive feedback may lead to different outcomes where treatment entry and retention is concerned. Nye, Agostinelli, and Smith (1999) found that with nonclient subjects, presentation of normative and self-focusing feedback can either increase problem recognition or generate defensiveness, depending on whether they are presented independently or together. Such studies may help to determine when feedback plays a key role in the effectiveness of AMIs, and how it interacts with other core components of motivational interviewing (e.g., counselor's style of communication), in order to maximize therapeutic impact.

A second prominent candidate for effective ingredient is the interpersonal style associated with motivational interviewing. The creation of a positive therapeutic relationship as a key ingredient in treatment success in general, and in motivational interviewing in particular, is reviewed elsewhere in this book. However, the specific question of how this "way of being with people" affects adherence is worth considering here. It would seem intuitively obvious that persons who leave an encounter feeling respected, valued, and deeply understood will want to return for more of the same, especially as such experiences may be relatively rare outside the therapeutic environment (Zuckoff & Daley, 2001). Empirical support for this intuition emerges in a comparative trial of "low-structure" (psychodynamic) and "high-structure" (cognitive-behavioral) treatments for alcohol problems, in which Nielson, Nielson, and Wraae (2000) found that irrespective of treatment assignment, having a counselor with a high "conceptual level" (CL) predicted greater likelihood of completion of the first four sessions than having a counselor with a low CL; this held true, contrary to prediction, whether the client's CL was high or low. Of interest is how conceptual level was defined: therapists with high CL were described as demonstrating empathy, flexibility, receptiveness, tolerance for ambiguity, intuitiveness, and a noncontrolling, nonauthoritarian stance—which the authors note could serve as an accurate summary of the interpersonal style proper to motivational interviewing. Research that clarifies how much the adherence effects of AMIs rest on counseling style, as opposed to specific strategies and techniques employed, would seem of central importance.

In What Ways Are We Called on to Go beyond the Research?

The research reviewed suggests core principles for motivational intervention and directions for future inquiry but it does not provide a specific answer to the question encountered by clinicians every day: what can I do to increase the likelihood that the clients I see will attend treatment and adhere to the plans we formulate? There are two main reasons for this. First, AMIs have been designed primarily to help people resolve ambivalence about change, with the presumption that doing so would lead to greater commitment to treatment. As discussed earlier, the question of how motivational interviewing can be adapted to address directly the specific task of enhancing adherence has been much less explored. Second, in everyday practice clinicians are unlikely to have access to the resources and infrastructure needed to provide the kinds of structured AMIs that have been most frequently tested. Guidelines for incorporating motivational adherence strategies in a variety of treatment types and settings would assist front-line clinicians in becoming more effective.

Therefore, we have developed an adherence model and intervention to assist clinicians in dealing with adherence issues. Based on the principles and practices of motivational interviewing and used in clinical contexts, this model views motivational readiness for treatment as consisting of two intertwined yet distinguishable dimensions: *problem acceptance* and *treatment acceptance* (Daley & Zuckoff, 1999; Zuckoff & Daley, 2001). Problem acceptance, the correlate of readiness to change, may be described as the extent to which an individual comes to experience change as *needed* (e.g., problem recognition or perceived severity), *wanted* (e.g., hope vs. fear), and *within reach* (e.g., self-efficacy). A high level of problem acceptance is taken to be necessary for a productive encounter with treatment, but it is not, however, seen as sufficient for treatment adherence. Individuals must also find treatment itself *acceptable* if they are to endure the often difficult or even distressing experiences of trying to improve their lives. Thus, what is typically described as client ambivalence about change may in some cases reflect a situation in which the individual clearly recognizes a problem and is ready and willing to work at resolving it (high level of problem acceptance) but feels hesitant to try to do so via the pathway being offered (low treatment acceptance).

The phenomenon of "spontaneous remission" or natural change in substance use and psychiatric disorders makes it clear that in many cases individuals have or can find the resources needed to succeed at self-change (Granfield & Cloud, 1996; Husby, 1985; Lambert, 1976; Malan, Heath, Bacal, & Balfour, 1975; McCollough et al., 1994; Miller, 2000; Pillay & Wassenaar, 1995; Sobell, Sobell, & Toneatto, 1992; Sobell, Sobell, Toneatto, & Leo, 1993; Stall & Biernacki, 1986; Vaillant, 1995; Waldorf, Reinarman, & Murphy, 1991). However, for those who make a series of unsuccessful self-change attempts, or who do not perceive their situation as subject to voluntary change, their level of treatment acceptance, or readiness to accept help, may be the determining factor in whether or not they achieve the changes they are considering or planning to make. In the sections that follow, we describe an adherence approach that employs principles of motivational interviewing for the purpose of recognizing and dealing with factors that typically cause clients to become ambivalent about needing, accepting, and using help—and thus to participate inconsistently or terminate treatment prematurely.

MOTIVATIONAL READINESS AND ADHERENCE

Box 20.1 links various sources or "risk factors" for nonadherence with the constructs of problem and treatment acceptance, and consequently represents an initial step toward furthering our understanding of how various motivational interviewing strategies can be employed systematically to facilitate treatment adherence. The proposed framework recognizes that the range of possible sources of nonadherence and related strategies may vary in accordance with different populations and/or settings and could be adapted and tested in a variety of programs.

Individuals low in problem acceptance often have reservations about the nature, extent, and severity of the presenting problems. They are uncertain or ambivalent about whether the "identified" problem really needs changing, as the perceived costs of maintaining the behaviors do not outweigh the familiar benefits. To illustrate, among drug-dependent clients, the long-term consequences of continued use (e.g., health effects, arrest, and incarceration) may not outweigh the immediate rewards or pleasures of "getting high." Some individuals may resolve the dilemma by minimizing the importance of the presenting problem, offering such comments as "I won't get caught since I use only on the weekends with friends."

Low problem acceptance may also reflect tension between an individual's hopes and fears about consequences of efforts at change. In some cases this conflict is concrete and specific; the hope of a problem drinker that life can be more rewarding by engaging in an abstinent lifestyle may conflict with the fear that a drinking significant other may leave once improvement in the problem begins to occur. More broadly, persons considering taking steps toward significant life changes may lack a significant sense of *safety* to be willing to risk giving up what is familiar for an uncertain future.

Finally, ambivalence about fully accepting the need for change may stem from doubts as to whether such change can really be accomplished. Faced with what seems an intolerable reality, a person has only three choices: deny that it is a reality, fall into a state of helplessness and despair, or find a way to change it. Problem acceptance rests in part on possession of the belief that the last of these is a real possibility, or on development of this belief.

A range of factors similarly influences treatment acceptance. Previous negative treatment experiences, negative relationship expectancies, external barriers to care, cultural attitudes, and ideological commitments may all have a negative impact on readiness to accept help; rapport-damaging interactions may reduce it further. In addition, individuals may find themselves being offered help in a form they find unacceptable, even though they are open to receiving help per se. For example, a patient may be interested only in taking medication for high blood pressure, while the clinician is recommending changes in diet and exercise.

Individuals who have had a series of unsuccessful treatment experiences may develop negative therapist and outcome expectancies. The latter may be a consequence of having had counterproductive relationships with clinicians resulting in a worsening of symptoms and other problems (e.g., marital separation or divorce, or medication side effects). In some cases, clients may begin treatment anticipating an authoritarian, neglectful, or manipulative interpersonal style on the part of the clinician; while these expectancies may be based on previous relationship experiences, their negative impact on treatment acceptance can be exacerbated if the clinician intentionally or unintentionally acts in ways that re-evoke them.

Ambivalence about treatment may also stem from cultural, ideological, or practical issues. Among some populations, stigma is attached to seeking help from mental health professionals, and help-seeking individuals may fear being labeled "crazy" by their peers. For others, issues about self-disclosure and confidentiality can become a major impediment in seeking and participating in therapy. Individuals with strong belief systems about the nature and source of their problems may bridle at perceived efforts of treatment providers to impose a different view—for example, members of twelve-step mutual support groups may resist psychiatric or psychological conceptualizations of their addictions and treatment needs. Yet others may be overwhelmed with everyday concerns (e.g., family hardships) or reside in unstable social environments, making it difficult to attend or participate in treatment; without adequate resources or support, such individuals may be unable to cope with or fulfill such task demands of treatment as attending sessions weekly, following a pill-taking regime, or doing homework assignments.

Individuals in these high-risk categories (i.e., low problem and/or treatment acceptance) have often been categorized as "unmotivated" and "untreatable" at worst, or "hard -to-reach" or "resistant" at best, resulting in large numbers being turned away from needed services (cf. Cooney, Zweben, & Fleming, 1995). Our model moves away from this "client driven" perspective and toward an interactional one (Carroll, 1997; Daley & Zuckoff, 1999; Mattson et al., 1998; Zweben & Barrett, 1993). Thus, the focus has shifted to eliminating provider practices that serve as roadblocks, and finding those that facilitate adherence in different populations and settings.

PRACTICAL MOTIVATIONAL INTERVIEWING STRATEGIES FOR IMPROVING TREATMENT ADHERENCE

Overview

Box 20.1 provides a repertoire of interventions believed to be effective in addressing the aforementioned adherence problems. These strategies are drawn

BOX 20.1. An Exploratory Framework for Addressing Adherence

Motivation category	Sources of nonadherence (risk factors)	Selected strategies
Problem acceptance	• Misperceptions, misunderstandings, and/or uncertainties about the significance of the presenting problem • Fears about unintended consequences of change • Doubts about whether change is possible or within reach	• Open questions • Empathic reflection • Providing feedback • Deploying discrepancy • Normalizing unclarities • Normalizing anxiety about change • Eliciting "change talk" • Exploring values • Reviewing past successes • Affirming small steps • Amplifying doubts
Treatment acceptance	• Uncertainty or ambivalence about change • Concerns about the suitability of the treatment modality offered • Misperceptions about treatment needs • Previous negative treatment experiences • Negative therapist or treatment outcome expectancies • Negative general relationship expectancies • Culture-specific differences • Stigma • Mandated treatment/coercion • High barriers to care (financial problems, family hardships) • Low self-efficacy in handling treatment demands	• Persistent empathy and nondefensiveness • Normalizing gradual development of trust • Exploring understandings of how treatment works • Providing information about how treatment works • Eliciting perceptions of treatment needs • Providing information on treatment needs • Decisional balancing • Reviewing past treatment experiences • Exploring and addressing previous and future barriers to change in treatment (e.g., immunizing) • Negotiating proximal goals (i.e., prioritizing and sequencing tasks) • Communicating a nonperfectionistic message • Recognizing nonadherence as a sign of damaged rapport • Addressing breeches in rapport • Involving a supportive other for motivational support • Identifying positive experiences of receiving help • Supporting self-efficacy or coping capacities • Displaying optimism about treatment effectiveness

from the research on motivational interviewing and our own clinical experiences. Though varied in intensity and style, these interventions share the same goal of enhancing problem and treatment acceptance.

Adherence strategies might be most broadly categorized as Phase 1 and Phase 2 strategies (see Chapters 6 and 10, this volume). Phase 1 strategies are focused on (1) assessing the individual's current levels of problem acceptance and treatment acceptance; (2) formulating hypotheses as to the wishes, beliefs, feelings, and experiences that are influencing each of these dimensions; and (3) considering options for resolving ambivalence about change and/or treatment.

Phase 2 strategies are aimed at helping clients develop an adherence plan appropriate to their capacities, resources, preferences, and treatment needs. This entails preparing clients to address sundry sources of nonadherence whenever they occur during the course of treatment. Clients may need to be helped to maintain participation via employment of the full array of adherence strategies.

Phase 1: Assessing and Understanding Influences on Adherence

Traditional adherence strategies involve telling, instructing, or showing clients what to expect from treatment and what they will need to do to make it successful (Zweben & Li, 1981). The underlying assumption is that clients are more likely to be engaged and retained if they are provided with the correct information about the respective roles and functions of clinician and client. This approach may be all that is necessary to gain the cooperation of clients who enter treatment with relatively high levels of problem and treatment acceptance; doubts or uncertainties these clients have about treatment may well stem from a lack of information about the proposed treatment rather than from underlying motivational issues.

In contrast, for clients with relatively low levels of problem and treatment acceptance, traditional induction techniques may be insufficient. The doubts or uncertainties these clients have about participation may stem from motivational matters (e.g., low self-efficacy, mistrust of the counselor, or ambivalence about change) rather than ignorance or misunderstanding of the proposed treatment. Measurement of initial treatment readiness might help to identify which clients might benefit from traditional adherence instruction and which might be helped more by a motivational interviewing-style intervention.

Phase 1 of our motivational adherence intervention begins with an empathic assessment, defined by Miller (1998b) as "getting to know the client well enough to be able to understand him/her from the inside while being able to provide a broader perspective." A major goal of the adherence assessment interview is to create a safe atmosphere in which to explore the client's thoughts and feelings.

The counselor seeks to discover clients' views about problems and expectations of treatment. Discovery may entail reviewing the chain of events that brought clients to treatment and eliciting their perceptions of the importance of addressing problems without offering interpretation. This process may be accomplished via the use of core motivational interviewing strategies, including open-ended questions, clarification and elaboration of client responses, and empathic reflection. Data on client perceptions may also be obtained through standardized measures; for example, in the alcohol treatment field, measures of clients' perceptions of their alcohol use are included on such instruments as the Inventory of Drinking Situations (IDS; Annis, Graham, & Davis, 1987) and the Desired Effects of Drinking questionnaire (Simpson, Arroyo, Miller, & Little, 1999).

Clinicians may ask about, reflect, and then summarize clients' past treatment experiences as they relate to adherence. Current beliefs about treatment may be influenced by previously unmet expectations ("I took the medication but I was still depressed"), unhappiness with therapist style ("My therapist didn't really seem to care about me"), or practical obstacles that were never resolved ("I could not find a reliable baby sitter," "I had no way to get to the clinic").

During the assessment process the clinician is also on the lookout for such "early warning signs" of nonadherence as client beliefs that are discrepant from what is being proposed in the treatment plan (e.g., a client beginning psychodynamic therapy for anxiety symptoms who believes that talking about the past is pointless). The clinician then communicates his or her observations and understandings about the confluence of factors that might have an impact on the client's participation in treatment through a process of information sharing, summarizing, and empathic reflection of both positive and negative reactions to information exchanged.

As mentioned earlier, there is a wide range of possible reasons for which clients might not participate in treatment; the clinician's goal is to help clients recognize or sort out some of these possible reasons.

This discussion often highlights and helps clients to recognize the discrepancy between their behavior, problems, or concerns and "where they want to be" (their goals) or "who they want to be" (their values). For example, a client revealed bitterly that despite a strong desire and commitment to reduce her drinking, she left therapy prematurely to avoid communicating feelings of anger and frustration about the program to her treating clinician—an abrupt departure that resulted in a full-blown relapse. Deploying the discrepancy between the personal importance of her goal and her reluctance to deal directly with an obstacle to achieving it led her to commit herself to learning other ways to cope with negative feelings toward others.

Once clients begin to engage in change talk regarding adherence to the treatment, the clinician asks them to rank the risk factors they have identified in order of importance. The value of such an exercise lies in helping to clarify which are the greatest threats and thus need to be addressed most urgently, to sensitize clients to any ongoing pattern of nonadherence (e.g., "I always avoid sources of bad feelings;" "I don't expect the therapist to want to see me after I stop doing well and miss an appointment"), and to help them to become committed to overcoming these major roadblocks.

Phase 2: Developing and Implementing an Adherence Plan

Phase 2 involves the negotiation of an adherence plan. This occurs only if a consensus is arrived at about the particular issues that need to be addressed. The clinician elicits ideas about how to resolve these issues and then (with permission) reviews alternatives to nonadherence; these alternatives may include talking things over in the sessions before acting on disappointed feelings, keeping a log to track negative feelings about the treatment process, identifying and involving significant others to provide additional support or to enhance motivation, or breaking down long-term treatment goals (which in many cases could feel overwhelming) into manageable tasks (e.g., sobriety sampling vs. long-term abstinence, taking medication on a limited trial basis, or improving communication with spouse before reinitiating a sexual relationship). Presenting a menu of options and reviewing their pros and cons (decisional balancing) gives clients the opportunity to choose one that is most appropriate to their needs, preferences, and capacities. In this way the counselor conveys confidence in clients' ability to take responsibility for making their own decisions and wishes to succeed.

Clinicians should avoid negotiating with individuals who still have lingering doubts about addressing adherence issues; otherwise, they might feel pressured into making an adherence plan before feeling ready or confident to implement it. Rather, the counselor might empathically reflect misgivings while normalizing the inaction—for example, it might be important to tell a client that many people prefer to find out how difficult it will be to remember to take their medication regularly before they decide whether to come up with ideas for enhancing their memory. Clients usually breathe a "sigh of relief" when this happens.

Individuals confronted with an aversive task, such as deciding whether to remain in treatment, may be better prepared to take action over time (Zweben et al., 1988). Such clients may benefit from hearing that treatment can focus initially on the question of whether treatment-based change is warranted or desired without necessitating immediate commitment to an extended treatment process. At the same time, the counselor needs to be prepared to shift out of the negotiating stance if conditions warrant it. In certain cases (e.g., clinically deteriorating clients) it may be necessary for the clinician to express his or her own concerns about the client's leaving before the decision is finalized. However, in accordance with the spirit of motivational interviewing, the clinician should obtain permission before stating his or her concerns.

It will be unsurprising that after they leave, some clients may have "second thoughts" or negative reactions about different matters that occurred during the treatment session. These thoughts or reactions may arise when clients do not feel comfortable with self-disclosure, especially to a person in a position of authority; some may feel that they do not have the "right" to question an authority, and/or may be fearful of retaliation, and thus decide that it is safer to appear cooperative even if such a stance is counterproductive to their treatment needs. For example, some clients might be seriously concerned that a prescribed medication is having little effect on their mood disorder; yet, rather than reveal their disappointment, they might prefer to stop taking the medication completely without first notifying the treating physician. This scenario, if repeated with different clinicians, could eventually become a major impediment to improvement.

Therefore, it is important for clinicians to focus clients' attention on possible future reactions by describing what these reactions might be and discussing ways to respond to them. The clinician reinforces the importance of dealing with these delayed reactions if or when they occur while expressing optimism about the client's efforts to cope with these challenges. Not doing so raises the danger of an individual's acting precipitously rather than after careful consideration and consultation with treatment providers.

To prepare a client to deal with delayed negative reactions, the counselor might deliver the following message at the close of a Phase 2 session: Mixed feelings or ongoing uncertainties about treatment, as well as setbacks or moments of struggle, are a normal part of the treatment process rather than signs of failure; discussing these matters openly can become a real opportunity for further learning and change. This "nonperfectionistic" message often helps to reduce the guilt, shame, or embarrassment that commonly occurs when an individual is unable to cope; just as important it also serves as mechanism to "immunize" the client against reacting impulsively to disappointment, frustration, or overall dissatisfaction with his or her own progress.

SUMMARY

Studies have revealed that clients who adhere to a treatment regime usually fare better than those who do not, and that motivational interviewing techniques can be effectively employed to facilitate adherence with various client groups and treatments across a variety of settings. Specifically, motivational interviewing appears to be helpful in decreasing ambivalence in order to maintain treatment participation. The current research allows us to be cautiously optimistic, but far more will be required before questions can be answered more definitely. Further work needs to be conducted not only in comparative outcome trials but also in process-focused research, to clarify the mechanisms of change and the optimization of the effective ingredients of AMIs.

Based on a review of the literature and our own clinical experience, we developed a framework for gaining a better understanding of interrelationships between motivational variables (problem acceptance and treatment acceptance) and adherence factors for the purpose of enhancing the delivery of motivational adherence strategies. We believe that we now have valuable tools to address adherence problems and that if they are applied systematically and in the spirit of motivational interviewing, at the beginning of treatment and throughout its course, we can enable a greater number of clients to take optimal advantage of therapy.

CHAPTER 21

Motivational Interviewing with Adolescents and Young Adults

JOHN S. BAER *and* PEGGY L. PETERSON

There is considerable interest in using motivational interviewing with younger populations. Much of this interest, we believe, is based on promising research outcomes using motivational interviewing with adult populations and the ongoing challenge of providing effective services for young people (Moskowitz, 1985). Some tailoring of the use of motivational interviewing may be necessary, however, when working with adolescents and young adults. Adolescents are different from adults in important ways. Clinical presentations of young people often differ from those noted among adults. Specific developmental and psychological factors influence the setting, content, style, and goals for interventions. This chapter reviews developmental issues and the rationale for the use of motivational interviewing and then briefly examines the relatively small existing evaluative literature. Finally, we present some clinical considerations and note what we consider to be key issues for future attention.

We believe that motivational interviewing describes a clinical style that is useful for a variety of health-related issues. Nevertheless, most efforts to apply motivational interviewing with adolescents and young adults have addressed substance use. This chapter thus focuses on substance use issues, despite any theoretical reason that motivational interviewing should be limited to this area of risk behavior.

DEVELOPMENTAL CONSIDERATIONS

Adolescence

Adolescence is a distinct life stage between childhood and adulthood characterized by changes in biological, psychological, and social processes. Individuals grow rapidly, develop secondary sex characteristics, develop higher-order cognitive abilities, and gradually adopt adult social behavior. The major psychological tasks of adolescence are the development of autonomy and identity and the social and personal competencies needed for the adoption of adult roles. Adolescence is commonly portrayed as a time of great turmoil that includes extreme parent–child conflict, mood swings, and irrationality on behalf of the adolescent. Such extreme turmoil has largely been debunked as a myth (Offer & Schonert-Reichl, 1992; Peterson, 1993). Although a significant minority of youth experience adolescence as tumultuous and troubled, problems for many are due to family, social, and mental health issues that predate adolescence. Over a third of adolescents transition to adulthood remaining well adjusted throughout, and only about a quarter are consistently troubled (Golombeck, Marton, Stein, & Korenblum, 1989).

Nevertheless, during adolescence there is an increase in activities that pose a risk to health and safety, including alcohol use, drug use, and sexual behavior. For example, by the 8th grade about a quarter of students report having been drunk. By 12th grade this proportion increases to 65% (Johnston, O'Malley, & Bachman, 2000a). The leading cause of death among youth and young adults age 10–24 is motor vehicle crashes (31%), followed by homicide (18%), suicide (12%), and other injury (11%) (Centers for Disease Control, 2000). Alcohol and other drug use have been implicated in all these causes of death (Cherpitel, 1994; Maio, Portnoy, Blow, & Hill, 1994). There is also a core group of young people who develop problems during adolescence that remain chronic into adulthood. Fortunately for the majority of adolescents, involvement in risk behaviors is time limited (Chen & Kandel, 1995). Furthermore, it is through testing boundaries and challenging social prohibitions that young people learn to develop internal control over their behavior (Jessor, 1991).

Young Adulthood

An end point for adolescence could be thought of as the point at which an individual is independently self-supporting and assumes adult roles. Arnett (2000) has recently suggested an intermediary developmental process that he calls "emerging adulthood." He argues that individuals within the rough age span of 18 to 25 are distinct demographically, subjectively, and psychologically from both younger (adolescent) and older (adult) age groups. Within emerging adulthood, individual identity explorations in the areas of love, work, and world view go beyond those initial formulations noted within adolescence but stop short of adulthood. This developmental process appears in cultures typically described as highly industrialized or postindustrial where young people tend to stay in educational systems longer (well into the 20s) and marriage and parenthood are often delayed. Like adolescence, emerging adulthood is noted for high levels of risk behavior (use of substances, sex, risky driving) as individuals explore their identities and roles. Rates of heavy episodic drinking, for example, peak between the ages of 19 and 21 (Johnston, O'Malley, & Bachman, 2000b). As Arnett (2000) states, "Emerging adults can pursue novel and intense experiences more freely than adolescents because they are less likely to be monitored by parents and can pursue them more freely than adults because they are less constrained by roles" (p. 475). Risky behavior can also be exacerbated by the highly social settings common within this age period. For example, increased drinking has been associated with residence in U.S. college dormitories (Gfroerer, Greenblatt, & Wright, 1997) and membership in collegiate social organizations (Cashin, Presley, & Meilman, 1998). Perceived social norms and peer use are strong predictors of drinking and substance use behavior in this age group (Baer, in press).

As a caveat, not all adolescents experience the process of emerging adulthood. It is the relatively successful adolescents who are more likely to extend educational processes toward more professional work. In fact, younger adolescents most involved in substance use and other risk behaviors may be least likely to extend role explorations. They are more likely to leave school earlier, assume adults jobs at younger ages, and marry and have children earlier than their less troubled peers (Baumrind & Moselle, 1985; Newcomb & Bentler, 1988). Thus, individuals characterized by a developmental process of emerging adulthood, and for whom motivational interviewing interventions might be designed, may not represent all members of the age group.

RATIONALE FOR MOTIVATIONAL INTERVIEWING WITH ADOLESCENTS AND YOUNG ADULTS

We see motivational interviewing as a promising style for working with adolescents and young adults. The tasks of adolescence—developing autonomy and individuation—require questioning and pushing against authority figures. For adolescents and young adults, ambivalence is common. And, ambivalence will extend beyond a specific risk behavior to quite general issues of identity and roles. Clinical styles that are respectful, acknowledge choices and ambivalence, and do not increase resistance seem to be logical choices. A clinical approach that not only minimizes arguing but also uses ambivalence to develop motivation for change should be a welcome addition. We also sense a common curiosity and openness to philosophical questions among young people, which might make motivational interviewing particularly helpful. Application of motivational interviewing tends to support personal change goals rather than institutional or counselor-based goals, which naturally supports explorations of world views and continued efforts toward autonomy. That motivational interviewing can be used consistent with harm reductive goals also seems well matched for younger individuals without chronic conditions.

Considerable resources have been devoted to universal prevention programs to prevent or delay initiation of risk behavior among young people. Yet prevention effects are typically small (Department of Health and Human Services, 2000; Pentz et al., 1989), and there is evidence that universal prevention programs are not effective for youth who have already initiated risk behavior (Brown & Horowitz, 1993; Ellickson & Bell, 1990). Motivational interviewing may be particularly appropriate for targeted or indicated prevention programs designed for young people already engaged in risk behaviors (see later).

We also see motivational interviewing as a promising approach for engaging youth in services. Few youth identify their risk behavior as a problem in need of treatment or other services. Motivational interviewing, with its nonjudgmental and nonconfrontational style, may be a useful approach for outreach or initial engagement (Slesnick, Meyers, Meade, & Segelken, 2000). Further, motivational interviewing's application in brief formats lends it to use in informal settings where youth tend to spend time (e.g., drop-in, recreational, or placement centers). Motivational interviewing may also be useful within existing treatment programs. Most adolescents enter drug treatment because someone else determined that they needed to be there (family member, court, school official), and treatment programs suffer from high noncompletion rates (20% to 50%; Winters, Latimer, & Stinchfield, 1999). Given encouraging results with adult populations, motivational interviewing may be helpful in improving treatment engagement and retention among adolescents and young adults.

EFFECTIVENESS OF MOTIVATIONAL INTERVIEWING WITH ADOLESCENTS AND YOUNG ADULTS

Conducting motivational interviewing with adolescents and young adults is relatively new, and to date there have been only a few well-designed studies. All the studies of which we are aware have examined brief interventions, typically the provision of personalized feedback about a specific risk behavior following an assessment (cf. Miller & Sovereign, 1989). As reviewed herein, brief interventions have been developed in several different settings for varied prevention or treatment goals. Most programs describe the counselors delivering the intervention in a style consistent with motivational interviewing, such as nonconfrontational, empathic, using reflections and open-ended questions, and developing discrepancies. These brief interventions typically are compared to a "no-treatment" or "standard treatment" control group.

We are not aware of studies where aspects of the clinical style of motivational interviewing have been compared to other styles of intervention. Furthermore, few studies have examined the content and delivery of the intervention; thus it is difficult to evaluate which aspects of motivational interviewing were specifically being tested.

Motivational Interviewing as an Indicated Preventive Intervention

A few studies have been conducted using motivational interviewing in what could be considered an indicated preventive intervention, that is, targeting youth who have already initiated risk behavior. Some have been small pilot studies (Colby et al., 1998; Roffman, 2000). Others are currently in the field (Peterson, 1998). An exception is a study by Monti and colleagues (1999) testing a brief motivational interviewing intervention conducted with adolescents admitted to the emergency room for an alcohol-related event. The hospital emergency room (ER) provides access to youth who are engaging in risk behavior who might otherwise not be identified and an opportunity for intervention with youth who have just experienced consequences due to their risk behavior (Barnett, Monti, & Wood, 2001).

In the study by Monti and colleagues (1999), youth age 13–19 were randomly assigned to either a brief (35–40-minute) interview with personalized feedback or to a standard care intervention (5 minutes), which provided handouts and referral lists regarding ways to prevent alcohol/related injuries and treatment resources. The interventionists' therapeutic style was described as having a "focus on empathy, not arguing, developing discrepancy, self-efficacy, and personal choice" (Monti et al., 1999, p. 991). Among the 18 to 19 year olds, those in the treatment condition reported reduced alcohol-related risk at a 6-month follow-up compared to those in the standard care condition (less likely to report drinking and driving, had fewer moving violations, and reported fewer alcohol-related injuries and fewer alcohol-related problems with family, friends, police, and school). Interestingly, among youth ages 13–17, no group differences were observed (Barnett et al., 2001). This result may in part be due to the fact that the younger adolescents did not report high levels of drinking or consequences to begin with, thus making it difficult to demonstrate change. The standard care treatment may also have been more intensive for younger adolescents due to the use of a separate emergency department that provided more social work intervention.

Three additional studies have been completed that tested brief interventions with personalized feedback delivered using a motivational interviewing style as indicated prevention. One study provided a similar intervention to that used by Monti and colleagues (1999) but targeted smoking cessation in a sample of youth admitted to a hospital ER or substance abuse treatment (Colby et al., 1998). Another study developed a "marijuana check-up" and was offered to volunteers within one high school (Roffman, 2000). A third study developed a brief intervention seeking to improve adherence to dieting goals (reduction of cholesterol and dietary fat consumption) among a sample of youth already participating in a longitudinal study (Berg-Smith et al., 1999). All these studies described their interventions as providing brief feedback on the risk behavior in a style consistent with motivational interviewing as described previously. All three of the studies found that that youth reduced their risk behavior at follow-up. Yet several qualifications limit confidence in findings. In the smoking cessation study, a clinically meaningful effect size (.28) for abstinence rates at the 3-month follow-up was observed between the motivational interviewing group and the brief advice control group (20% vs. 10%), but with a sample of only 40, this difference was not statistically significant. The other two pilot studies (Berg-Smith et al., 1999; Roffman, 2000) did not have comparison groups.

Our own ongoing research effort, Project STARRS (Street Teen Assessment and Risk Reduction Study) also seeks to test an indicated prevention model but goes one step further by actually doing street intercepts of high-risk youth. Homeless, or "street," youth present some of the highest rates of substance use, as well as mental and health-related problems, among all adolescents (Adlaf, Zadnowicz, & Smart, 1996; McCaskill, Toro, & Wolfe, 1998). Yet only a small proportion of street youth seek help for alcohol or drug problems. Like those studies just described, in Project STARRS street youth are randomly assigned to receive personalized feedback on risk behavior assessed using a baseline interview. Motivational interviewing guides the clinical style. The goal is to encourage youth to contemplate making changes in their substance use behavior and, if possible, facilitate linking youth to available social services. Although preliminary results appear promising, formal evaluation awaits larger sample recruitment.

Motivational Interviewing with Adolescents in Other Treatment

We are aware of two studies that included motivational interviewing in conjunction with other adolescent treatment services. The Cannabis Youth Treatment project (CYT) is a large ($n = 600$) multisite study comparing five outpatient treatment modules for marijuana use (Dennis, 2000). Motivational enhancement therapy (MET) conducted in two sessions was part of two of the five treatments, combined with either 3 or 10 additional sessions of group cognitive-behavioral (CBT) sessions (MET/CBT5 and MET/CBT12, respectively). The other therapies that were compared were multidimensional family therapy (MDFT), adolescent community reinforcement approach (ACRA), and a treatment that added a family support component (FSN) to the MET/CBT12. The study used two treatment arms, one that compared incremental increases in treatment intensity (MET/CBT5, MET/CBT12, and MET/CBT12 plus FSN) and the other that compared alternative treatments (MET/CBT5, MDFT, and ACRA). Youth were randomly assigned to one of three treatments offered within a given site. The specifics of the MET therapy were not reported in the published paper, although treatment manuals are in preparation.

Although motivational interviewing was not evaluated as a stand-alone treatment, there were some interesting findings. First, brief MET/CBT resulted in similar outcomes to lengthier or more intensive therapies at 6-month follow-up. For example, in the alternate treatment arm, MET/CBT5 had a similar percentage of youth reporting abstinence and no symptoms as did longer programs (ACRA and MDFT). Second, any differences observed in outcomes between MET/CBT5 and MET/CBT12 were in the direction of MET/CBT5 showing better outcomes. Thus, adding more cognitive-behavioral group sessions did not appear to increase treatment effectiveness in terms of substance use or substance use problems.

A second study that added motivational interviewing to existing treatment services was conducted by Aubrey (1998). Youth were randomly assigned to receive or not receive one 30–60-minute motivational interviewing session prior to residential treatment. The session provided youth with structured feedback on their drug use using an "empathic and motivational therapeutic style" (Aubrey, 1998 p. 22). Youth who received the motivational interviewing session showed fewer days of alcohol use following treatment, although there was no difference in days of other drug use. The motivational interviewing session also appeared to impact treatment retention. Youth in the motivational interviewing condition also showed greater treatment attendance (17 sessions vs. 6 sessions).

Motivational Interviewing with Parents of Adolescents

The role of the family is critical in both prevention and successful treatment of adolescent risk behavior. Dishion (in press) has developed a brief intervention for parents of adolescents called the Family Check-Up. The check-up is a three-session intervention to strengthen and support parenting practices to reduce adolescent risk behavior. The three sessions include an initial interview with parents and the adolescent, a family assessment session, and a feedback session. The motivational intervention incorporates FRAMES components of brief interventions: feedback, responsibility, advice, menu of options, and self-efficacy. The style is one of building rapport with the client using techniques of open-ended questioning, empathy, and reflections (Dishion, in press). An initial test of the Family Check-Up (Rao, 1999) involved 40 families with high-risk youth ages 11–14. Youth in families randomized into the motivational interviewing condition showed reduced problem behavior at follow-up as reported by youth, parents, and teachers compared to youth assigned to a wait-list control condition. Further, parents reported improved parent management skills. In another application, Dishion and Kavanaugh (in press) reported that the motivational interviewing intervention provided in a school context resulted in reduced escalation of deviant peer involvement, drug use, and antisocial behavior (cited in Dishion, in press).

Motivational Interviewing with College Students and Alcohol Use

To date there have been several published studies of brief interventions using motivational interviewing with U.S. college students targeting heavy alcohol use. In a study conducted at the University of Washington (Marlatt et al., 1998), heavy drinking college freshmen were recruited for a longitudinal study of alcohol-related risk reduction throughout college. High-risk students, defined as individuals in the top quartile of recent heavy drinking in high school, were recruited for the study and completed a baseline assessment within the first few weeks of the autumn academic term. These students were then randomly assigned to receive a personal feedback interview using motivational interviewing principles. The personalized feedback was designed to address issues of interest to college freshman. Feedback materials provided data of typical and episodic drinking rates, normative comparisons to same-age peers, perceived benefits and risks of drinking, and mythology about alcohol effects (placebo and expectancy, tolerance). Dimeff, Baer, Kivlahan, and Marlatt (1999) describe the content of this program, Brief Alcohol Screening and Advice for College Students (BASICS), in detail. Trained interviewers not only used motivational interviewing and feedback to develop discrepancies between behavior and standards but also provided education if the participant was receptive.

Results of the study indicated that college students who received the motivational preventive intervention fared better than those who did not (Marlatt et al., 1998). At a 2-year follow-up, small effects were noted with respect to drinking rates and more moderate effects were observed with respect to alcohol-related negative consequences. Differences between control and motivational intervention groups with respect to negative consequences continued through a 4-year post-baseline assessment (Baer, Kivlahan, Blume, McKnight, & Marlatt, 2001). Longitudinal analyses indicated that prevention effects appear to function, on average, by accelerating a normative pattern of reduced drinking over time. Yet, the course of drinking varies a great deal from one student to another. Further analyses suggested that the motivational interviewing intervention may also have slowed drinking escalation over time relative to those who did not receive the intervention (Baer et al., 2001; Roberts, Neal, Kivlahan, Baer, & Marlatt, 2000).

The effectiveness of the BASICs curriculum has been replicated with other samples of general college students (Borsari & Carey, 2000; Murphy et al., 2000), as well as in a program that tailored the motivational program specifically for members of fraternities (Larimer et al., 2001). A key control condition—that of a standard alcohol-education curriculum—was added to the replication study by Murphy and colleagues (2000). This condition not only provides an "attention control" not previously tested but also mimics typical educational programming found on college campuses. The inclusion of a standard educational control group further strengthens the conclusion that personalized feedback is a critical part of the BASICS program.

As with much research using motivational interviewing (Rollnick & Miller, 1995), what is not clear is how and under what conditions the programs are most effective. Risk reduction for college student alcohol use may be possible based on mailed personalized feedback of a form consistent with those used in drinkers' checkup protocols (Agostinelli, Brown, & Miller, 1995). Two recent studies further suggest that group discussions by college students about alcohol risk reduction not only fail to enhance the impact of mailed feedback but may actually interfere with it (Walters, Bennett, & Miller, 2000).

CLINICAL CONSIDERATIONS

Motivational interviewing with adolescents and young adults does present certain clinical challenges. Ingersoll, Wagner, Gharib (2000), for example, note several dimensions thought to be characteristic of adolescents encountered in clinical settings for alcohol and drug problems: a history of controlling interactions with adults, previous exposure to exaggerated drug education messages, a sense of invulnerability, coercion by justice systems, the need to establish identity, and the likelihood that they have not progressed to substance dependence. Note that with this list, the prevailing result of each characteristic is in the direction of *more* resistance to influence.

Such resistance can cut two ways. It makes motivational interviewing all the more logical as a choice for a style of intervention. But it does not make the use of motivational interviewing particularly easy. Ingersoll and colleagues (2000) suggest that the counselor's first task is to distinguish him- or herself from other adults with more traditional messages. This may be accomplished by providing information that is indeed different from that to which the young person has previously been exposed. Counselors may also acknowledge and reflect doubts the adolescent may have about of the motivational interviewing session. Advice about options for change or for treatment, although still an important component of brief interventions, should come only after great care is made to develop alliances.

Implicit contracts about clinical relationships are important. It is the exceptional case where the adolescent or young adult *seeks* services. Young people are often coerced into treatment and are often angry. These feelings will conflict with engagement in any interview. Although this problem with engagement can not be eliminated, there are strategies for minimizing its harm. Counselors can openly acknowledge common thoughts and feelings and, if appropriate, encourage the young person to see if he or she can benefit from or enjoy the interview despite the circumstances (having to be there).

Indicated and targeted prevention programs suffer from a particular form of this odd therapeutic contract. Prevention programs are seldom requested or sought and often benefit from incentive systems to facilitate participation. Thus the participation of young people may be less coerced but nevertheless may be easily attributed to incentives such as payment, course credit, or, at best, curiosity. In this situation, a fundamental difference exists between the goals of the interviewer and interviewee. Young people may assume a "show me" attitude: they are willing to go through the motions of participation but not to engage in a therapeutic dialogue. Counselors can and should address these concerns openly and try to provide some basis for a shared goal within an interview. We often state, "You may be wondering if this interview will be of any interest or use to you. I appreciate that. Let me know if and when we hit on something that fits with your experiences." In our work we have found it critical to be sensitive to a young person's doubts but also not to belabor the issue. Essentially, rapport and alliance will develop when the *experience* of the interview is different rather than by hearing the counselor's intentions that it will be so. Often gently launching into material and feedback with a warm and nonjudgmental tone is more effective than reflecting resistance. Indeed, one reason for using feedback in motivational interviewing interventions with young people is that it provides a structure for the interview and material to interact about. It is through such discussion that rapport can be developed. Protocols described in our foregoing review have attempted to provide feedback on dimensions of substance use that are most relevant to young people's experiences. It is also helpful to seek responses from young people about their evaluation of the relevance of feedback content and not to pursue areas of disinterest.

We also encounter many young people who are not particularly verbal. Even open-ended questions often result with the response "I dunno." As noted elsewhere in this book, motivational interviewing, and reflective listening in particular, may be particularly useful for less verbal clients. Yet practitioners need to be prepared to roll with this form of resistance with adolescents. We find ourselves providing a great deal of structure by describing what is to be expected in the interview, how long it will take, and that we are curious about their thoughts even if they disagree. Close-ended questions become more common as well, as simple yes–no responses can at least orient discussion in a direction. Therapists are sometimes slower and quieter with less verbal clients but not so quiet as to raise the discomfort of the interviewee.

We explore and *support* personal goals, even those goals that are peripheral or even contrary to the point of the intervention. Many adolescents and young adults may come to the attention of a health care provider because of substance use but have personal goals, and even concerns, about quite different issues (e.g., peer relations or sexuality). Counselors need to be quite flexible about topics of conversation and seek to develop discrepancies between widely diverging topics.

We keep language nonjudgmental and must be attuned to highly sensitive concerns about criticism and judgment among young people. For example, in a treatment setting with adults, it does not usually raise resistance to use the word "problem." Yet with young people, particularly when participating in preventive programs, merely referring to alcohol or drug use as a "problem" can elicit a defensive reaction. We strive to talk with young people about their "choices," their "behaviors," and, perhaps, their "risks," but we do not label behaviors "problems," "issues," or even "concerns" unless the young person does so first.

It is noteworthy that these clinical issues likely vary from one group to the next, from one culture to another, and as a function of age and context for clinical services. Young adolescents with many problems and histories of involvement with criminal justice systems may feel considerable distrust for almost any adult. High school and college students without other difficulties, however, often appear curious about learning about risk reduction options. Yet this interest is often expressed only after participants have been informed that the program seeks to be different from other health education programs.

DIRECTIONS FOR THE FUTURE

Using motivational interviewing with adolescents is still relatively new. The evaluations that have been conducted to date have largely been small pilot studies, and not all have used control groups. As noted previously, the central components of the style of motivational interviewing have not been evaluated specifically. Thus, any conclusions that are drawn about the appropriateness and effectiveness of motivational interviewing with adolescents are necessarily tentative.

That said, the consistency among the studies reviewed earlier warrants some optimism. Taken together, existing studies suggest that brief intervention using motivational interviewing for adolescents and young adults may reduce risk behavior, improve program retention, and improve substance abuse treatment outcomes. Changes in behavior have been noted within randomized clinical trials with longitudinal follow-up. One study reports significant effects at a 4-year follow-up (Baer et al., 2001). Studies to date have focused on only a few clinical problems. The current focus on alcohol use is reasonable given the associated risk to health and safety. Yet many other health risk behaviors, such as drug use, risky sexual practices, and physical risk taking, could be targeted for interventions. Studies to date have also exclusively used "check-up" protocols as tests of motivational interviewing. Clearly, personalized feedback and the Drinker's Check-Up are but one application of motivational interviewing.

Motivational interviewing appears particularly promising as an intervention method to reach youth and young adults who are engaging in risk behavior. Thus, motivational interviewing may be most helpful for the development of selected or indicated prevention programs. However, motivational interviewing may also work well as a component within comprehensive universal prevention programs that integrate both primary prevention and indicated prevention. For example, one recent university program on a college campus combined media campaigns to increase perceptions of risk and lower perceptions of drinking norms for the general college community and provided brief motivational interventions targeting drinking students (Miller, Toscova, Miller, & Sanchez, 2000). However, for younger adolescents and those who have not initiated risk behavior, it is unclear how motivational interviewing might be used in universal prevention programs. School-based prevention programs that are most effective avoid values clarification but rather develop resistance and other life skills in conjunction with modifying drug use norms (Botvin, Baker, Dusenbury, Tortu, & Botvin, 1990; Hansen & Graham, 1991).

It is noteworthy that when used for indicated prevention, motivational interviewing may also prove to be controversial. Alcohol consumption by people under the age of 21 is illegal in the United States, as is true of the use of other nonprescribed drugs. At least in some contexts, goal setting and risk reduction messages may run counter to commonly held beliefs that young people simply should abstain from illegal behavior, and professionals should tell young people to do so. Clearly, we disagree with this model of preventive messages. Yet all prevention work is completed within a cultural and community context. And most drug and alcohol use prevention programs make use of social processes and integrated social influences from many quarters (Mrazek & Haggerty, 1994). Those using motivational interviewing in a prevention context will need to carefully provide rationale and garner support from other important influences in young people's lives.

As with research on motivational interviewing generally (see Chapter 16, this volume), there is much we do not know about how it works and what may be the necessary and sufficient conditions for positive outcomes. Research is needed that examines the structure and cognitive complexity of motivational interviewing interventions for adolescents of different ages. Younger adolescents may require more simple or structured feedback within "checkup"-type interventions. It is also possible that there is a lower bound in adolescence in terms of cognitive complexity (abstract reasoning) where motivational interviewing would not be expected to be beneficial. Research is needed that examines values commonly held among adolescents and young adults. For example, motivation to change substance use might be based on quite different values (avoiding parental conflict) than among adults. Most programs already focus on short-term consequences, rather than long-term ones. Arnett's (2000) model of role explorations for emerging adults suggests specific values to be addressed with motivational interviewing for many young adults. Relational issues between adolescents and motivational interviewing clinicians (i.e., therapeutic alliance) deserve research and clinical attention as well. We suspect that there may be great variability in this dimension among youth, as some youth are quite alienated from traditional social systems. As noted previously, therapeutic alliances with adolescents and young adults may require more time, energy, and technique compared to those with adults.

Finally, we are not naïve to the "file drawer problem" in clinical research. The literature reviewed earlier for the most part includes published studies with positive outcomes. We are aware of at least one dissertation testing motivational interviewing in college populations, with a normative (not high-risk) sample of college students (Miller, 1999) that did not result in treatment effects favoring a motivational interviewing treatment condition. And, there are several tests of motivational interviewing with young people in progress (including our own) as we write. Perhaps in another 10 years with the third edition of motivational interviewing, a review of applications with adolescents and young adults will reveal different conclusions and we hope a much more refined knowledge base for clinical application.

ACKNOWLEDGMENT

Work on this chapter was funded in part by Grant No. 5 R01 AA12167 from the National Institute on Alcohol Abuse and Alcoholism.

CHAPTER 22

Motivational Interviewing with Criminal Justice Populations

JOEL I. D. GINSBURG, RUTH E. MANN, FREDERICK ROTGERS, *and* JOHN R. WEEKES

Few would argue that the goal of maintaining a criminal justice system is to contribute to society's protection by identifying and intervening with individuals engaging in criminal behavior. Notions of punishment and retribution understandably exist within this perspective, but, at the same time, public opinion polls indicate support for offender rehabilitation. Another role of the criminal justice system is to assist offenders in changing behaviors (e.g., substance use and inappropriate sexual behavior) that contribute to their criminality, thereby reducing their risk to reoffend. In addressing these multiple tasks, criminal justice jurisdictions around the world have developed and implemented a variety of interventions to address offenders' needs (e.g., antisocial attitudes and inadequate problem-solving skills (Andrews, Bonta, & Hoge, 1990). Cursory examination of these interventions suggests that they vary widely in their theoretical base, approach, and likely effectiveness in facilitating behavior change.

Despite this variety, since the 1980s great strides have been made in delineating the hallmark characteristics of effective correctional programs. Spe-

333

cific program recommendations have been detailed in several meta-analytic studies, which overall support the effectiveness of programs that target criminal behavior (Andrews, Zinger, et. al., 1990; Dowden & Andrews, 2000; Lipsey & Wilson, 1993). Many of these social learning and cognitive-behavioral skills-oriented programs are delivered to higher-risk offenders. Instead of responding to the question, "What works?" this chapter addresses the question "What can be done to help offenders engage and remain in programs that focus on changing criminal behavior?" Motivational interviewing, it appears, might provide one answer to this question.

Most criminal justice workers acknowledge that offender motivation is a critical component to the behavior change process, but our experience with the criminal justice fields in Canada, the United Kingdom, and the United States indicates that definitions of offender motivation and intervention practices are wide ranging. In this chapter, we first discuss motivational issues in criminal justice settings. Second, we examine the use of motivational interviewing with offenders. Emphasis is placed on applications with sexual offenders and offenders with substance abuse problems. A review of selected research and clinical literature is provided. Third, we discuss using motivational interviewing as a treatment adjunct. Fourth, some possible drawbacks to using motivational interviewing with criminal justice populations are covered. And, finally, we suggest some of the future directions that criminal justice workers might take in this field.

MOTIVATIONAL ISSUES IN CRIMINAL JUSTICE SETTINGS

In this section we discuss issues that affect motivation for behavior change in criminal justice clients. Motivation can be conceptualized both broadly as readiness to change criminal behavior and more narrowly as readiness to engage and participate in treatment programs. Although many longer-term outcomes can be measured following intervention, the measure of primary interest to society, and ideally the offender, is the reduction in the likelihood of future criminal behavior.

Motivation and the Criminal Justice Culture

The overarching culture that exists within criminal justice systems often hinders offenders' motivation. Traditionally, the view has been that society must "get tough" with offenders and treat them accordingly. Many citizens view offenders as less than human and thus undeserving of respect and dignity. These sentiments, coupled with the widely and strongly held misconception that punishment reduces recidivism, has led to "boot camp" and "scared straight" treatment programs and regimes, which maximize the level of confrontation and external control.

Similarly, in some correctional facilities there is a palpable adversarial relationship between staff and inmates. Within these systems, there is little meaningful social interaction. Gestures of warmth and respect (e.g., eye contact, smiling, and greetings) used by institutional personnel can lead colleagues to label them "con lovers" or "bleeding hearts." For instance, Larivière and Robinson (1996) found that only 23% of Canadian federal correctional officers exhibited empathic views toward offenders. Moreover, 76% of the sample endorsed punishment as an important correctional goal. Only 54% of the officers believed in the efficacy of rehabilitation. Similar attitudes can be found among correctional officers in the United Kingdom (Hogue & Mann, 2000).

In contrast, our opinion is that this strong adversarial culture tends to lead to a "them versus us" situation, which is the antithesis to the collaborative spirit of motivational interviewing. Moreover, the belief that harsh treatment will be good for offenders is simply untrue (Andrews, Zinger, et al., 1990). Rather, we believe that motivational interviewing and its focus on reducing resistance has the potential to provide criminal justice workers with skills that could increase the effectiveness of their interactions with offenders and improve the climate of the criminal justice system which has traditionally been moralistic, judgmental, punitive, and demeaning.

Although there will undoubtedly be some technical considerations that may alter the practice of motivational interviewing (see Chapter 18, this volume), its basic principles remain the same: eliciting client concerns, reflecting ambivalence, and allowing the client to develop a plan for change that best suits him or her. In this way, the respectful, humanistic ethos that characterizes motivational interviewing might enhance the climate of criminal justice settings.

However, training criminal justice personnel in motivational interviewing cannot be done halfheartedly or with scarce resources, nor will this cultural shift occur overnight. Like other successful interventions, it will require the support and practice of the organization, including all levels of senior management. Indeed, the widespread adoption of motivational interviewing in criminal justice settings would, in many instances, necessitate a major shift in corporate perspective from a belief in coercive control to a philosophy that espouses treating offenders with more respect.

Self-Determination Theory and the Criminal Justice Culture

Self-determination theory (SDT; Ryan & Deci, 2000) provides a helpful way of conceptualizing the motivational problems inherent in a typical criminal justice culture that emphasizes coercive control and authoritarianism. This theory postulates that human motivation lies along a continuum anchored at one end by "amotivation," where there is a distinct lack of motivation to engage in new behavior, through "extrinsic motivation," where behavior change may occur in response to specific environmental contingencies, to "autonomous (or "intrinsic") motivation," where behavior change occurs in response to the individual's self-determined reasons and desires. Research on SDT has shown that when behavior change is autonomously motivated, changes are more lasting than when change is extrinsically or nonautonomously motivated. Extrinsically motivated changes tend to persist only as long as the change-focused contingencies that prompted the changes remain in place.

According to SDT, change agents can create environments supportive of intrinsic motivation to change by addressing three basic human needs: (1) the need for personal autonomy or experiencing one's behavior as determined by oneself and under one's own control rather than the control of external forces; (2) the need for relatedness or believing that others value and respect one's thoughts, beliefs, and feelings as part of a supportive, caring group; and (3) the need for competence or coming to believe that one's behavior is efficacious in producing desired outcomes.

This theoretical analysis parallels the tripartite (i.e., autonomy, collaboration, and evocation) spirit of motivational interviewing discussed in Chapter 4 (this volume), in that it emphasizes a framework within which to understand how change occurs. Further, it provides clinicians with guidelines to specific strategies that can provide a context in which motivation can become more intrinsic and new behavior more lasting. The basic behaviors the clinician should employ map onto the foregoing three basic human needs outlined. In terms of autonomy, personal responsibility is emphasized—where the individual always has a choice of how to respond to internal and external demands. The need for relatedness is addressed through an empathic context in which autonomy is supported and a genuine attempt is made to consider the individual's views, beliefs, and behavior as valid and making sense from that individual's perspective. And, finally, competence is enhanced by reinforcing the attempts and commitments the individual makes toward positive change.

Some offenders, particularly repeat offenders, are well prepared to resist all the criminal justice system's threats to needs for autonomy, relatedness, and competence. They demonstrate massive reactance and become more refractory to change, rather than less. But Miller (1999b) contests the opinion that most offenders will respond only to coercive control. He compares this mind-set with that of counselors who advocated using confrontational approaches with "alcoholics" in the recent past. Many people believe that offenders are likewise an "unmotivated" group who persist in their lies and denial. Thus, it follows that one would need to confront and take control, but to what end? Offenders, like the previously misunderstood "alcoholics," may respond much better to motivational interviewing than to confrontation.

By understanding the principles of SDT and implementing strategies to enhance autonomy, relatedness, and competence, criminal justice workers might be able to reverse some of the damage done to offender motivation by the criminal justice culture that is supposed to be effecting change. As Miller (1987) noted, motivational interviewing may be a welcome alternative to a practice in forensic settings in which problem drinkers are coerced into traditional abstinence-focused, disease-model treatment programs.

Motivation and Treatment Uptake

Criminal justice contexts present several challenges to those who assist offenders with behavior change, challenges quite different than the ones most counselors might encounter. First, offenders are frequently mandated for treatment. Some clients view a court order as prima facie coercion and an infringement upon their rights and thus steadfastly refuse to consider behavior change. This is not surprising given the phenomenon of reactance (Brehm & Brehm, 1981; Miller & Rollnick, 1991). When the idea of change or treatment is forced on an unwilling recipient it is not uncommon for the individual to engage in the problem behavior to a greater extent in an attempt to assert his or her freedom. Others simply "jump through the hoops" by participating in programs but show little personal investment in behavior change. For example, quite often we see clients who participate minimally in group discussions and fail to complete assignments.

Second, there is the widely held notion of the captive client—that offenders are imprisoned and therefore collaborating with them is unnecessary. This perspective obviously threatens the development of rapport between offenders and criminal justice personnel and, we think, ignores the fact that most incarcerated persons will be released back into society. In addition, in many cases, the client is not the offender. The offender may receive intervention, but the client can be the court, government, or society in general. It is important to be aware of the client and the stakeholders in the criminal justice context because they can have an impact on the practitioner's work. For example, ethical concerns like dual roles can arise.

Third, "correctional plans" often dictate the therapeutic goals, giving the offender little input. These documents mandate programs to be completed by the offender, which by definition diminish freedom of choice and responsibility, and may even contain pejorative descriptors (e.g., substance abuser and psychopath). For example, a program recommendation might be worded as follows: "Inmate Smith will participate in the substance abuse program because he is an alcoholic and he will change his harmful behavior by learning to abstain from drinking and practice relapse prevention." After reading statements such as this, it is not difficult to see why offenders would be reluctant to contemplate behavior change. Of course, labeling and treatment prescription are not unique to criminal justice settings. But they do become more salient in an authoritarian setting that too clearly differentiates the keeper from the kept.

Fourth, there is the temptation to "fix" offenders by telling them what they "should" do in such an environment. We believe that this power dynamic tends to move individuals away from collaboration and consideration of change. By arguing for change and telling offenders what to do, we engender resistance behavior. This is coupled with the fact that many outside agencies may be implicitly impinging upon the therapy session, threatening to punish clients who do not follow correctional plans or meet imposed treatment goals.

Further, peers may reinforce antisocial attitudes and behavior in an offender, resulting in program refusal. Thus, the courts, the institutional milieu, and the criminal population all exert unique pressures on offenders which may reduce the likelihood that they will consider changing criminal behavior. Conversely, consistent with the motivational interviewing style, we view resistance as an invitation to try a different approach and work within the offender's agenda rather than the state's or his or her peers'.

Finally, internal factors also make incarcerated clients unique. For example, some offenders categorically deny committing an offense. Sefarbi (1990) found that 50% of sexual offenders denied committing their offense, and Barbaree (1991) found categorical denial in 54% of rapists and 66% of child molesters. For these types of individuals, treatment options can be limited (Marshall, Thornton, Marshall, Fernandez, & Mann, 2001), but Mann and Rollnick (1996) have suggested that motivational interviewing may be a useful strategy in engaging clients in some of these cases. Indeed, many offenders welcome motivational interviewing because it respects their viewpoint and does not force change. In our experience, badgering a client to change his or her perspective does little to encourage behavior change, whereas respecting the client always leaves the possibility of movement toward change.

Motivation and Treatment Progress

Understanding the role of motivation in behavior change among forensic clients is a vital clinical issue and might have large social implications. Similar to findings in studies with alcohol-dependent persons (e.g., Ryan, Plant, & O'Malley, 1995), Stewart and Montplaisir (1999) found that "inadequate motivation" was most frequently the reason that offenders drop out of some programs. Forensic practitioners have been eager to decrease program attrition because evidence indicates that failure to complete treatment increases the risk of recidivism (e.g., Hanson & Bussière, 1998). Stewart and Millson (1995), for example, found that as motivation to address treatment needs increased, release suspensions decreased. These findings underscore the conclusion that treatment motivation can influence release.

A principle of effective correctional rehabilitation that has been discussed in the context of motivation is treatment responsivity (Andrews, Bonta, et al., 1990). Responsivity refers to treatment delivery using approaches and modalities that are matched to client characteristics such as intellectual ability and cognitive style. Unfortunately, motivation is sometimes conceptualized as a client trait rather than a reaction to the therapist's style. This misconception is complicated by the widely held expectation that criminal justice personnel are "supposed to" motivate offenders. (To us this conjures an image of a cheerleader or a "personal power guru" who will energize the client and spur him or her on to great achievements.) But, at best, criminal justice personnel can work with offenders to create a situation in which the probabilities that they will engage in self-exploration, contemplation of change, and change talk are increased. And in this process, we believe that motivation to change is best elicited from clients rather than imposed on them.

An example of the impact of offender motivation on recidivism comes from Marques, Nelson, Alarcon, and Day (2000). They examined the effectiveness of the SOTEP, an inpatient sexual offender program based heavily on the relapse prevention model, to determine why the program did not seem to work for some individuals. Case reviews indicated that offenders who were unsuccessful in the program exhibited a high level of motivation to avoid rearrest and imprisonment but little motivation that was not fear-based. "Even after considerable exposure to treatment, some offenders were still in the early stages of change" (Marques et al., 2000, p. 326). In reality, a strong internal commitment to abstain from sexual offending was lacking, and although participants left the program with skills and strategies for avoiding reoffending, they lacked the motivation to actually apply such strategies.

Mann (2000) has hypothesized why relapse prevention fails to affect sexual offenders' motivation to change. She noted that the conditions needed for relapse prevention assume that motivation is already present. That is, the client must want to avoid relapse before he or she will apply whatever skills were learned. Thus, without a focus on motivation as a treatment target, as many as 50% of sexual offenders can complete lengthy relapse prevention interventions without any apparent increase in motivation to change their behavior. The message is clear: Motivation must be a critical component of offender treatment.

MOTIVATIONAL INTERVIEWING WITH OFFENDERS

Research over the past decade, particularly the secondary findings from Project MATCH (Project MATCH Research Group, 1997b), have begun to suggest that the authoritarian approach to prompting behavior change is less effective than those approaches that target internal motivation. One of the few matching variables that emerged from Project MATCH suggests that relative to other interventions used in the study, motivational enhancement therapy (National Institute on Alcohol Abuse and Alcoholism, 1995) is well suited for use with clients who are initially angry.

Project MATCH is an example of a large study that included offenders in its sample; however, separate analyses have not been reported for the offender subgroup. Results from this subsample might support our contention that it seems reasonable that motivational interviewing has applications with offenders in forensic settings. Miller (1991) endorses using motivational interviewing in criminal justice settings because it is brief and inexpensive relative to other interventions and has demonstrated significant benefit in treating alcohol abuse and other addictive behaviors. Furthermore, motivational interviewing is adaptable for use in criminal justice settings because its fundamentals can be taught to a variety of professionals (Rollnick & Bell, 1991; see Chapter 18).

Motivational interviewing has been used with offenders in clinical trials, but its history is brief. Much of the literature consists of recommendations rather than empirical reports. For example, McMurran and Hollin (1993) suggest using motivational interviewing with alcohol-abusing young offenders. Annis and Chan (1983) indirectly recommend motivational interviewing by questioning the value of intensive and highly confrontive group treatment of offenders with alcohol and other drug problems. Murphy and Baxter (1997) came to a similar conclusion in their discussion of treatment programs for domestic abuse perpetrators that focus on confrontation of client defenses. In their discussion of stage-specific interventions for batterers, Walker Daniels and Murphy (1997) also recommend motivational interviewing strategies. In short, motivational interviewing is being considered by some individuals as a viable treatment alternative to confrontational strategies in criminal justice settings.

In terms of published curricula, in the most comprehensive application of which we are aware, Graves and Rotgers developed a group program for substance-abusing offenders known as motivational enhancement treatment (Jamieson, Beals, Lalonde, & Associates, 2000). This intervention was designed as a precursor to a cognitive-behavioral treatment program in settings in which the detailed information needed for individualized feedback is absent or incomplete, and in which constraints on staff availability limit the use of individual treatment sessions. Group exercises include "Drugs on Trial," a mock trial that examines the pros and cons of substance use, and "The Inner Struggle" in which participants role-play the "Devil" and an "Angel" and attempt to influence a participant who is trying to maintain changes in his or her substance-using behavior. In motivational enhancement treatment, the facilitator's role is to enhance autonomy, relatedness, and competence in a group setting where substance use and its consequences can be discussed and offenders can explore whether they want to change their substance use.

Motivational Interviewing with Sexual Offenders

The forensic population for whom motivational interviewing has most often been recommended is sexual offenders. These clients share a number of characteristics with substance- abusing individuals, not the least of which is a high rate of relapse to the problem behavior. George and Marlatt (1989) set the stage for using motivational interviewing with sexual offenders by comparing sexual offending to addictive behaviors. Other addictions treatment approaches (e.g., relapse prevention) have been successfully imported into the sexual offender treatment field (Laws, 1989), and motivational interviewing may be equally applicable. Garland and Dougher (1991) first suggested that motivational interventions could occupy a crucial role in sexual offender treatment, and others (e.g., Kear-Colwell & Pollock, 1997) have supported this recommendation, although empirical studies are limited.

There are two reasons why motivational interviewing might make a significant contribution to the field of sexual offender treatment. First, motivational interviewing is a respectful, humanistic approach to working with clients, which seems particularly important for sexual offenders (Marshall, Anderson, & Fernandez, 1999). Sexual offenders are usually the most despised group of the criminal population, facing condemnation from the public, many criminal justice personnel, and other offenders. Sexual offenders know that they are vilified and respond by developing self-serving biases (Bradley, 1978) such as denying or minimizing their crimes, seeing themselves as victims, and resisting trust and collaboration with others. Thus, a successful intervention for sexual offenders needs to communicate clearly that the client is respected despite his or her harmful behaviors. Only with such an approach can a sexual offender recover the self-esteem necessary to contemplate behavior change (see, e.g., Marshall et al., 1999).

Second, sexual offenders often present in treatment with the same motivational issues as do substance abusers. They feel angry about attending compulsory treatment, frightened about what might happen, reluctant to examine their abusive behavior and the feelings which surround it, and unwilling to relinquish their only sense of control in a judgmental environment, and they have difficulty accepting responsibility for their behavior (Mann, 1996).

In other words, sexual offenders are ambivalent about engaging in treatment and behavior change. Mann and Rollnick (1996) report a case study of this type. The client did not believe that he committed an offense despite admitting to engaging in sexual intercourse with the complainant. Further, he believed that sexual offender treatment was irrelevant. Motivational interviewing was used to reevaluate his involvement in the offense, including having him determine whether he thought he could benefit from treatment. The intervention included assessment feedback, a shift away from labeling, an emphasis on personal choice, and control in deciding whether to participate in treatment. At follow-up the client was participating in treatment and meeting treatment goals.

Posttreatment assessment indicated a decrease in precontemplation and increases in contemplation and action. Similarities between sexual offending and other addictive behaviors were noted, primarily the vulnerability of the perpetrator to blame and labeling and the need to avoid using a confrontational approach. Indeed, several such case studies have been documented in a manual published by the U.K.-based National Organisation for the Treatment of Abusers (Mann, 1996), where sexual offenders responded well to the motivational interviewing approach. Based on these case studies, the manual also suggests initial strategies for incorporating motivational interviewing into assessment and treatment. Farrall (2001) also describes an application of motivational interviewing with this population.

Mann (1996) identified a range of situations in sexual offender work where motivational interviewing might be relevant:

1. *With sexual offenders in the precontemplation stage of change.* These offenders may be mandated to treatment, but they can be unwilling to enter treatment or they completely deny committing their offenses. Using mo-

tivational interviewing to create a safe environment for exploration could enhance contemplation in such offenders.

2. *In conjunction with assessment feedback.* Sophisticated tools exist for assessing sexual offenders, such as penile plethysmography (see, e.g., Konopasky & Konopasky, 2000) and structured risk assessment procedures (see, e.g., Thornton, in press). These provide valuable information about risk and treatment needs, but they do not usually incorporate the client's agenda. Instead, they are often used as tools to label the offender and provide some measure of public protection. We contend that motivational interviewing can engage sexual offenders collaboratively in risk assessment procedures (see, e.g., Mann, Ginsburg, & Weekes, 2002; Mann & Shingler, 2001) so that the offenders' interests are served and the public is protected.

3. *With sexual offenders who drop out of treatment or those at risk to drop out.* Mann (1996) described a case in which a sexual offender became increasingly resistant to what he felt was the stigmatization of being in a sexual offender program. Components of motivational interviewing such as empathy and emphasis on personal choice were used to help the client work through his ambivalence and continue with treatment.

4. *With sexual offenders who want to change.* Given the fluid nature of motivation, even offenders who are distressed by their behavior and want to change might benefit from motivational interviewing. The reexamination of ambivalence and other strategies to enhance motivation could be incorporated into treatment programs (see, e.g., Dempsey, 1996).

Motivational Interviewing with Offenders with Substance Abuse Problems

Substance abuse has long been linked to criminal behavior. This is most obviously so because users of drugs such as heroin and cocaine are, by definition, offenders because of the illegal nature of these drugs. Moreover, some users engage in theft and other criminal activity so they can procure these substances. In attempting to reduce substance abuse among offenders, available studies provide only modest evidence for the efficacy of motivational interviewing.

On the one hand, some studies have shown no impact of the intervention relative to the control condition. Amrod (1997) studied the effect of motivational enhancement therapy (National Institute on Alcohol Abuse and Alcoholism, 1995) on motivation to change heavy drinking in a sample of randomly assigned incarcerated alcohol abusers. Group sessions focused on resolving discrepancies between past behavior and future goals, and eliciting change talk. At follow-up, there was no differential effect on motivation between the intervention and no-treatment control condition. Similar null findings were reported by Ferguson (1998) after using motivational interviewing in a double-blind, randomized, attention-placebo controlled study of mandated DUI offenders. At follow-up, there were no significant differences between the intervention and control groups in alcohol consumption. Easton, Swan, and Sinha (2000) targeted motivation to change substance use among perpetrators of domestic violence. Random assignment was only mentioned with respect to the treatment group in which subjects participated in motivational enhancement therapy (National Institute on Alcohol Abuse and Alcoholism, 1995). Posttest data indicated that participants in the intervention and control groups showed increases in taking steps to change their substance-abusing behavior. Finally, the anticipated effects of using motivational interviewing with offenders were also not observed by Kennerley (2000) when he used a motivational intervention as a pretreatment primer for randomly assigned domestic abuse perpetrators. No significant differences were found between the intervention and control groups on measures of treatment attendance, participation, and likelihood of graduation.

On the other hand, some studies have shown modest effects of motivational interviewing relative to control comparison groups. Ginsburg (2000) used motivational interviewing in a prison reception and assessment center for recently adjudicated offenders. The aim was to enhance treatment readiness (stage of change) in randomly assigned offenders with symptoms of alcohol dependence. The intervention included the use of objective assessment feedback and a decisional balance exercise. Relative to control participants, offenders participating in a motivational interview showed increases in problem recognition, and precontemplators showed increased contemplation of their drinking behavior. The assessment center seems to be a promising setting for using motivational interviewing because offenders are at the front end of their sentence. Early intervention might prime them for future treatment. The alternative is to refrain from intervening and to miss a potentially important opportunity while offenders wait to be placed in a facility to serve their sentence. Harper and Hardy (2000) reported on the use of motivational interviewing by probation officers supervising substance-abusing offenders. They found modest positive effects of the intervention on participants' attitudes toward their offending, although random assignment was not mentioned and control group participants also showed some attitudinal improvement.

The absence of clear effects in the first series of studies might suggest that motivational interviewing and motivational enhancement therapy might be ineffective with substance-using offenders. However, it is also possible that the interventions were not delivered as intended. Treatment fidelity is an extremely important consideration because it has a direct effect on treatment outcome (see Chapter 16, this volume). It is often difficult to determine the expertise of practitioners and the integrity of their interventions from the journal description. Moreover, it is sometimes a leap of faith to assume that practitioners are competent and that interventions are delivered as intended. Similarly, a host of other methodological issues, such as inadequate statistical power, might have minimized the likelihood of obtaining significant findings. This area of research is clearly in a relatively early stage of development, as is the case with so many studies of motivational interviewing in other settings (see Chapter 16, this volume).

MOTIVATIONAL INTERVIEWING AS A TREATMENT ADJUNCT

Earlier in this chapter we noted that many offenders resist engaging in treatment programs, sometimes due to poor intrinsic motivation and sometimes due to negative external factors. One promising avenue has been related by Saunders, Wilkinson, and Phillips (1995) who suggest that using motivational interviewing adjunctively with other treatments can enhance the potency of the intervention. For instance, a useful feature of motivational interviewing is its ease of integration with existing programs such as cognitive-behavioral relapse prevention to form a broader treatment framework (Bien, Miller, & Boroughs, 1993; Miller & Rollnick, 1991; Rollnick & Morgan, 1995). Bien and colleagues (1993) characterize brief interventions as focusing on increasing problem awareness and advising change in a way that complements more extensive cognitive-behavioral interventions. A natural progression might be to initiate treatment with a brief intervention such as motivational interviewing and follow with cognitive-behavioral skills training. Indeed, Baer, Kivlahan, and Donovan (1999) suggest exactly this approach, where skills training and motivational interviewing are integrated. Chapter 18 notes some of the necessary skills involved.

Of course, combining the style of motivational interviewing with other approaches would necessitate that program delivery staff learn how, for example, to "roll with resistance." Although difficult for many, these recommendations are consistent with current thinking on treatment style for offenders (e.g., Marshall et al., 1999). In adopting the motivational interviewing style, it is thought that resistance and reactance will be minimized and attrition rates reduced.

POSSIBLE DRAWBACKS TO USING MOTIVATIONAL INTERVIEWING WITH CRIMINAL JUSTICE POPULATIONS

Motivational interviewing is directive but still a client-centered approach. Its use with offenders might be of concern in light of findings discussed by Gendreau (1996). He noted that nondirective/client-centered therapies have generally been ineffective in reducing recidivism, but it is unclear to what extent motivational interviewing falls under this rubric. Cognitive-behavioral skills-based programs are generally accepted as being "appropriate" for use in criminal justice settings (Gendreau, 1996; Ross & Lightfoot, 1985), and it bears repeating that although motivational interviewing is client centered, it is also directive in its use of reflective listening to selectively reinforce certain client statements such as statements of concern and change talk. Moreover, the use of motivational interviewing with offenders does not have to be geared toward reducing recidivism, though this would be a welcome outcome. Other uses of motivational interviewing include helping offenders consider change, commit to change, engage in treatment, and remain in treatment (see Chapter 20, this volume). If any of these aims are achieved they could ultimately contribute to reducing recidivism.

Another possible concern about using motivational interviewing with offenders is ethical (Miller, 1994; Rollnick & Morgan, 1995). Under what circumstances should one not use motivational interviewing? For example, is it acceptable to use it with individuals who are not contemplating change when we believe this to be in their best interest? If our motive is to reduce the risk of reoffense and thereby contribute to societal protection, is this acceptable? Chapter 12 in this volume provides a more detailed discussion of these issues, including the case of parole and probation personnel who must take special care in using motivational interviewing because of the power inherent in their relationships with offenders.

Central to the ethical practice of motivational interviewing is ensuring that those who use it are properly trained. As Chapters 13 and 14 indicate, this requires reflection, patience, and practice. One of its limitations might be its relative complexity, in which case consideration might be given to training practitioners in other methods closely related to motivational interviewing (e.g., behavior change counseling) (see Chapter 18).

CONCLUSION

As the field of criminal justice continues to evolve, agencies are looking for innovative and effective ways of reducing recidivism by helping offenders change their criminal behavior. Alternatives to incarceration such as drug courts, restorative justice, and alternative dispute resolution are being examined by jurisdictions concerned about rising prison populations, the increasing cost of prison warehousing, and the failure of incarceration as a deterrent to criminal behavior. But, at the same time, when incarceration must be used, an increasing number of correctional jurisdictions have begun to look critically at their mandate and mission and the approaches they use to effect behavior change. Offender motivation remains a priority in the criminal justice system given the competing motives, incentives, and punishment that face offenders.

In this process, motivational interviewing is a theoretically relevant approach that has shown some evidence of efficacy in terms of behavioral change in this population. At this point there is a great need for further examination, implementation, and evaluation of the approach in criminal justice settings. In this chapter, we have discussed some of the motivational issues affecting offender engagement in, and completion of, treatment. More generally, we have also been concerned with issues affecting motivation to change criminal behavior. Although low intrinsic motivation is often observed in forensic clients, we ignore at our peril the problems caused by external pressures such as mandated treatment, antitreatment peer approval, and, antirehabilitation criminal justice cultures. Perhaps the biggest contribution that motivational interviewing has to offer the criminal justice domain is its focus on building supportive relationships. These are key ingredients to the success of any intervention that attempts to foster internally motivated behavior change.

Motivational interviewing holds promise for enhancing offender motivation to change criminal behavior. When used by practitioners with knowledge of SDT, this approach highlights therapist behavior and environmental conditions that could allow motivation to flourish and change to be embraced. Motivational interviewing can be used with incarcerated offenders and offenders under community supervision. Temporary detention units provide a promising milieu for using this approach with offenders who have violated their release conditions. Successful use of motivational interviewing by parole and probation officers, correctional officers, and other criminal justice personnel might help offenders reintegrate more quickly and successfully in our communities.

The motivational interviewing "spirit" of encouraging choice about behavior change in an accepting therapeutic environment is not yet a staple of the criminal justice landscape, but it is beginning to flourish in some quarters. Despite the promise that this approach holds for use with criminal justice populations, we must remain cognizant that it will not work equally well with all offenders. However, if motivational interviewing is applied with care in criminal justice settings, and scientifically evaluated, it might demonstrate that change can be promoted in difficult circumstances.

ACKNOWLEDGMENTS

The opinions expressed in this chapter are those of the authors and do not necessarily represent the Correctional Service of Canada, the Solicitor General of Canada, and Her Majesty's Prison Service of England and Wales. We wish to thank Jeff Allison, Greg Graves, Chantal Langevin, Andrea Moser, Susan Vanderburg, and Scott Walters for their helpful comments on an earlier version of this chapter.

CHAPTER 23

Motivational Interviewing with Couples

BRIAN L. BURKE, GEORGY VASSILEV,
ALEXANDER KANTCHELOV, *and* ALLEN ZWEBEN

> Philosophers can tell us that it doesn't matter what the world
> thinks of us, that nothing matters but what we really are. . . . But
> as long as we live with other people, we are only what other
> people consider us to be. . . . It's naïve to believe that our image
> is only an illusion that conceals our selves, as the one true essence
> independent of the eyes of the world. . . . Our self is a mere
> illusion, ungraspable, indescribable, misty, while the only reality,
> all too easily graspable and describable, is our image in the eyes
> of others.
>
> —MILAN KUNDERA, *Immortality*

As highlighted in the first chapter of this book, putting the pieces of the puzzle together regarding why people change leads to the conception of *motivation* as fundamental to the process. Motivation for change not only can be influenced by but, in a very real sense, arises from an interpersonal context (Chapter 3, this volume). A counselor's skilled use of motivational interviewing can certainly affect a client, but other people in the client's life—significant others[1]—can have an even greater influence on the client's motivation for change. This chapter presents a rationale for including significant others in the course of motivational interviewing. Treatments designed specifically for use with couples that have paralleled the development of motivational interviewing are then discussed. Finally, the chapter paints a picture, using clinical examples, of what motivational interviewing with couples might look like, including some practical recommendations for involving the significant other in the treatment process.

RATIONALE FOR INVOLVING SIGNIFICANT OTHERS IN MOTIVATIONAL INTERVIEWING

Empirical Support

Allen Zweben (1991), in the first edition of this book, explored the idea of applying motivational interviewing principles in working with couples. Although there has been no specific research to date on motivational interviewing with couples, there is evidence that involving significant others in treatment is beneficial for a wide variety of clinical problems (e.g., Barlow, 1988). In the domain of substance abuse, including a significant other in the therapy process leads to better retention and more favorable outcomes overall (Miller & Heather, 1998; Zweben & Pearlman, 1983).

Social Support

The wide-reaching benefits of social support have been demonstrated empirically, including its relation to improved physical health (Cohen, Doyle, Skoner, Rabin, & Gwaltney, 1997) and its ability to function as a general buffer that shields people from the detrimental imprints of life stress (Cohen & Willis, 1985). In accordance, it is becoming increasingly evident that social support may be a critical variable to target in therapy, beyond the session as well as within it. Although motivational interviewing takes support within the session seriously, it has not yet begun to address how to extend the client's support system beyond the few sessions with the counselor. One way of doing this would be to enlist the aid of the significant other in the client's life, who can be encouraged to provide social support by commenting favorably on the client's efforts to deal with the problem as well as providing ongoing help for targeted behavior changes.

Uncovering "Hidden" Information

Involving the significant other in the client's initial assessment may provide valuable information about the real context of the client's life, the problematic behavior, and the natural communication patterns of both the client and the couple that may remain hidden in individual motivational interviewing. Moreover, the significant other can be used to provide ongoing information about the client's progress, which can serve as an indicator of clinical significance—the extent to which important others are noticing the client's behavior change. Although research studies often make use of such collateral assessment (see Chapter 16, this volume), this information is generally lacking in clinical practice.

The Importance of Client Context

One possible shortcoming of traditional motivational interviewing is that is does not fully take into account client context, which could be essential in view of growing evidence linking individual problems to the interpersonal situations in which they occur (e.g., Jacob & Leonard, 1988; McCrady & Epstein, 1995). In some cases, the client is involved in a social network or relationship that is a maintaining factor for the current problem behavior (Shoham, Rohrbaugh, Stickle, & Jacob, 1998).

For example, the demand–withdraw couple interaction is one that has been widely studied (Christensen & Shenk, 1991) and appears to be especially prevalent when one partner has a drinking problem (Bepko & Krestan, 1985). In a common scenario, a nondrinking wife pursues, criticizes, or requests change from her drinking husband, who then withdraws or defends himself, which leads to more demands from the wife and fuels the problem-maintaining cycle (Shoham et al., 1998). One can easily see the potential frustration of doing motivational interviewing with a client in this situation, only to have him[2] return home to be confronted by his partner and immediately resume the pattern of "resistant" behavior and drinking. Involving the partner in treatment could afford the therapist with an opportunity to address the specific interactional sequences that maintain the client's problem behavior and undermine motivation for change. Many clinical problems show evidence that therapeutic benefit accrues by including a specific focus on the individual's interpersonal relations outside therapy as a fundamental component of the treatment (Borkovec & Whisman, 1996).

The client's significant other can deflate motivation for change in yet another way: Instead of demanding that the client cease the problem behavior, significant others in the client's life may actively encourage him to continue such behavior (and even engage in it with him). In Project MATCH (1997a, 1997b, 1998a), twelve-step facilitation was more efficacious than motivational enhancement therapy for clients whose social networks were highly supportive of drinking, whereas the opposite was true for clients whose social networks were low in support for their drinking.[3] In other words, motivational interviewing was least therapeutic when clients had important others in their lives to reinforce the problem behavior. When individuals try to change, the system often pushes back against them to resist such change. Working directly with client context—in the form of a significant other—could remedy this potential shortcoming of individual motivational interviewing.

Even if the significant other is not interfering in the client's change process as described previously (i.e., by explicitly demanding change or supporting no change), she may still be helpful in identifying and removing other practical barriers to the client's progress. It is clear that motivation does not lie solely within the individual but is affected by the person's relations and environment. If those around the person express concern, offer help, and reinforce the negative consequences of the problem in a nondemanding way, motivation for change is increased (Miller & Rollnick, 1991).

Amplifying the Four Principles of Motivational Interviewing

Involving the significant other in treatment may provide critical leverage for the therapist in enacting each of the key principles of motivational interviewing: expressing empathy, developing discrepancy, rolling with resistance, and supporting self-efficacy (Chapter 4, this volume). For example, the significant other may help develop discrepancy for the client by providing him with constructive feedback (i.e., information presented in a nonblaming manner) on the costs and benefits of the problem behavior for himself as well as for important others. One spouse, for instance, pointed out in session that her husband's inability to participate in family outings as a result of his drinking might be causing their children to become alienated from him; she also expressed concern about the stability of their marriage if the drinking did not change (Zweben, 1991). The underlying assumption here is that the client may become more committed to change when highly valued interpersonal relationships are threatened (Longabaugh & Beattie, 1985).

Further, conditions conducive to self-efficacy—and thus personal change—can be reliably achieved by enlisting the assistance of significant others in treatment (Bandura, 1988, 1997). With appropriate guidance, significant others can become better than professionals at guiding the client through self-efficacy-building mastery experiences (Moss & Arend, 1977). In addition, significant others can remind the client of personally relevant past successes while supporting his current efforts to change. The significant other's role in working with resistance in motivational interviewing is discussed in some detail later.

Motivational Interviewing with Couples in the Action Stage and Beyond

In the client transition from the action stage to the maintenance stage (Prochaska & DiClemente, 1982), Project MATCH (1997a) found that the greatest number of clients chose spousal support as the factor most helpful in maintaining their resolution for change. These findings are consistent with a number of other treatment outcome and natural recovery studies (Azrin, Sisson, Meyers, & Godley, 1982; Sobell, Sobell, & Leo, 1993). Significant others can facilitate change plan implementation and bolster the client's perception of self-efficacy by encouraging him to make internal attributions for progress. In maintenance activities, significant others may learn to recognize the triggers and signs of problem relapse, thereby providing the client with an early warning system and helping him recycle through the stages of change if relapse does occur.

Summary

It may be beneficial to include significant others in the motivational interviewing process for a number of reasons. There is empirical support for involving significant others in treatment for a wide variety of clinical problems, and the significant other can boost the client's social support both within and outside the sessions, as well as provide the therapist with access to critical client information that might otherwise remain hidden. Further, the inclusion of the significant other in treatment allows for a careful consideration of client context and removal of possible barriers to client change while taking into account the interpersonal nature of motivation. Finally, the significant other can furnish the therapist with a prime opportunity to put the four main principles of motivational interviewing into practice and can continue to be helpful for the client through the action stage and beyond.

MOTIVATIONAL INTERVIEWING AND COUPLE THERAPIES

Motivational Interviewing and Systems Therapies

Most couple therapies place significant therapeutic accent on such clinical practices as direct confrontation with a client's problematic behavior, use of skills training, and analysis of cognitive distortions. Nevertheless, there are two systems approaches to working with couples that explicitly apply techniques for influencing client motivation and commitment for change: the MRI model (named for the research institute at which the model was developed; Fisch, Weakland, & Segal, 1982; Weakland & Fisch, 1992) and solution-focused therapy (deShazer et al., 1986; O'Hanlon & Weiner-Davis, 1989). These approaches feature several techniques and strategies that resemble those employed in motivational interviewing. Four key similarities between these therapies and motivational interviewing are outlined herein.

- *Responding to resistance (Chapter 8, this volume)*. These approaches view resistance as an interpersonal rather than an individual variable, emphasizing the importance of avoiding argument and using the couple's values and concerns to elicit motivation for change. Specific techniques for rolling with resistance include reframing and therapeutic paradox (which in motivational interviewing takes the altered form of "coming alongside").
- *Honoring ambivalence (Chapter 2, this volume)*. These approaches often examine the symptom–system fit (i.e., how a client's problem behavior may be serving a vital function within the couple). In the MRI style, this generally leads to a consideration of the positive (as well as the negative) aspects

of the problem, akin to the decisional balance often used in motivational interviewing.

  • *Supporting self-efficacy (Chapter 9, this volume)*. The main goal of solution-focused therapy is to focus client attention on exceptions, solutions, and strengths as much as possible, thereby enhancing self-efficacy for change. As in motivational interviewing, confidence (i.e., whether the person is *able* to change) may be specifically addressed by techniques such as repeated affirmations of the client's efforts, reviewing past successes, and imagining what making the change might look like (termed "hypothetical change" in motivational interviewing).

  • *Eliciting change talk (Chapter 6, this volume)*. In solution-focused therapy, change talk is evoked early and often as the therapist helps clients paint a vivid picture of change. This change is accomplished by strategies that are also widely used in motivational interviewing, such as looking back ("Tell me about a time when the problem did not exist"), looking forward (envisioning a different future), and scaling questions (eliciting the client's rating on key variables).

Although motivational interviewing and systems therapies adopt similar strategies, there are major differences between the approaches that lie beyond the scope of this chapter, such as the skilled use of reflective listening emphasized in motivational interviewing but not in systems therapies and the common use of paradox in MRI but not motivational interviewing. The similarities, however, serve to bring out a key point: If strategies consistent with motivational interviewing are already being applied successfully in couple therapies, then motivational interviewing itself can be readily adapted for use in this domain.

Motivational Interviewing and Acceptance-Based Couple Therapies

Ideas that parallel those espoused in motivational interviewing are also being applied to couple therapies beyond systems approaches. Client-centered therapy, one of the foundational elements of motivational interviewing (Chapter 3, this volume), has been widely used with couples for several decades (Gaylin, Esser, Schneider, Rombauts, & Devriendt, 1990). Furthermore, there is a new approach to working with couples that embraces both techniques for fostering acceptance and techniques for fostering change: integrative couple therapy (ICT; Jacobson & Christensen, 1996). The emphasis on acceptance in ICT—through strategies such as empathic joining around the problem and tolerance building—represents the application of a core motivational interviewing construct to the field of couple therapy.

Motivational Interviewing: Integration with Action-Oriented Couple Therapies

Virtually all empirically supported couple therapies to date (Baucom et al., 1998) focus on the application of specific behavioral techniques that are best suited for clients in the action stage of change (Prochaska & DiClemente, 1982), with little emphasis on how to prepare couples for change (i.e., how to enhance motivation in clients who are not yet in the action stage). In light of this, motivational interviewing can be a potentially valuable addition to the field of couple therapy. Just as individual motivational interviewing can be integrated with behavioral strategies once readiness for change is augmented, in working with couples it is also possible to combine motivational interviewing with more action-oriented behavioral approaches.

THREE ROUTES TO MOTIVATIONAL INTERVIEWING WITH COUPLES

There are many ways to apply the principles of motivational interviewing in working with couples, but it appears to us that there are basically three formats such a treatment approach could take: the significant other as a participant in the client's individual motivational interviewing, motivational interviewing applied to both partners separately in session, and motivational interviewing specifically targeting couple interactions. Each of these possibilities is discussed further herein.

Significant Other as a Participant in the Client's Motivational Interviewing

One approach to adapting motivational interviewing for use with couples is to continue practicing individual motivational interviewing with the client while the significant other observes or participates. Using motivational interviewing with both partners present can help each one listen to and better understand the other's perspective and point of view. Motivational enhancement therapy (MET; Miller, Zweben, DiClemente, & Rychtarik, 1992) in Project MATCH (1997a) took essentially this approach, with the significant other included in a maximum of two (out of four) therapy sessions.

The role of the significant other in treatment depends in part on the couple's degree of interpersonal commitment to resolve the problematic behavior. When the client does not perceive significant other support as important in dealing with the problem or the significant other herself has little investment in whether the client changes, extensive involvement of the significant other may have little impact on subsequent outcome. In these situations, it may still be useful for her to be a "witness" in the sessions, with her involvement limited to sharing and receiving information about the client's problem and progress. This use of the significant other as collateral verification may help uncover "hidden" information and enhance the truthfulness of the client's talk, thereby bolstering the treatment process.

In contrast, in circumstances in which interpersonal commitment is high, it may be beneficial for the significant other to play a more active role in the individual-focused motivational interviewing sessions. The significant other may be asked to share relevant information in the planning and development of treatment goals; to collaborate constructively with the client in determining how to attain the established goals; and, in general, to help promote the client's commitment to change.

Motivational Interviewing with Both Partners

Another way to use motivational interviewing in working with couples is to do motivational interviewing with both partners during the course of the treatment. This approach might be useful in three different situations:

- If both partners see themselves as clients (e.g., both have the same or a similar problem that might be treated with motivational interviewing). A modified form of this usage has been employed by Allsop and Saunders (1991), who found clear advantages to working with two clients simultaneously.
- If the stress and impairment experienced by the significant other in attempting to cope with the client's problem precludes her participation in the *client's* motivational interviewing (Moos, Finney, & Cronkite, 1990). In this case, she may first need to attend to her own difficulties (which can done with motivational interviewing) before she can be a support to the client.
- If the significant other is ambivalent about some of her own behaviors that maintain the client's problem (contributing to his depression by not spending any time with him; protecting him from the negative consequences of substance use; etc.). In this case, motivational interviewing with the significant other may help resolve her ambivalence and allow her to alter these problem-maintaining behaviors.

The following mock session transcript illustrates what this approach to motivational interviewing with couples might look like:

INTERVIEWER: (*to significant other*) We've spent some time today discussing your husband's concerns about his weight. Now I want to hear your perspective. What are some of *your* concerns about his weight?

SIGNIFICANT OTHER: Well, the worst part for me is that he's never home lately. We used to enjoy doing things together, but now he's always out with his buddies, eating fast food and watching sports.

INTERVIEWER: (*to significant other*) You don't spend as much time together anymore.

SIGNIFICANT OTHER: We're both off doing our own things. He goes out for food, and I go to the library to study. When we first met, we did things together all the time. We went to the movies a few times a week and had dinner together almost every night.

INTERVIEWER: But things have changed.

CLIENT: She went back to school—that's what changed. She studies all the time and leaves me to fend for myself.

INTERVIEWER: (*to client*) So you see your wife's returning to school as quite a big change.

INTERVIEWER: (*to significant other*) And how do *you* see it?

SIGNIFICANT OTHER: I guess it's true . . . I've become a bit of a "studyholic." I find it really hard to clear time for things other than school—and now he's never around anyways.

The interviewer might continue on this road and elicit change talk from the wife to alter her own behaviors that may facilitate her husband's poor eating habits, leading to an eventual summary statement to the wife as follows:

> "So you're concerned about your husband's weight, and what worries you most is that you don't spend quality time together anymore like you used to. You think it might help if you started doing things as a couple again—perhaps going to movies or having dinner together. Part of you feels like your husband's going out for food with his buddies prevents you from spending time together, but part of you feels like your own studying sometimes gets in the way too. You really want to help your husband, and you think that it might be an important first step for you to clear some time to do things together once in awhile, especially around dinnertime. You indicated that you want to try this idea over the next few weeks and see what happens."

The foregoing session transcript is a hypothetical (and oversimplified) example of how motivational interviewing might be used with a significant other to get her to change a behavior (i.e., studying all the time) that might be contributing to the client's problem while allowing her to share her own perspective on the situation. In its use with couples, motivational interviewing can target not only a single significant other behavior but also a complex pattern of interconnected behaviors, as described further below.

Motivational Interviewing Targeting Couple Interactions

A third approach to motivational interviewing with a couple is to focus on the dyadic interaction sequences that maintain the problem behavior. One way to target problematic patterns of communication within the couple is to explore alternate ways of interacting, which can be accomplished by teaching the couple *how to practice motivational interviewing with each other*. For instance, frequently neither partner in the distressed couple feels listened to or supported by the other. Teaching each member of the couple how to communicate in a motivational interviewing style can help break this and other dysfunctional patterns, like the demand–withdraw interaction described earlier.

There is a mounting body of knowledge regarding how people learn the interpersonal style of motivational interviewing (Chapters 13 and 14, this volume) that suggests how to incorporate it as a component of treatment. As usual, it is not forced onto clients but, rather, gently introduced as one viable option to consider. Here is a hypothetical session transcript of how this might proceed:

INTERVIEWER: (*to significant other*) So far, we have talked about your husband's smoking and his concerns. I would also like to know: What do *you* do when your husband smokes?

SIGNIFICANT OTHER: Usually I talk to him about it. . . . If I keep quiet, I end up feeling resentful. So I try to convince him that he shouldn't smoke so much, that it's not the right thing to do.

CLIENT: She can be a real nag sometimes.

INTERVIEWER: (*to significant other*) And what happens when you do that?

SIGNIFICANT OTHER: Well, he often goes away—into the basement or his study—and I suppose he keeps smoking.

INTERVIEWER: (*to significant other*) It's difficult for you to know how to help him with this.

SIGNIFICANT OTHER: Exactly—it's very frustrating sometimes.

INTERVIEWER: (*to significant other*) I have another idea that people sometimes find useful for bringing about change in situations like this. Would you like to hear it?

In this session, once the interviewer has identified a demand–withdraw sequence, it might be helpful to introduce alternate, motivational interviewing-consistent ways of responding for both members of the couple—for example, teaching the wife to support instead of demand, which might decrease the husband's withdrawing ("resistant") behaviors, or teaching the husband to provide empathy and support to his wife and see behind the "nagging." Note, however, that there does not have to be a demand–withdraw or any negative interaction sequence present for significant others to learn the skills and techniques of motivational interviewing and become more effective partners in the change process (Miller & Heather, 1998).

These new patterns and ways of interacting might be taught to the couple in much the same way as motivational interviewing is taught to counselors. It is not merely a technical matter but a matter of eliciting the learner's own perspective on the potential value of motivational interviewing, listening to their concerns and reservations about the method, and addressing the heart of their everyday experiences (e.g., their basic interactions with their partners). In other words, the intrinsic motivations of both client and significant other to learn motivational interviewing need to be attended to and enhanced. Once this is accomplished, the learning can take place through practice (such as role-play exercises in session) with recurrent feedback from the therapist to guide the couple's progress.

Teaching a client's significant other how to use motivational interviewing is far more complex than teaching the same approach to a counselor. In the former case, the significant other may have difficulty being detached from the client's outcome because it has a direct effect on her own life. As discussed elsewhere in this volume (Chapter 12), motivational interviewing must be used with care when someone has a personal investment in which direction the client takes, even if that investment is not in conflict with what is in the client's best interest.

Summary

Motivational interviewing can be used with couples in various formats: the significant other as a participant in the client's individual motivational interviewing, motivational interviewing applied to both partners separately in session, and motivational interviewing specifically targeting couple interactions. Because many cases involve a combination of an individual with a problem (e.g., substance abuse) and an interactional, couple-level variable (e.g., demand–withdraw sequence), these three formats can be used in conjunction with one another as well as in combination with a more traditional (i.e., one-on-one) motivational interviewing approach.

PRACTICAL RECOMMENDATIONS FOR MOTIVATIONAL INTERVIEWING WITH COUPLES

Regardless of how motivational interviewing is used with a couple, there are similar decisions to be made and challenges to be met throughout the process. This section offers practical recommendations for doing motivational interviewing with a couple, addressing whether to invite the significant other into the treatment and how to join with the couple, form a consensus about goals, promote relationship cohesion, and work with different types of resistance that may arise along the way.

Inviting the Significant Other into Treatment

The practicalities of involving the significant other in the treatment process are of the utmost importance. The first determination to be made is whether there is a suitable significant other in the client's life, someone the client values and with whom he is interpersonally invested (Longabaugh, Beattie, Noel, Stout, & Malley, 1993). Because clients often have more than one significant other[1] in their lives, it is essential to explore all potential candidates so that the possibility of involving a detrimental person in the treatment can be diminished. Once an appropriate candidate has been identified, the client is asked for permission to involve her in the treatment process with a careful explanation of the associated rationale. Motivational interviewing strategies can be employed to address client concerns about such involvement, using open-ended questions followed by reflective listening, as well as decision balancing (e.g., "What is the worst and best thing that could happen if your significant other attends the session?").

Significant other involvement is generally postponed if the client remains ambivalent about it, although one option is to invite the candidate into treatment on a limited (trial) basis, with the opportunity to reconsider if it does not prove helpful. Finally, the timing of the significant other's involvement in treatment may be critical; for instance, such involvement may not be beneficial for precontemplative clients, as these clients might feel pressured and overwhelmed if both counselor *and* significant other offer feedback about their problem.

During the initial meeting with a couple, it is important to compliment their commitment to work together and clarify the roles and expectations of each partner. The rationale for including the significant other in treatment is reviewed, while stressing the client's personal choices and responsibility for behavior change. This first session also creates a unique opportunity to observe the couple's interactional patterns and test the real level of the significant other's commitment to support the client's process of change.

Joining with the Couple

The same early methods employed in individual motivational interviewing are also useful in attempting to join with a couple: asking open questions, listening reflectively, affirming, summarizing, and eliciting change talk. In working with a couple, these methods are used with both partners while the counselor expresses empathy to each one. The therapist can affirm the significant other's efforts to help the client in the past as well as, if appropriate, the steps she undertook to initiate the current treatment process. While the significant other's own concerns are specifically addressed, she can also be enlisted as a support to the client throughout the session. For example, in building self-efficacy for change, the counselor can ask the significant other of an agoraphobic client the following:

> "Have you noticed any changes in your husband that you believe to be encouraging?"
> "Are you aware of times when your husband has been able to successfully conquer his fears?"
> "What have you found to be most helpful to your husband in terms of changing his agoraphobic behavior?"

In exploring these areas with the couple, the therapist strives to make the significant other feel involved and valued in the treatment process and to instill an optimistic attitude toward change in both partners.

Forming a Consensus about Treatment Goals

There comes a point in motivational interviewing—whether with an individual or a couple—when it is time to shift approach, with the goal changing from enhancing importance and confidence to strengthening commitment to a change plan (Chapter 10, this volume). When a supportive significant other is being asked to assist the client in changing his problem behavior, it is valuable to forge a consensus between the two partners at this critical stage. The techniques and style of motivational interviewing are particularly warranted at this step, because the development of the change plan is a process of shared decision making and negotiation—between three people now rather than two—that involves setting goals, considering options, arriving at a plan, and eliciting commitment. Though consensus is valuable, it is by no means essential: The chief role of the significant other is to assist the client in generating his *own solutions* for change by providing constructive input and support, thereby helping the client derive maximum benefit from treatment.

Promoting Relationship Cohesion

As discussed previously, the client's significant other is especially helpful in the treatment process if she can function as a source of social support, thereby providing a natural helping relationship in the client's life. An ongoing aim of motivational interviewing with a couple, therefore, is to promote relationship cohesion and satisfaction—particularly between partners who already evidence strong interpersonal ties—in order to consolidate the client's commitment to change (Edwards & Orford, 1977). Specific goals for the relationship can be explicitly addressed, such as engaging in shared activities (e.g., vacations) that can improve the quantity and quality of couple interactions.

Working with Resistance

A basic difference between motivational interviewing with one individual and with a couple is that in the latter case there are three possible sources of resistance: the client, the significant other, and the couple as a whole.

Using the Significant Other in Working with the Client's Resistance

Because resistance is shaped by interpersonal interactions, it is critical to assess the significant other's role in evoking resistance from the client during the session. If necessary, the treatment can include a specific focus on any resistance-promoting relational patterns (e.g., demand–withdraw and confront–resist), teaching the couple how to do motivational interviewing with one another as described previously.

If the significant other is not contributing to the client's resistance in session, she can often play an important role in helping him become more committed to change. For instance, feedback is usually more meaningful to the client when it is verbalized by the significant other rather than the therapist. This feedback can be elicited by the following questions:

> "What have *you* noticed about [the client's] problem?"
>
> "How has the problem behavior affected the situation at home?"
>
> "Has anything changed to cause you to become more concerned about the problem?"

Having the significant other deliver these important messages in a nonconfrontational manner can be valuable in diminishing the client's resistance and enhancing motivation for change.

There may be instances, however, in which the significant other is full of "action" talk while the client remains ambivalent. In these cases, it may be useful for the therapist to soften the significant other's feedback and prevent the session from proceeding into the action stage before the client is ready.

A Resistant Significant Other

The significant other's involvement in treatment may be counterproductive if she is uncommitted to change (Longabaugh et al., 1993) or overburdened with anger and resentment. Relationship problems (e.g., marital discord) that might be affecting the client's problem behavior can be addressed in a motivational interviewing style, but preferably after the main treatment target is thoroughly examined. In a situation in which the involvement of the significant other may be interfering with the motivational process, her role can be limited to being a bystander or "witness" in the client's individual sessions.

A Resistant Couple

Couples who appear to be unresponsive to motivational interviewing usually evidence a negative pattern of interaction (Zweben, 1991), tending to blame, criticize, and harass each other in the sessions—a situation that can increase the client's resistance to change or cause him to leave treatment prematurely. A primary objective in this case is to reduce the negative interactions by teaching the couple how to do motivational interviewing with one another, as discussed in detail earlier.

CONCLUSIONS

This chapter has provided an overview of the current state of motivational interviewing strategies for working with couples. Empirical and clinical evidence so far suggest that significant other involvement may lead to improved retention in treatment and better outcomes for a wide variety of clinical problems.

This is consistent with the motivational interviewing conception of the importance of the social context in achieving and maintaining change.

For motivational interviewing to fulfill its potential in working with couples, this area requires further clinical precision and development. Key issues remain, such as whether and how to involve the significant other in treatment for a given client, as well as the specifics of using motivational interviewing to address interactional sequences rather than merely individual behaviors. Research efforts are needed to evaluate the efficacy of motivational interviewing with couples, to better understand the influence of the significant other's presence on the dynamics of client motivation, and to further delineate the therapeutic traps specific for motivational interviewing in this domain.

NOTES

1. A significant other can be a spouse, partner, or any other key member in the client's life, such as a family member or friend. In this chapter, we use the term "couple" to denote any of the foregoing relationships.
2. A note on pronoun use: For convenience, we will be referring to the client as "he" and the significant other as "she" in this chapter, as this is the most common scenario in the case of substance abuse and dependence (where motivational interviewing was first developed). However, the principles outlined in this chapter are meant to apply to clients or significant others of any gender, as well as to a broad range of clinical problems.
3. For more details on Project MATCH, see Chapter 16 in this volume.

CHAPTER 24

Motivational Interviewing in the Treatment of Dual Disorders

NANCY HANDMAKER, MICHELE PACKARD, *and* KELLY CONFORTI

Problems with adherence are common complaints among treatment providers. Few client populations show more serious problems with adherence than do persons with either addictions or mental illness, evidenced by the necessity for such extreme interventions as involuntary commitment, incarceration, and court-mandated treatment. When persons have *both* substance use and mental illness simultaneously, the problems with treatment adherence are compounded. Recent studies on applications of motivational interviewing show promise for enhancing treatment adherence and retention among persons with comorbid substance use and mental disorders. This chapter reviews developments in motivational interviewing with this challenging population.

The coexistence of psychiatric and substance use disorders is commonly referred to as dual disorders. Epidemiological studies have shown that the likelihood of having a substance use disorder is higher among persons with a mental health disorder than in the general population. The rates are highest among persons with severe and chronic mental illness such as schizophrenia and bipolar affective disorder. Lifetime prevalence rates of substance use disorders among persons with schizophrenia (48%) or bipolar affective disorders (58%) are more than three times the rate for the general population (Regier et al., 1990). Estimates of recent or current substance use disorders among mentally ill treatment samples have ranged from 20 to 65% (Mueser, Bennett, & Kushner, 1995; Regier et al., 1990). These high rates of comorbidity are of concern as substance abuse compromises the efficacy of neuroleptic medication and enhances the activity of the dopaminergic system, thereby exacerbating psychiatric symptoms and often causing hospitalization (Bellack, 1992). Substance abuse also increases the risk for adverse drug reactions, including accidental overdoses. Moreover, the use of alcohol and illicit drugs impairs cognitive functioning. Because most psychiatric disorders have attendant problems with judgment, attention, and memory, substance use further impairs already compromised reasoning abilities, increasing the risk for harm among persons with mental disorders (Bellack & DiClemente, 1999). Alcohol and drug use among the mentally ill exacerbates all the negative outcomes associated with severe mental illness such as homelessness, incarceration, joblessness, poverty, infectious diseases, violence, and suicide (Mueser, Drake, & Noordsy, 1998). Persons with substance use disorders are less adherent with psychosocial and pharmacological interventions (Jerrell & Ridgely, 1995) than others who are engaged in mental health care. Consequently, they tend to use more costly services such as emergency room visits and hospitalizations.

Despite the high rates of comorbidity of mental and substance use disorders and related problems and costs, historically there has been a lack of coordination in the treatment of dual disorders. For years substance use disorders have been treated by professionals in systems that were separate from mental health treatment. Separate treatment systems have been largely ineffective in treating dual disorders. Prospective studies of alcohol and drug treatment have consistently reported poorer outcomes for persons with psychiatric symptoms (e.g., Project MATCH Research Group, 1997a). Similarly, persons with severe mental disorders who abuse alcohol or drugs show worse outcomes in mental health treatment settings (Mueser & Noordsy, 1996). The lack of coordination between the two (substance abuse and mental health treatment) service systems has led to poor treatment engagement, high dropout rates, and relapse among the dually diagnosed.

Experts have generally agreed since the mid-1980s that persons with dual disorders are served best by care that integrates substance abuse treatment with mental health treatment. In an integrated approach, alcohol and drug treatments are incorporated into existing psychiatric, nursing, counseling, and case management services provided by multidisciplinary teams within community mental health treatment programs (Mercer-McFadden, Drake, Brown, & Fox, 1997). A primary assumption of integrated treatment is that long-term care leads to the greatest improvement and stabilization among persons with dual disorders. A second assumption of an integrated treatment approach for dual disorders is that treatment should address the ongoing changes in client motivation to reduce substance use. Thus, recommendations for integrated treatment include a longitudinal perspective that accommodates shifts in client commitment to treatment and/or sobriety.

A comprehensive review of treatment outcomes over the past decade (Drake, Mercer-McFadden, Mueser, McHugo, & Bond, 1998) revealed that integrated care shows only a modest advantage over nonintegrated treatment. Although integrated models are arguably the best models of treatment, engagement and retention remain issues and treatment programs continue to show high dropout rates, as great as 83% in one study of residential treatment (Drake et al., 1998). However, when dually disordered clients were successfully engaged in an integrated treatment program, they showed significant improvement. Furthermore with the benefits of mental health care increased, clients remain in treatment longer. Extended participation in treatment of 18 months or longer was associated with significant reductions of substance abuse, reductions in hospital use, and improvements in psychosocial outcomes. Therefore, a major focus for increasing success in treatment of dual disorders is engaging clients in long-term outpatient care.

MOTIVATIONAL INTERVIEWING WITH THE DUALLY DIAGNOSED

Recent pilot research in motivational interviewing has shown positive results in increasing treatment engagement and adherence with dual disorders. Motivational interviewing has been applied in at least three areas of adherence that affect engagement in outpatient care: inpatient settings, outpatient settings, and medication adherence. Although findings are mixed in studies of medication adherence, other studies have shown the potential benefits of motivational interviewing. Overall, application of these methods are yet to be fully tested, but initial findings are thus far consistent with reported effects of motivational interviewing.

Transitioning from Inpatient to Outpatient

Individuals with dual disorders are more frequently hospitalized and spend more days in inpatient units than do individuals with mental disorders who do not drink or use drugs. After becoming stabilized in a psychiatric hospital, clients with dual disorders are less likely to follow through with initial outpatient sessions (Axelrod & Wetzler, 1989; see Chapter 20). For example, as part of a quality assurance review, clinicians found that persons with comorbid depression and a substance use disorder complied with their initial outpatient appointment at half the rate as those who did not have a substance use disorder (Daley & Zuckoff, 1998), which was about half the rate of referrals directly from the community. Thus, clients with the worst symptomalogy and impairment have been shown to be at the greatest risk of failing to enter treatment following discharge. This pattern of service use is costly and frustrates providers because the lack of engagement in outpatient care increases the risk for relapse and future inpatient admissions.

Three studies published in the late 1990s have shown that a motivational interview session during a psychiatric hospitalization increased rates of client engagement with outpatient treatment (Daley, Salloum, Zuckoff, Kirisci, & Thase, 1998; Daley & Zuckoff, 1998; Swanson, Pantalon, & Cohen, 1999). Daley and Zuckoff (1998) found that a motivational interview several days prior to discharge from a psychiatric inpatient unit nearly doubled the rate of adherence with the initial outpatient session from 35% to 67% among dually disordered clients during their study period. Daley and his colleagues (1998) replicated these findings in a pilot study of motivational interviewing for a group at significant risk for rehospitalization—individuals with comorbid depressive disorder and cocaine dependence. As in the earlier study, results showed that clients with comorbid depression and cocaine dependence who were consecutively assigned to receive a motivational interview session prior to discharge were more likely to attend their first session. The third study showed an effect of motivational interviewing on adherence with aftercare among 121 psychiatric inpatients, 77% of whom had concomitant substance use disorders (Swanson et al., 1999). In this study, a two-session motivational intervention more than doubled (42% vs. 16%) the rate of adherence with an initial outpatient session following discharge. Inpatients randomly assigned to the motivational interview group completed the University of Rhode Island Change Assessment Scale (URICA; McConnaughy, DiClemente, Prochaska, & Velicer, 1989), a measure of treatment readiness at intake. They were then provided a 15-minute scripted feedback session on their URICA scores. Prior to discharge, the motivational interview group received a second hour-long session. The second session was an open-ended motivational interview that focused on the relationship between the patient's current mental conditions and treatment readiness at the onset of hospitalization.

The three foregoing studies showed significant increases in adherence with outpatient treatment following a motivational interview as part of inpatient care. Aftercare attendance rates were doubled by addressing readiness for outpatient treatment and obstacles to treatment as part of inpatient care in a motivational interviewing style. The lack of randomly assigned control groups in two of these studies and the small sample sizes limit their generalizability. However, these findings suggest that a motivational interview session prior to discharge is likely to increase client engagement in an initial outpatient session.

Enhancing Treatment Adherence

In a pilot study with dually diagnosed outpatients (Martino, Caroll, O'Malley, & Rounsaville, 2000), subjects randomly assigned to receive a preadmission

45–60-minute motivational interview as a prelude to a partial hospitalization program (outpatient day hospital program) showed better attendance patterns than did subjects who received the standard preadmission interview. The motivational interview included feedback from preadmission questionnaires, which included measures of psychiatric symptoms, ratings on severity of alcohol and drug use, and recent alcohol and drug use, and a decisional balance activity. A second pilot study (Graeber, Moyers, Griffith, Guajardo, & Tonigan, 2000) compared three 60-minute motivational interviewing sessions with three educational treatment sessions for persons with concomitant alcohol disorders and schizophrenia who were already engaged in either outpatient or inpatient programs. The motivational interview included "check-up" feedback and when appropriate, strategies for initiating and maintaining changes in drinking. The didactic sessions focused on phases and signs of alcoholism, cognitive-behavioral strategies for improving self-esteem and self-efficacy to reduce drinking. At 4- and 8-week follow-ups, both groups reduced their alcohol consumption, but the group that received the motivational sessions had significantly fewer drinking days than did the educational intervention group during the follow-up periods. No differences were found between groups on total drinks consumed or estimated peak blood alcohol levels. Despite the small sample size, moderate to large treatment effects ($d = .53$) were found for the motivational intervention. These clients were more likely to complete 30 and 90 days of outpatient treatment. They also attended more treatment sessions and were rehospitalized less often than a treatment-as-usual group consisting of clients with the same diagnoses. Furthermore, 9 of the 11 motivational interview clients had continuous sobriety and lower self-reports of depressive symptoms during the first 30 days of outpatient treatment.

These two studies suggest that the motivational interviewing holds promise for improving outpatient treatment engagement and related outcomes. The impact on attendance rates was only modest in the first study, but previous research suggests that abstinence-oriented, restrictive programs, such as partial hospitalization, generally have poorer adherence rates for this population (Drake et al., 1998). The second study (Graeber et al., 2000) is the first to demonstrate that motivational interviewing as an adjunct to outpatient treatment improves short-term drinking outcomes with persons with severe and chronic mental disorders. Both studies were limited by small sample sizes. However, the moderate to large effect size of motivational interviewing on drinking days is noteworthy given the limited sample size and that the participants were significantly impaired.

Medication Adherence

Medication adherence is an important determinant of treatment outcome for individuals with a serious mental illness (Kemp, Hayward, Applewhaite,

Everitt, & David, 1996). Individuals with serious mental illness are often more ambivalent about taking medication than any other issue. Obstacles to medication adherence include lack of patient recognition of the need for medication, side effects of medications, ongoing substance abuse, cognitive impairment, and motivational deficits (Bellack & DiClemente, 1999; Owen, Fischer, Booth, & Cuffel, 1996).

At least two studies have failed to show that motivational interventions increased the rate of adherence in mentally ill individuals. In one study, a dually diagnosed group of psychotic and mood-disordered clients received either a preadmission motivational interview or a standard preadmission interview. There were no differences between the two groups on medication adherence (Martino et al., 2000). In another study, 21 hospitalized patients were randomly assigned to receive two to three half-hour sessions of medication self-management conducted in a motivational interviewing framework. Physicians rated patient compliance at 1 to 2 months after discharge. Again no differences were noted between the group that received the motivation-based intervention and those that did not.

Other studies conducted in the United Kingdom with larger sample sizes did find that an adapted motivational interviewing intervention produced better outcomes. In one study, 47 male and female hospitalized subjects were randomly assigned to receive "compliance therapy" or routine supportive counseling. The "compliance therapy" intervention was drawn from the principles of motivational interviewing and cognitive treatment of psychosis. The authors felt it was not fair to label their intervention "motivational interviewing" because the subject of medication compliance was brought up regardless of whether the patient saw it as a problem. Nevertheless, elements of motivational interviewing used in the study included the decisional balance, exploration of ambivalence, development of discrepancy, and affirmation of adaptive behaviors. As such, the study fits the rubric identified by Burke, Arkowitz, and Dunn (Chapter 16, this volume) as an adaptation of motivational interviewing. Subjects in the intervention group received four to six sessions of compliance therapy, twice weekly, for 20–60 minutes. Outcome measures were collected at discharge from the hospital and at 3-month and 6-month follow-up. Compliance rates in the intervention group steadily improved over time, while those of the control group remained relatively unchanged through the three follow-up periods. At the 6-month follow-up, the intervention group had 23% higher rates of compliance. Attitudes toward medication were at their highest right after the intervention and had begun to decline in both groups by 1-month follow-up, though the intervention group did have significantly better attitudes toward medication. The intervention group steadily gained in insight at 3- and 6-month follow-up, while the control group had begun to decline by 6-month follow-up. There were no differences in global assessment of functioning (GAF) between the two groups at the point at which they were discharged from the hospital. However, GAF in the intervention group continued to improve at 3-month follow-up, while that of the control group had begun to decline. GAF in both groups was beginning to decline by 6-month follow-up, though the intervention group fared significantly better (Kemp et al., 1996). A subsequent study by the same group confirmed findings of the earlier study. The second study randomly assigned 74 patients to compliance therapy versus a control condition. At 18-month follow-up the compliance-therapy group had greater rates of retention, better insight, better attitudes to treatment, better compliance, lower rates of rehospitalization, and more improvement in GAF over time (Kemp, Kirov, Everitt, Hayward, & David, 1998).

STRATEGIES FOR INCREASING ADHERENCE WITH OUTPATIENT TREATMENT

Raising Awareness of Nonadherence on Psychiatric Symptoms

During an inpatient hospitalization, a client has time to explore his or her life events without the complicating effects of alcohol or illicit drugs. This provides an opportunity for the clinician to raise awareness of the relation of treatment nonadherence and the resulting crisis. Common elements of successful pilot studies of motivational interviewing with inpatients included the following to increase treatment adherence:

- Affirming the recognition of problems and the need for help.
- Exploring the client's reasons for not using treatment services.
- Exploring client role in improving.
- Discussing treatment options.

Eliciting Pros and Cons of Treatment Nonadherence

Client commitment to attending a first session can also be elicited by examining the pros and cons of treatment nonadherence. Emphasizing the preservation of personal liberties through the use of outpatient services versus the restrictions of inpatient hospitalization have been shown to elicit statements of intent or desire to engage in less invasive outpatient care (e.g., "When you are hospitalized, you lose your freedom to act and move about. What is that like for you? How can this be avoided in the future?"). Another strategy for evoking self-motivational statements about attending an initial outpatient session is to ask open-ended questions about how the recent crisis was related to nonadherence with an ongoing treatment program, ("Who or what could have helped you prevent this setback?"). The process of such an interview might be summarized in a decisional balance exercise, which elicits the reasons for using treatment versus not using treatment, including obstacles to care. Box 24.1 illustrates a decisional balance summary during an inpatient hospitalization.

BOX 24.1. Decisional Balance Exercise

Reasons for not attending treatment		Reasons for attending treatment	
Benefits	Costs	Benefits	Costs
No one "checks up" on me.	Bus money	Support from staff	Relapse
	Interferes with other activities	Medication	Disappoint family
	Giving up drinking	Stay sober	Incarceration
		Fewer symptoms	Rehospitalization
			Loss of self-respect
			Depression

BUILDING MOTIVATION FOR CHANGE IN SUBSTANCE USE

Open-Ended Interview

Phase 1 of an open-ended interview may proceed simply with asking questions, reflections, and summary statements of the client's change talk toward increasing a discrepancy between psychosocial well-being and substance use. Using these strategies, the emphasis is on eliciting recognition of how alcohol and drug use interacts with mental disorders. Asking open-ended questions can elicit self-motivational statements of the effects of alcohol and drug use on cognitive symptoms or other problems. Following is an example of how a therapist might conduct this session with a client who was recently hospitalized.

COUNSELOR: You've told me about how when you were in a manic state, you drank more than you usual, got into a fight, and the police were called to step in. What happened next?

CLIENT: I was brought here to the hospital.

COUNSELOR: What was the worst part of all of this?

CLIENT: Feeling like I do now which is miserable.

COUNSELOR: You're feeling really bad. What are some of the things that you are thinking about while you are here?

CLIENT: How I let my family down.

COUNSELOR: In what ways?

CLIENT: Last time I was here they felt so bad. I told them I wouldn't put them through this again.

COUNSELOR: But something changed.

CLIENT: I started drinking again.

COUNSELOR: You think that the drinking played a role in this set back.

CLIENT: I stopped coming in for my doctor's appointments. Then the drinking went from one or two beers to hanging out at the bars all day. After awhile, I didn't remember to take my medication.

COUNSELOR: Your drinking eventually led to your missing appointments and forgetting to take your medication.

Feedback

When appropriate, the therapist might elicit the hazards or complicating psychopharmacological effects of alcohol and drugs in an "elicit–provide–elicit" interview format described by Rollnick, Mason, and Butler (1999). For example, a client might say the following in response to how drinking affects his or her depression:

CLIENT: Well, at first I feel pretty good, but after drinking all day I just pass out. Then I feel terrible.

COUNSELOR: So drinking helps improve your mood initially, but later, the bad feelings are there again.

CLIENT: Yeah. Like today I feel like it's hopeless.

COUNSELOR: Today, you're really feeling down. You know last week you were feeling more hopeful. What was different then?

CLIENT: Well I wasn't drinking, for one thing.

COUNSELOR: That's right. You hadn't had any alcohol for three days and your mood improved. How much do you know about how drinking affects moods?

CLIENT: Only that I feel bad.

COUNSELOR: Would it be OK if I told you a bit of what I know?

CLIENT: Sure.

COUNSELOR: Ethanol is a central nervous system depressant. Its chemical effect is depression.

CLIENT: Huh?

COUNSELOR: You're not sure what to make of this.

CLIENT: Well, I'm taking this medication to feel better.

COUNSELOR: Uh huh.

CLIENT: It probably doesn't give it a chance to work.

COUNSELOR: Yes, that's right. You're taking one medication for reducing depression while also taking alcohol, which has the chemical effect of increasing depression. What do you make of that?

CLIENT: I won't feel better if I keep drinking.

A "check-up" approach used by Graeber and his colleagues (2000) led to decreased drinking among schizophrenic outpatients. Check-up feedback may be modified to include measures of emotional problems for the dually disordered clients. For example, measures of severity of psychiatric symptoms might be included as personalized feedback to raise the awareness of how symptoms are related to changes in substance use. Graphic presentations patterns of use over an entire lifetime or the past month or week are concrete strategies to elicit talk about change. They may also be useful in pointing out the relationship between the substance use and increased psychosocial or psychiatric symptom escalation and hospitalizations. Measures of expectancy effects that assess a client's cognitions about the expected benefits of a given substance are especially relevant for this population. Persons with dual disorders frequently believe that drugs and/or alcohol are the best means for alleviating their psychiatric symptoms (depression, auditory hallucinations, social anxiety, loneliness from isolation, etc.). Clarifying the relationship between beliefs and substance use opens the door to challenging beliefs, modifying cognitions, and increasing commitment for skills training.

Drop-In Motivational Groups

A novel approach for increasing treatment adherence among dually disordered outpatients is being practiced at the University of New Mexico Mental Health Center's dual-diagnosis program. Drop-in groups may affect engagement of dually disordered clients within a clinic setting. The drop-in motivational groups can be incorporated into a broader, stage-matched program of skills training and relapse prevention. The advantages of a drop-in group are that the clients can "sample" substance abuse treatment with minimal commitment toward change and that groups are accessible and available. The drop-in group format recognizes the lack of structure in actively drinking or drug using clients who are less likely to remember and follow through with scheduled appointments. To encourage attendance, the groups are offered during the medication clinics when dually disordered clients are likely to be present. The drop-in motivational groups provide an innovative opportunity for clients to explore their ambivalence about change. The therapist gently guides the clients with exercises that evoke change talk. Although this format has not been tested, the enduring popularity of the group in the New Mexico clinic suggests that this mechanism may match an important treatment need of dually disordered clients at the initial stages of change. In the early stages of client engagement, the goal is group attendance, not cognitive or behavioral changes. The commitment to abstain from substance use or change in any way is optional. It is explained to the client that others in the group are similar to him or her in that they are ambivalent about change and merely want a nonpressured, safe environment to explore their thoughts about drinking and using drugs.

SPECIAL ISSUES WITH DUAL DISORDERS

Harm Reduction or Abstinence?

Because even relatively infrequent or low amounts of substance abuse disrupt behavior and lead to severe consequences, such as loss of housing, an early focus of treatment is substance use. However, persons with comorbid mental and substance use disorders are generally not seeking to change their alcohol and drug use in the initial stages of psychiatric treatment. Thus, it is likely that in the initial stages of engagement or even throughout the course of treatment, persons with dual disorders will continue to drink or use drugs. Increasing motivation for harm reduction and "sampling sobriety" are frequently the best options for the therapist.

Where to Begin?

Those with concomitant alcohol and drug use disorders typically have multiple disabling conditions and complications. Consequently, motivational interventions may focus on multiple behavior change such as adherence with appointments, medication compliance, and substance use reduction concurrently or single goals such as medication compliance and symptom stabilization. A team initiates a treatment plan that addresses multiple domains such as psychiatric services, case management, nursing, psychotherapy services, and substance abuse. Treatment providers develop a hierarchy of treatment goals, considering meeting basic needs and safety as priorities. Ultimately, it is the client's responsibility to choose how to proceed, which is determined by readiness for action. A tool for measuring multiple behaviors might be employed to assist in the decision-making process, such as the example in Box 24.2.

Cognitive Impairment

Individuals with severe mental illness are known to have problems with abstract reasoning, concentration, and working memory. Consequently, it is important to adapt intervention strategies to accommodate these problems. Writing on a chalkboard, repeating, and making lists for clients are examples of such strategies. A concrete method for conducting the process of exploring pros and cons to alcohol and drug use is helpful. For example, using colored cards (e.g., red for reasons to stop) handed to clients to take with them after the session is a strategy for evoking self-regulatory behavior after the session. A schizophrenic client who wrote his reasons for abstaining from methamphetamine on an index card, which he kept in his wallet, used this external cue to resist acting on urges to use drugs. Another concrete method for conducting this exercise would be to stack blocks into two piles and review "which has more?" When possible, using visual aids such as graphs or charts assists in understanding normative feedback. With more cognitively impaired

BOX 24.2. Readiness to Change Measure

How ready are you to do something to change?	Not ready	Unsure	Thinking about it	Ready	Very ready
Write in possible areas:					
Stopping drinking			✓		
Quitting smoking	✓				
Taking medication					✓
Finding a safe place to live					✓
Making new sober friends			✓		

individuals, it is a good idea to offer the feedback across multiple, brief sessions so that it is delivered in small, assimilated units. In general, a slower pace with more pauses for questions and clarifications is indicated.

Because schizophrenics possess a variety of cognitive, neurobiological, and social deficits, particularly in executive functioning, Bellack and DiClemente (1999) provide a compelling argument that schizophrenics would be incapable of sustaining intentional behavior (i.e., following through with commitment elicited in a motivational interview) before they acquired the skills to do so. A model of treatment such as the one described in the section "Putting It Together: A Clinical Program Example," which provides skill training such as drug refusal skills even before a commitment for sobriety is reached, may enhance goal attainment when the desire or intent for change increases.

Heterogeneity in Groups

Most treatment populations in any clinical setting of persons with dual disorders are diverse. Clients differ in the number and nature of mental disorders, severity of substance use, medical disabilities, cognitive functioning, and many other variables not considered here. Consequently, it is challenge to provide services in a group format (see Chapter 25). A young man with an addiction to crack cocaine who recently engaged in mental health treatment following his first psychotic episode and who has no desire to change his lifestyle will present different treatment issues from a 50-year-old male with liver disease who is maintained on methadone for his heroin addiction and alcohol dependence. The common theme of ambivalence to changing their substance use might place both of these clients together in a group for precontemplators or contemplators. It is this commonality that can be drawn on in the group content. Naturally, there are many individuals who cannot benefit from group treatment, and individual interventions (e.g., case management) should be available as an alternative.

Involving Significant Others/Case Managers

Strategies shown to be effective in engaging and retaining clients with dual disorders include assertive community outreach, removal of barriers through practical assistance such as stable housing and transportation, case management, contingency management through reinforcers such as the use of vouchers, and social supports. Applying motivational interviewing principles in the treatment components shown to be effective in engaging and maintaining clients with dual disorders is likely to enhance their efficacy. Specifically, case managers or supportive significant others might participate in the motivational interviews (e.g., feedback sessions; see Chapter 23, this volume). Moreover, including significant others or case managers increases the likelihood that dually disordered clients will follow through with their plans to change. Significant others or case managers can offer the "scaffolding" in the community to support change efforts. This is especially relevant for persons who have concomitant attention and memory problems or "frontal–temporal" impairments associated with schizophrenia, which make it difficult to initiate and follow through with intentions or plans for behavior change.

PUTTING IT TOGETHER: A CLINICAL PROGRAM EXAMPLE

A program initiated several years ago at the University of New Mexico serves as one example of an integrated, stage-matched approach. Outpatient group treatment serves as a core for treating substance use and related problems among persons with severe mental illness within a community mental health center (see Box 24.3). Group referrals are made on the basis of (1) the patient's general readiness to change for substances that present the greatest problems, based on Stages of Change Readiness and Treatment Eagerness Scale (SOCRATES); (2) willingness to participate in a group; (3) ability to benefit from the treatment; and (4) coping skills deficits (i.e., whether patients are "ready, willing, and able").

The program relies on a social learning model for treating substance use disorders. Patient needs for skills training are identified through a functional analysis of substance use and related problems (e.g., social skills training to

---

BOX 24.3. Stage-Matched Outpatient Abuse Treatment Model

Precontemplation	Contemplation Preparation	Action	Maintenance
Individual "check-up" interviews "Talking about change" groups		Tools for change Practicing change	Maintaining change

---

BOX 24.4. Group Model for Stage-Matched Integrated Dual Disorders Treatment

- *Talking about change.* Individuals in the precontemplation or contemplation stage of change are referred to this group. The goal can be simply attendance versus other cognitive or behavioral changes. The groups are described to clients as "talking about" change to appeal to those without problem recognition or intentions of changing. Structured motivational exercises are implemented. For example, working through a pros-and-cons list on a dry erase board is often helpful. Another exercise is to engage the group in a discussion of the stages of change, drawing a wheel of change on the board and asking group participants where they feel they are in the wheel and what it would take to make them move. Finally, a change plan worksheet is often constructed in the group as a means of transitioning individuals into the more action-oriented groups when appropriate (i.e., when self-motivational statements indicate stage movement).

- *Tools for change.* Once individuals begin to espouse self-motivational statements and it becomes clear that they are moving into the preparation stage of change, the didactic cognitive-behavioral coping skills classes are offered. These 6-week classes target skill deficits that are associated with both mental and substance use disorders. For example, a dually diagnosed individual with a depressive disorder might be assigned to a cognitive restructuring class, an assertiveness class, and a problem-solving class.

- *Practicing change.* Often simultaneous with the Tools for Change classes, individuals in the action stage of change are encouraged to attend one or more of the Practicing Change groups. The facilitator in these groups assists clients in applying their newly honed skills to their own behaviors and life circumstances.

- *Maintaining change.* A 6-week relapse prevention curriculum based on Marlatt and Gordon's model is offered to individuals in the maintenance stage of change (defined as 30 days clean and sober within the past 90 days). Graduation from Tools for Change and some participation in the Practicing Change groups is a prerequisite for this group as well.

---

decrease drinking as coping strategy in social situations) at the onset of treatment as well as from input from clients or team members and are incorporated into a psychosocial treatment plan. Treatment goals include specific behavior changes (e.g., abstain from crack cocaine for 90% of next 90 days). Treatment involvement (e.g., number of groups to attend per week) is negotiated with the client. In an effort to abstain from crack cocaine, a patient may attend group daily toward achieving that goal. The group program is structured so that patients may join in action stage or maintenance groups at any time as they cycle through their readiness for change in specific behaviors. Box 24.4 describes the stage-specific groups to which individuals are assigned. Clients who drink and/or use multiple drugs can be in different stages of readiness for drinking and other drugs and/or other problem behaviors (e.g., social skills deficits). Consequently, they may simultaneously attend the drop-in groups for alcohol while attending skills training modules for other substances or problems. For example, a client may perceive his crack cocaine use as more destructive as it has been associated with arrests and involuntary hospitalizations but continues to drink excessively on occasion and has ambivalence about changing his drinking because it is a big part of his social interactions. Another example is a client who believes that his anxiety is related to social skills deficits and is motivated to engage in skills training for social skills but has no plan for his substance use reduction. However, the learning and practicing of assertiveness may generalize to the practice of refusing substances, or the increased self-efficacy in social contexts may lessen cravings/urges for alcohol and drugs.

The advantages of this approach include flexibility and a long-term perspective—clients can participate in multiple groups simultaneously—and recognizes the cyclic nature of change and overlap among stages. The major disadvantage is that this treatment model has not been studied. The separate components of motivational interventions, motivational interviewing as a counseling style, and skills training were developed from empirically based methods, but the efficacy of these approaches for dual disorders has not yet been determined.

SUMMARY AND CONCLUSIONS

Recent research in motivational interviewing suggests that this is an effective approach for engaging and retaining clients who have comorbid mental and substance use disorders in treatment. This is important as dually disordered clients who engage in and remain in treatment over extended periods show significant improvements in both psychiatric and substance use problems (Drake et al., 1998).

Motivational interviewing strategies adapted to explore ambivalence about attending an initial inpatient session have doubled the rates of adherence with an initial outpatient session. Also, modifications of the "check-up" intervention to explore the relationship between substance use and emotional disorders in one preliminary study yielded significantly fewer drinking days among schizophrenic clients already engaged in treatment. Thus, motivational interviewing shows potential for increasing adherence to treatment and behavior change when integrated into mental health or other treatment services.

Future research is needed to elucidate the benefits of motivational interviewing in a group format, which is the typical mechanism of providing therapeutic interventions in most mental health treatment settings. Empirical support for the impact of motivational interviewing with dually disordered treatment samples is modest. The available research is limited by small study samples and lack of control groups. Larger, more comprehensive, and controlled studies will determine the benefits of motivational interviewing as part of integrated treatment for dual disorders.

CHAPTER 25

Perils and Possibilities of Group-Based Motivational Interviewing

SCOTT T. WALTERS, RICHARD OGLE, *and* JOHN E. MARTIN

Is group motivational interviewing a half-baked or fully baked idea? We are now at a point in the investigation and application of individual motivational interviewing at which a fork in the road has been reached. Is this something that can—or should—be done in a group? The question has significant implications: Group treatment is less expensive and can serve more patients with fewer providers than can individual treatment. The presence of the group also provides participants with additional opportunities for role playing and social support. For these reasons, there has been a push to adapt efficacious individual approaches—motivational interviewing not excepting—to a group format, despite many unresolved issues. For instance, the resistance we might try to "roll with" in individual motivational interviewing might be both amplified and complicated in the presence of others, whereas other factors we hope to promote, such as discrepancy, may be minimized.

This chapter addresses the perils and possibilities of a group-based motivational interviewing (GMI) through four sections. We begin with a review and analysis of the early empirical findings of group-based motivational applications. This review is followed by a discussion of evidence that one might be able to conduct motivational interviewing in the context of a group with minimal loss of fidelity. We then turn to the process itself, including a detailed discussion of how GMI might be implemented to work in different populations and contexts, as well as the questions that inevitably arise when structuring the motivational group. We conclude by providing recommendations and critical suggestions for future research and clinical applications.

THE CASE FOR GROUP MOTIVATIONAL INTERVIEWING

College Student Drinking

Among heavy-drinking college students, we are aware of three studies using GMI, with results that have proved puzzling. All three were structured as a single-session intervention with personalized feedback. In the first study, Walters, Bennett, and Miller (2000) recruited heavy-drinking college students in an effort to determine the incremental effectiveness of adding a mailed feedback component to a 2-hour psychoeducational group delivered in a motivational style. Elements of the group included norm comparisons, a discussion of pros and cons of use, and role playing, whereas the feedback included quantity/frequency information, norm comparisons, and risk indicators and offered nonjudgmental advice on risk reduction. At a 6-week follow-up, participants who received only the mailed feedback reported the largest decrease, an average quantity reduction of 53.1%, as compared to those in the control group who remained nearly unchanged. Those who attended the group and also received feedback showed a lesser decrease of 23.2%. Although the group treatment in this trial was primarily psychoeducational in content, the findings are intriguing in that they suggest a possible deleterious effect of attending the group prior to receiving the mailed information. The success of the mailed feedback led to a second study (Walters, 2000), where identical feedback was given to participants in a group or via mail. The group was delivered in a similar way to the single-session Drinker's Check-up (Miller, Sovereign, & Krege, 1988). As in the previous study, participants in the mailed feedback condition again showed the largest quantity decrease (33.3%) at a 6-week follow-up, compared to those in the group feedback (decrease of 1.8%) and control conditions (decrease of 10.6%). Finally, in a third study (Martin, Noto, & Walters, 2000), students in six residential houses (i.e., fraternities and sororities) were randomized by house to receive feedback in a group or via mail or to a control condition. Consistent with previous findings, the GMI was not associated with reductions in drinking outcomes (increase of 12.3%) as compared to control (increase of 4.1%). Although there was a small reduction in the feedback-only group (decrease of 4.9%), this trend did not reach significance.

In sum, the available studies provide little evidence for the efficacy of GMI among heavy-drinking college students. On the contrary, they seem to provide much better overall support for the use of mailed feedback in this population. In the first study, although the group-plus-feedback condition showed some reduction over control, the superiority of the feedback-only condition suggests the feedback to be the more salient component. Also supporting this view are the findings of the second study, where group and mailed feedback were directly compared. Finally, in the last study, the "mailed" feedback was, in fact, distributed to individuals after a group meeting, unlike in previous studies where feedback was mailed to participants at their separate residences. Using this method of distribution meant that most recipients immediately opened their feedback and shared it with other members of the group, which may have minimized the discrepancy of the feedback.

Adult Outpatients

Among adults receiving outpatient treatment for alcohol dependence, we found four studies that used GMI. Studies varied from a single session to a 6-week group, and GMI was offered in each as a prelude to more extensive treatment. In the first study, Foote and colleagues (1999) report process effects of a four-session GMI versus treatment as usual when delivered prior to outpatient treatment. At follow-up, the authors found that GMI participants perceived more support for autonomy, and these feelings seemed to be positively related to treatment attendance. In addition, group participants seemed to be more realistically assessing the costs and benefits of quitting, though no behavioral outcome data were reported for this study. In a similar vein, Noonan (1995b) compared the effectiveness of a single-session GMI with feedback to an equivalent educational group for a group of outpatient, alcohol-dependent male veterans. The GMI was structured using elements of the Drinkers' Check-up (Miller et al., 1988) and consisted of an exploration of reasons for drinking, pros and cons of use, and a discussion of each participant's reactions to items in the feedback. Both groups showed significant reductions in drinking at 3 and 6 months with no consistent differences between them. After a 6-month period, the number of drinking days for those in the GMI had decreased 77% from baseline levels, whereas those in the educational group showed a mean decrease of 84.7%. The third study (Lincourt, Kuettel, & Bombardier, in press), targeting substance abusers mandated to attend, used a six-session GMI prior to standard treatment. Sessions were designed following procedures similar to the motivational enhancement therapy developed for Project MATCH (Miller, Zweben, DiClemente, & Rychtarik, 1992) and included an introduction to the transtheoretical model of change (Prochaska, DiClemente, & Norcross, 1992), a decisional balance exercise, personalized drinking feedback, and a discussion of past change success stories. Although not randomly assigned, those who attended the GMI had higher rates of attendance and treatment completion. After equalizing the two groups on baseline variables, the GMI group assignment still accounted for a small but significant proportion of the variance in treatment completion (3.5%) and percent of sessions attended (2.3%). Finally, Sobell, Sobell,

Brown, Cleland, and Buchan (1995) compared a four-session motivationally based cognitive-behavioral intervention to a similar individually administered intervention for alcohol and drug abusers. At 12 months posttreatment, significant reductions were found in alcohol and drug use measures, with no differences between the treatment groups in outcome or attrition. As one indicator, mean percent days abstinent for the group condition increased by 81%, while those in the individual condition increased by 93.6%. Those in the GMI missed significantly less sessions (25 vs. 210 missed session), but there were no differences between the formats in terms of overall satisfaction with the program,

In sum, these studies with outpatients provide some slim evidence for the utility and efficacy of GMI. In the two studies that measured changes in motivation and treatment compliance, GMI seemed to produce some changes. One study that measured changes in consumption did not find an effect relative to an educational control, but another found it to be as good as individually delivered care. In the final study, the relative efficacy of the group format led to a 41% cost savings in terms of therapist time. The cost savings of this format, coupled with the fact that group members missed fewer sessions, offer the best support for the efficacy of GMI.

Other Health Behaviors

Besides addictions treatment, GMI has been attempted in three health intervention studies. First, Carey, Kalichman, Forsyth, Wright, and Johnson (1997) employed a four-session behavioral-skills training (BST) program combined with motivational enhancement strategies to reduce the risk of HIV infection. Motivational techniques included personalized feedback on HIV risk, eliciting members' concerns about their behavior, a decisional balance exercise, and an action plan. At a 3-month follow-up, participants had increased both their knowledge and intention to practice safe behaviors as compared to those from a control group. A mean increase in partner communication, observed immediately after the intervention, had disappeared by this time. Although this intervention showed some meaningful effects, because of the combination of the two approaches, it is impossible to determine the incremental effectiveness of the motivational versus BST components. In a later study, Carey and colleagues (2000) included a health promotion control group and found essentially the same effect, where BST/GMI tended to increase knowledge and strengthen risk-reduction intentions, most of which were maintained at follow-up. Finally, Murphy, Cameron, Sharp, and colleagues (2000) collected data from inpatient veterans with posttraumatic stress disorder (PTSD) on whether they felt a particular symptom was one they "might have," "definitely have," or "definitely don't have." The intervention was a six-session, open group that explored such topics as "rationale for the group," "comparison to the average guy," "pros and cons," and "roadblocks." Results from a postintervention follow-up showed that 40% of the behaviors classified as "might have" prior to the group were now classified into one of the other two categories and more behaviors were now classified as "definitely have" than "definitely don't have," suggesting that the GMI may have facilitated disclosure of traumatic events.

When considering these other areas of health promotion, GMI seems to have been somewhat more efficacious, leading to decreases in risky behavior and resolution of ambivalence, at least in the short term. The findings related to HIV risk are intriguing in that they seem to provide an alternative to a problem typically addressed through psychoeducational channels. In terms of the PTSD study, the value of GMI appears less clear. During a group discussion of an issue, members' opinions tend to polarize (Brauer, Judd, & Gliner, 1995), and because the authors did not include a control group, we again cannot determine what part the motivational aspect played in this. In addition, because this study included only self-perceptions of psychiatric symptoms, it is difficult to say whether an increased belief that one does (or does not) meet diagnostic criteria is an advantage. For all these studies, it must be noted that the lack of process accounts and fidelity checks are major limitations. Moreover, the format and activities outlined in the GMI manuals available to us appear to be essentially transplanted from those of individual motivational interviewing, and because this "easy translation" has not reliably demonstrated results on par with those of individual motivational interviewing (Sobell et al., 1995, being the exception), we must consider the more difficult task of creating a GMI that is *fundamentally* group based.

POSSIBILITIES

In adapting motivational interviewing to work in a group, it is important to consider why and how motivational interviewing works at all. In the first edition of this book, Miller and Rollnick (1991) speculate on the possibility of therapist variables, change talk, and faith/hope concepts as mechanisms underlying the dramatic shifts in behavior often seen following motivational interviewing. But whatever the true mechanisms, the notion that this process would work equally well in the presence of others may be reminiscent of a knowledge dissemination model. However, unlike patient education, motivational interviewing is more a navigation process than a transmission of information: Behavior change happens when the individual weighs relevant reasons in relation to the short-term rewards of the behavior. Because of the complexity of interactions in a group, there is more potential for discrepancy diffusion, nonparticipation, resistance, and collective argumentation. Moreover, the limited talk time allotted by the group would seem to be a problem if Amrhein, Miller, Yahne, Palmer, and Fulcher (2000) are correct in their hypothesis that behavior change is initiated by increasingly strong change statements elicited during the therapy session.

These caveats not withstanding, there are also some reasons to believe that motivational interviewing might be particularly suited for groups of individuals. First, the interpersonal pressure of the majority might have a pull on those less interested in change and draw the less ready toward a mutual public commitment, especially under the guidance of a skillful GMI facilitator. The presence of the group in other contexts provides a powerful support system which assures the individual that he or she is not isolated in the desire for action. In addition, because of group diffusion there is added reason to think that individual resistance might be minimized. Unlike the intensive, one-on-one encounter in individual therapy, the group "automatically" wins any debate by virtue of its superior numbers. And if vocal group members hold the status quo and argue against change, this might actually promote the opposite reaction in others by highlighting a discrepancy between the negativity of the outspoken member(s) and the empathy and motivational style of the facilitator.

PROCESS

There have been several attempts to translate the activities used with individual motivational interviewing into the group setting. In the most comprehensive effort of which we are aware, Ingersoll, Wagner, and Gharib (2000) outline a 10-session GMI that uses activities borrowed from the procedures of individual motivational interviewing. Similarly, Foote and colleagues (1999) discuss a four-session group based on the FRAMES approach that consists of a discussion of problems, decision-making exercises, identification of roadblocks, and strategies for change. There are also several unpublished manuscripts (e.g., Apodaca & Martin, 1996; Noonan, 1995a; Walters, 1998) outlining groups that are essentially variations on the individual approach. But before applying these main processes, much less the spirit of motivational interviewing, one is faced with at least seven considerations in determining what format the group will take.

1. *Will the group be an adjunct to treatment or a stand-alone intervention?* As an individual intervention, motivational interviewing has been used both as an adjunct to treatment and a stand-alone intervention (Noonan & Moyers 1997). As a prelude or booster to more extensive treatment, it has typically consisted of one or two sessions. As a stand-alone treatment, the number of sessions has varied and becomes a programmatic choice due to the lack of evidence for differential efficacy based on number of sessions.

2. *Will the group be psychoeducational or process in nature?* In a psychoeducational group such as that described by Walters, Gruenewald, Bennett, and Miller (2001), the focus is didactic, though elements of the motivational process are considered. This type of group has a focal topic and is facilitated by a counselor who takes an expert role. What sets this format apart from purely didactic education is that group process, discussion, and role-play

are integral elements. In contrast, process groups (Yalom, 1995) primarily rely on the interactions of the group to guide members toward a "corrective emotional experience." Motivational interviewing in this format involves the exploration of ambivalence, elucidation of value discrepancies, and the exploration of options. The counselor selectively reflects, questions, and summarizes group content so that individual motivation is enhanced.

3. *Will the group have a fixed length or will it be ongoing?* Time-limited groups with a specific content have ranged from a single session to 10 or more sessions and are typically used when the group is expected to change little during the course of treatment. In contrast, an ongoing group may be more appropriate when the membership of a group is expected to change daily (e.g., a waiting-list intervention), where client turnover is high, or as an addition to an ongoing multimodal program. An ongoing format has no particular number of sessions and may not even have a specific agenda but is used to support change efforts on a continuing basis (see Chapter 24).

4. *Will groups be open or closed to new members?* A closed group begins with a cohort of clients and continues without the addition of new ones. The regularity of membership in closed groups tends to promote trust as the team works on change together. An open format such as that outlined by Murphy, Cameron, Rosen, and Thompson (2000), on the other hand, uses a rotating curriculum that allows individuals to join at any time in the group process and still participate in all sessions.

5. *Will the intervention provide feedback or not?* As we have previously indicated, few individual treatment studies (and no group studies) have examined the differential effectiveness of motivational interviewing with and without feedback, so the basis for a decision at this point would seem to involve the assessment time available and character of the group. If giving feedback, one must further decide whether the feedback will be given to the group as a whole, to one individual at a time, at some separate time (e.g., mailed before or after group attendance), or in some combination at multiple time points.

6. *Will the group be mixed or homogeneous in terms of readiness to change?* "Stacked" groups, selected on the basis of their readiness to change, can be used advantageously to encourage less ready members and solidify those who are more ready. For instance, the narratives of individuals at more advanced stages might help those less motivated to build discrepancy and resolve ambivalence. Groups that are relatively equal in their advanced stages of readiness can also create a sense of efficacy and mutual support. In contrast, groups equalized at less advanced stages might pose a particular difficulty through the strengthening of a deviant norm.

7. *Will it be a motivational group or will it be group motivational interviewing?* A final complication is that many of what have been called "motivational" groups in the literature may actually be more psychoeducational in approach. As such they attempt to correct deficient knowledge in a fashion other than that prescribed by classic motivational interviewing. Many of the aforementioned studies appear to have used methods closer to motivational

groups rather than a truly adapted motivational interviewing. In its "pure form" GMI is more a process of following the concerns of the group and reflecting points of individual and group discrepancy to enhance motivation.

PERILS

Although the process of individual motivational interviewing is well established, the dynamics of a group seem to suggest additional considerations. The process expands from a dance involving two people to look more like a dance production held by a company. Can you imagine a dance production consisting of multiple individuals doing different dances to different tunes? (In recalling one early group, one of us lamented, "This is like herding cats to the tune of a junior high orchestra, without a conductor!") What was once the joining of therapist–patient is now the simultaneous joining of therapist–patient, therapist–group, patient–patient, and patient–group. Thus, in the same spirit that prompted Miller and Rollnick (1991) to discuss the spirit and traps of individual motivational interviewing, we suggest the following as complications and modifications in adapting motivational interviewing and its core component processes to the group context.

Express Empathy

The "nest" for effective discrepancy building seems to be expressed empathy, but there are numerous difficulties with conveying this attitude in a group. Not only is the number of necessary interactions multiplied, but one must also consider that in the presence of others, there is a greater potential to defend oneself against real or imagined criticism (Diwan & Littrell, 1996). Affect is amplified in this context: Individuals may state opinions more strongly or introduce issues purely for the sake of bravado. As with individual motivational interviewing, the counselor partially addresses this issue through differential attention, reflection, and summary statements. We have found in our GMI experience that with two counselors, one can be expressing empathy while the second monitors and rolls with resistance. There may also be a tendency for the empathic flavor of the group to become diluted by other members who play therapist by proxy—for example, give advice and confront and label other members' behavior. Most Alcoholics Anonymous groups, for instance, have rules against such "cross-talk," allowing participants to only talk about themselves. The counselor can explain the different types of cross-talk that are appropriate and inappropriate in the group, and this should further increase the level of change talk in the group. If an inappropriate comment is made, the counselor can reframe to indicate that comments from the group are appreciated and often helpful, but ultimately it will be up the individual to decide what to do. Thus, the corrections and reframes of the counselor, coupled with the positive comments given by group members, might potentially outweigh the predicted loss of empathic fidelity to each individual.

Enhance Discrepancies

People consider change when they become uncomfortable with the status quo, whether privately or (presumably) in a group. Given more than one facilitator, the group might be broken into smaller working groups with co-facilitators present. These smaller, more personal groups might be especially useful when dealing with high-risk or coerced populations, where deviancy may be the norm. In settings such as this, a mix of deviant and prosocial members would seem to be the most desirable approach. Alternatively, one or two "veteran" peers might be included in each group to dispel deviant talk by virtue of their experience (e.g., the use of recovering smokers as facilitators in treatment groups; cf. Martin et al., 1997).

To further highlight individual discrepancies in a group format, we have sometimes used a values card-sort activity. In one variation, each client is given an assortment of cards, each of which contains a potentially important life value. Clients are asked to select the 10 values that are most important to them, prioritize these "top 10" from most to least important, and elaborate on their relevance in their lives (Miller & C'de Baca, 2001). One advantage of prefacing a change discussion with an activity like this is that it personalizes a relatively generic discussion to the more specific needs of the individual and encourages honesty. As an adjunct, we sometimes ask members to sort their cards into three piles based on how each value relates to the problem behavior (i.e., my problem behavior helps me to get, has no relation to, or hinders me from getting this value), producing a sort of decisional continuum. With groups that have some initial motivation, this activity works well as a prelude to a decisional balance discussion. On the other hand, we have also found that with groups initially low on motivation, this may actually solidify commitment to a problematic behavior. (In one group that ended with this exercise, the overwhelming rate of pro-alcohol commentary left us with the impression that group members would be reconvening at a local bar that evening!)

Finally, most formats of motivational interviewing have used normative feedback as one mechanism for building discrepancy. Although the evidence is strong that feedback can be an effective component for individuals, for groups the evidence is limited at best. Indeed, in our work with high-risk college drinkers, there is a constant attempt to "abduct" the norm and replace it with one that is more comfortable. For instance, when general population norms were presented to our high-risk drinkers, there was a tendency to devalue the discrepant norm as irrelevant. This makes sense when one considers that the greater the perceived difference between them, the more one group (e.g., the treatment group) will tend to devalue another (e.g., the normative group to which the treatment group is being compared). To avoid this situation, the counselor must not only highlight the difference between the two groups but also their many similarities in terms of goals and other relevant norms. It might also be more effective to have members privately estimate norms (e.g., "What percent of U.S. college students drink more than you?") before providing the correct figures, which highlights a true discrepancy between belief and fact, rather than presenting information initially (e.g., "You are at the 99th percentile of college students).

Avoid Argument and Confrontation

In our experience, therapy with one resistant individual is infinitely easier than with a group of such persons, who seem to have an endless supply of resistant talk. In addition, the resistance of the strongest personalities in a group seem to have a disproportionate influence over the direction of other members. Dominant persons may discourage others from voicing their opinions through their overt behavior and comments, by stating their positions with confidence, or simply by monopolizing group time (Diwan & Littrell, 1996). In our own groups, these argumentative, highly resistant persons have not only confounded the motivational process but also supported a deviant "renorming" effect. In discouraging such disruptions, the ground rules of the group should be explicit in prohibiting hostile or dominating speech, and group members can be gently reminded of this rule. The counselor can also reframe negative comments in a friendlier, more cooperative style, affirming the objector with a "twist." Quieter members or those who are more experienced can be asked for their reactions, to permit an alternate viewpoint. The most relevant comments are, in turn, selectively emphasized in a group summary reflection. In dealing with continued dominance, group leaders can use standard motivational techniques to handle resistance: empathic reflection, asking for elaboration on statements that are consistent with the direction of the group, and validating personal choice and responsibility. Strategic use of the simple time out (e.g., ignoring argumentative comments) or differential reinforcement (e.g., attending to positive, nonargumentative, or change talk) may also be useful in modeling and maintaining a positive motivational style. Such selective reflection allows individuals to be reinforced and heard within the context of increasingly constructive comments.

One exception to the "do not argue" rule is the paradoxical debate exercise, where the client plays the role of arguing for change while the therapist argues against it. In our experience, this is an activity that works especially well for highly resistant groups or those low on motivation for change. For example, as a variation on the "Good Things, Not-So-Good-Things" activity (Miller et al., 1992), we have asked group members to brainstorm a list of reasons for not making a change (i.e., all the good things about the present behavior). One facilitator uses the group's list to argue *against* change and invites the rest of the group to take the counterargument (i.e., why change would be a good thing). During this debate, a second facilitator can be recording the group's reasons, reinforcing comments and encouraging group members to argue their point even more forcefully. In this way, the natural antagonism of resistant groups is channeled into talk for change. When the debate is over, the first facilitator uses the list the group has generated to summarize the main points of the argument for change and asks specific members to elaborate on their expressed reasons. Change talk is thereby reinforced in the group's own words.

Encourage Self-Efficacy and Change Talk

In the "Ready, Willing and Able" triumvirate suggested by Rollnick (1998), no amount of readiness and willingness will make up for perceived inability. Individuals are encouraged to talk about the steps they plan to take. However, members of a group are more prone to "social loafing"—assuming that others will comment for them, or that the leader will provide answers for them. To prime participants to begin to talk about change, we sometimes begin with a "forced choice" exercise where group members must strongly agree, agree, disagree, or strongly disagree with a series of position statements related to the behavior of interest (e.g., "It's OK for people to smoke, as long as its not every day). An activity such as this sets the stage for self-disclosure in a nonjudgmental atmosphere and allows facilitators to identify the relative interest in change of various participants. Statements for this activity should be picked to suit the unique aims of the group but should be ones that will not further solidify positions contrary to those of the group. For instance, a forced choice, such as "Marijuana should be legalized," may have the unintended consequence for those who endorse it of solidifying a view the therapist would rather discourage. Better, forced questions such as "Which of these posted drugs is the most addictive to the user/dangerous to society?" allows participants to voice an opinion within appropriate boundaries. In this case, participants can also hear their peers voice opinions against the use of a drug they themselves did not endorse.

We have discussed some reasons why confidence and importance might be supported in a group format. On the other hand, an inherent roadblock, no matter what the structure, would seem to be the limited "talk time" of members. We know from Amrhein and colleagues (2000) that an increasing amount of talk about change during the session is a predictor of outcome. In a group, however, it is unclear to what extent these rules apply: Can change talk be done "by proxy" where some individuals listen to *others* talk about their increased motivation? If so, groups could be asked to consider the implications of another's session for their own individual process. For instance, in a group, certain individuals tend to cluster at the center of the social structure, indicating their centrality to the decision-making process. When such a leader is identified, the "proxy" motivational interviewing session can be conducted with this individual and either presented via videotape or in a "fishbowl" where the rest of the group watches the session as it is conducted. This might be used to prime participants before giving feedback, such that they first see an admired person struggling with personal discrepancy and modeling appropriate talk.

A final caveat relates to a group's tendency to "follow" and then resist the leader. In classic motivational interviewing, we are cautioned to avoid the expert trap. Yet, in a group setting, resistance may focus on knocking the leader off his or her pedestal. Although many group members expect the facilitator to tell them what to do, we suggest that the facilitator avoid giving unsolicited advice, especially early in the session. Rather, demands for answers should be used as opportunities for group comment and reflection, so that solutions emerge from group members rather than the therapist (see also the "expert trap" in Chapter 6).

FURTHER POSSIBILITIES

What should our future directions be, providing that GMI is an approach that holds significant, albeit unrealized, potential? The following represent some clinical and research suggestions to help answer two questions: (1) Does group-based motivational interviewing work, and for whom? (2) Under what conditions might it work best?

Does GMI Work and for Whom?

As we have previously discussed, little is known about how motivational interviewing works within a group setting. There is significant room and need at this early stage for even uncontrolled studies integrating motivational interviewing with group processes and demonstrating changes in cognitive readiness and behavior. Controlled investigations will also be required, where a complete GMI might be compared to other approaches or a nontreated control. As indicated earlier, this also might be represented by an add-on to an existing intervention, including individual motivational interviewing. Imagine a GMI that meets daily, much as a process group, as part of an inpatient, partial hospitalization, or outpatient format. For this "preferred" GMI evaluation, we would suggest using two group leaders, a group of no more than 10 to 12 participants, and screening for a group that is not overloaded with precontemplators. (We certainly learned a hard lesson in one of our college studies where we did the opposite of each of these suggestions, with pitiful results.) From this point, there are a number of group applications (e.g., Ingersoll et al., 2000), which provide additional structure for a multisession group and a good start toward a manualized "standard" for GMI research comparisons.

Studies are also needed to determine the populations that might most benefit from such an approach. Although the efficacy of individual motivational interviewing is well established in the addictions field, there is some evidence for its appropriateness in other behavior change areas as well (cf. Chapter 16). Conversely, when considering group applications, we have only scant evidence of empirical efficacy outside alcohol treatment and wide room for applications to other populations and settings such as smoking, diet, exercise, and medication compliance.

How Can GMI be Implemented to Work Best?

Once these questions have been addressed, we might turn our attention to the many possible interactive effects. Process variables to be experimentally manipulated include factors such as optimal group size, motivational (stage of change) profile, number of leader-facilitators, whether and how feedback might be used, structured versus unstructured groups, and the use of live or videotaped peer leader interview. When approaching the question of group size, depending on the context and problem area, we suggest a general guideline akin to that used in motivational interviewing training (Miller & Rollnick, 1991) of no more than 20 participants per facilitator, although half that number might be more appropriate based on the nature, severity, and chronicity of the problem area (e.g., morbid obesity and chronic smoking). But still the overriding question seems to be, What is the process and leadership structure that will most facilitate verbal participation (i.e., personal change talk) within the group setting? A solution, only partly facetious, has been made to develop a kind of motivational interviewing "language lab" analogue where individuals are simultaneously prompted but individually responded to via personal earphones in separate cubicles. In this process, the role of motivational feedback presented in a group also deserves consideration. Although this technique has good empirical support when used as an adjunct to individual motivational interviewing, when added to a group there appear to be additional complicating factors.

In terms of readiness for change profile, our difficulties with college drinkers led us to believe that the groups might have been more effective if we had selected participants based on stage of change—contemplators and above. For those low on the readiness-for-change scale, the personalized feedback alone might have been sufficient. We also suspect that having group members quietly view an individual motivational interviewing session would have better engaged precontemplators.

Finally, when further matching individuals to treatment approaches, we would suggest a consideration of the stepwise approaches used for some medical and psychological conditions (e.g., antihypertensive medications). Given limited resources, a stepped intensity program might begin with the most cost-effective approach, a general screening measure (e.g., the AUDIT; Claussen, & Aasland, 1993) and motivational feedback material, delivered either via mail (Agostinelli, Brown, & Miller, 1995) or computer (R. K. Hester, personal communication, January 15, 2001). The second step for individuals not effectively "reached" by this approach might include one of the group interventions discussed here. Those who continue to exhibit problematic behavior might be referred to the more costly (but also more effective) individual motivational counseling session and/or a small support group meeting.

THE FORK TO GROUP MOTIVATIONAL INTERVIEWING

In our venture down this basically uncharted path, the transfer of motivational interviewing into a group format seems anything but straightforward. Group-based approaches have been implemented by people quite experienced with individual approaches and thus far have yielded disappointing results. Furthermore, there is the possibility that individual motivational interviewing (e.g., via a single session) may actually prove to be more cost-effective than group applications in the long run (e.g., multiple sessions with multiple therapists). Yet, as we have discussed, there are also many reasons why GMI is being and should be attempted. A number of ideas have thus been outlined to suggest how motivational interviewing might be adapted to a more general group intervention, including caveats and traps to avoid. Finally, we have proposed directions for future research and applications of GMI while including specific study questions and designs. For those brave (or perhaps foolish) enough to take up these challenges, there are many future paths, as well as dead ends, to be explored in what will surely become one of the next directions that motivational interviewing will take.

References

Adlaf, E. M., Zdanowicz, Y. M., & Smart, R. G. (1996). Alcohol and other drug use among street-involved youth in Toronto. *Addiction Research, 4*(1), 11–24.

Agostinelli, G., Brown, J. M., & Miller, W. R. (1995). Effects of normative feedback on consumption among heavy drinking college students. *Journal of Drug Education, 25*(1), 31–40.

Allsop, S., & Saunders, B. (1991). Reinforcing robust resolutions: Motivation in relapse prevention with severely dependent problem drinkers. In W. R. Miller & S. Rollnick, *Motivational interviewing: Preparing people to change addictive behavior* (pp. 236–247). New York: Guilford Press.

American Psychiatric Association. (1987). *Diagnostic and statistical manual of mental disorders* (3rd ed., rev.). Washington, DC: Author.

American Psychiatric Association. (1994). *Diagnostic and statistical manual of mental disorders* (4th ed.). Washington, DC: Author.

Amrhein, P. C. (1992). The comprehension of quasi-performative verbs in verbal commitments: New evidence for componential theories of lexical meaning. *Journal of Memory and Language, 31,* 756–784.

Amrhein, P. C., Miller, W. R., Yahne, C. E., Palmer, M., & Fulcher, L. (2000, September). *Committing language emergent from a motivational interview predicts behavioral change in drug-addicted clients.* Paper presented at the international conference on Treatment of Addictive Behaviors, Cape Town, South Africa.

Amrod, J. (1997). The effect of motivational enhancement therapy and coping skills training on the self-efficacy and motivation of incarcerated male alcohol abusers. *Dissertation Abstracts International, 57*(9–B), 5904.

Andrews, D. A., Bonta, J., & Hoge, R. D. (1990). Classification for effective rehabilitation. Rediscovering psychology. *Criminal Justice and Behavior, 17*(1), 19–52.

Andrews, D. A., Zinger, I., Hoge, R. D., Bonta, J., Gendreau, P., & Cullen, F. T. (1990).

Does correctional treatment work? A clinically relevant and psychologically informed meta-analysis. *Criminology, 28*(3), 369–404.

Annis, H. M., & Chan, D. (1983). The differential treatment model. Empirical evidence from a personality typology of adult offenders. *Criminal Justice and Behavior, 10*(2), 159–173.

Annis, H. M., Graham, J. M., & Davis, C. S. (1987). *Inventory of Drinking Situations (IDS): User's guide.* Toronto: Addiction Research Foundation.

Apodaca, X., & Martin, J. E. (1996). *Alcohol information and motivation.* Unpublished manuscript.

Arnett, J. J. (2000). Emerging adulthood: A theory of development from the late teens through the twenties. *American Psychologist, 55*(5), 469–480.

Aubrey, L. L. (1998). *Motivational interviewing with adolescents presenting for outpatient substance abuse treatment.* Doctoral dissertation, University of New Mexico.

Avants, S. K., Singer, J. L., & Margolin, A. (1993–1994). Self-representations and negative affect in cocaine-dependent individuals. *Imagination, Cognition and Personality, 13*(1), 3–24.

Axelrod, S., & Wetzler, S. (1989). Factors associated with better compliance with psychiatric aftercare. *Hospital and Community Psychiatry, 40,* 397–401.

Azrin, N. H., Sisson, R. W., Meyers, R. J., & Godley, M. D. (1982). Alcoholism treatment by disulfiram and community reinforcement therapy. *Journal of Behavior Therapy and Experimental Psychiatry, 13*(2), 105–112.

Baekeland, F., & Lundwall, L. (1975). Dropping out of treatment: A clinical review. *Psychological Bulletin, 82,* 738–783.

Baer, J. S. (in press). Student factors: Understanding individual variation in college drinking. *Journal of Studies of Alcohol.*

Baer, J. S., Kivlahan, D. K., Blume, A. W., McKnight, P., & Marlatt, G. A. (2001). Brief intervention for heavy drinking college students: Four-year follow-up and natural history. *American Journal of Public Health, 91*(8), 1310–1316.

Baer, J. S., Kivlahan, D. R., & Donovan, D. M. (1999). Integrating skills training and motivational therapies: Implications for the treatment of substance dependence. *Journal of Substance Abuse Treatment, 17*(1–2), 15–23.

Baker, A., & Dixon, J. (1991). Motivational interviewing for HIV risk reduction. In W. R. Miller & S. Rollnick (Eds.), *Motivational interviewing: Preparing people to change addictive behavior* (pp. 293–302). New York: Guilford Press.

Baker, A., Heather, N., Wodak, A., Dixon, J., & Holt, P. (1993). Evaluation of a cognitive-behavioural intervention for HIV prevention among injecting drug users. *AIDS, 7,* 247–256.

Baker, A., Kochan, N., Dixon, J., Heather, N., & Wodak, A. (1994). Controlled evaluation of a brief intervention for HIV prevention among injecting drug users not in treatment. *AIDS Care, 6*(5), 559–570.

Bandura, A. (1986). *Social foundations of thought and action: A social cognitive theory.* Englewood Cliffs, NJ: Prentice Hall.

Bandura, A. (1988). Self-efficacy conception of anxiety. *Anxiety Research, 1*(2), 77–98.

Bandura, A. (1997). *Self-efficacy: The exercise of control.* New York: Freeman.

Barbaree, H. E. (1991). Denial and minimization among sex offenders: Assessment and treatment outcome. *Forum on Corrections Research, 3*(4), 30–33.

Barlow, D. H. (1988). *Anxiety and its disorders: The nature and treatment of anxiety and panic.* New York: Guilford Press.

Barnett, N. P., Monti, P. M., & Wood, M. D. (2001). Motivational interviewing for alcohol-involved adolescents in the emergency room. In E. F. Wagner & H. B. Waldron (Eds.), *Innovations in adolescent substance abuse* (pp. 143–168). New York: Pergamon Press.

Basch, C. E., Sliepcevich, E. M., Gold, R. S., Duncan, D., & Kolbe, L. (1985). Avoiding Type III errors in health education program evaluations: A case study. *Health Education Quarterly, 12*, 315–331.

Baucom, D. H., Shoham, V., Mueser, K. T., Daiuto, A. D., & Stickle, T. R. (1998). Empirically supported couple and family interventions for marital distress and adult mental health problems. *Journal of Consulting and Clinical Psychology, 66*(1), 53–88.

Baumrind, D., & Moselle, K. A. (1985). A developmental perspective on adolescent drug abuse. *Advances in Alcohol and Substance Abuse, 4*(3–4), 41–67.

Belcher, L., Kalichman, S., Topping, M., Smith, S., Emshoff, J., Norris, F., & Nurss, J. (1998). A randomized trial of a brief HIV risk reduction counseling intervention for women. *Journal of Consulting and Clinical Psychology, 66*, 856–861.

Bellack, A. S. (1992). Cognitive rehabilitation for schizophrenia: Is it possible? Is it necessary? *Schizophrenia Bulletin, 18*, 43–50.

Bellack, A. S., & DiClemente, C. C. (1999). Treating substance abuse among patients with schizophrenia. *Psychiatric Services, 50*, 75–80.

Bem, D. J. (1967). Self-perception: An alternative interpretation of cognitive dissonance phenomena. *Psychological Review, 74*, 183–200.

Bem, D. J. (1972). Self-perception theory. In L. Berkowitz (Ed.), *Advances in experimental social psychology* (Vol. 6, pp. 1–62). New York: Academic Press.

Bepko, C., & Krestan, J. (1985). *The responsibility trap: A blueprint for treating the alcoholic family.* New York: Free Press.

Berg-Smith, S. M., Stevens, V. J., Brown, K. M., Van Horn, L., Gernhofer, N., Peters, E., Greenberg, R., Snetselaar, L., Ahrens, L., & Smith, K. (1999). A brief motivational intervention to improve dietary adherence in adolescents. *Health Education Research, 14*(3), 399–410.

Bien, T. H., Miller, W. R., & Boroughs, J. M. (1993). Motivational interviewing with alcohol outpatients. *Behavioural and Cognitive Psychotherapy, 21*, 347–356.

Bien, T. H., Miller, W. R., & Tonigan, J. S. (1993). Brief interventions for alcohol problems: A review. *Addiction, 88*, 315–336.

Blackwell, B. (1976). Treatment adherence. *British Journal of Psychiatry, 129*, 513–531.

Blackwell, B. (1997). From compliance to alliance: A quarter century of research. In B. Blackwell (Ed.), *Treatment compliance and the therapeutic alliance* (pp. 1–15). Amsterdam: Harwood Academic.

Booth, R. E., Kwiatkowski, C., Iguchi, M. Y., Pinto, F., & John, D. (1998). Facilitating treatment entry among out-of-treatment injection drug users. *Public Health Reports, 113*(Suppl. 1), 116–128.

Borkovec, T. D., & Castonguay, L. G. (1998). What is the scientific meaning of empirically supported therapy? *Journal of Consulting and Clinical Psychology, 66*(1), 136–142.

Borkovec, T. D., & Whisman, M. A. (1996). Psychosocial treatment for generalized anxiety disorder. In M. R. Mavissakalian & R. F. Prien (Eds.), *Long-term treatments of anxiety disorders* (pp. 171–199). Washington, DC: American Psychiatric Press.

Borrelli, B., Hecht, J., Enright, K., Hooper, S., Emmons, K., & Abrams, D. (1998). *A new channel for behavioral health intervention: The Visiting Nurse Association.* Paper presented at the meeting of the Association for Advancement of Behavior Therapy, Washington, DC.

Borsari, B., & Carey, K. B. (2000). Effects of a brief motivational intervention with college student drinkers. *Journal of Consulting and Clinical Psychology, 68*(4), 728–733.

Botvin, G. J., Baker, E., Dusenbury, L., Tortu, S., & Botvin, E. (1990). Preventing adolescent drug abuse through a multimodal cognitive-behavioral approach: Results of a 3-year study. *Journal of Consulting and Clinical Psychology, 58*(4), 437–446.

Bradley, G. W. (1978). Self-serving biases in the attribution process: A re-examination of the fact or fiction question. *Journal of Personality and Social Psychology, 36*(1), 56–71.

Brauer, M., Judd, C. M., & Gliner, M. D. (1995). The effects of repeated expressions on attitude polarization during group discussions. *Journal of Personality and Social Psychology, 68*(6), 1014–1029

Brehm, S. S., & Brehm, J. W. (1981). *Psychological reactance: A theory of freedom and control.* New York: Academic Press.

Brown, D., & Crace, R. K. (1996). Values in life role choices and outcomes: A conceptual model. *Career Development Quarterly, 44,* 211–223.

Brown, H. P., & Peterson, J. H. (1990). Rationale and procedural suggestions for defining and actualizing spiritual values in the treatment of dependency. *Alcoholism Treatment Quarterly, 7,* 17–46.

Brown, J. H., & Horowitz, J. E. (1993). Deviance and deviants: Why adolescent substance use prevention programs do not work. *Evaluation Review, 17*(5), 529–555.

Brown, J. M.(1998). Self-regulation and the addictive behaviors. In W. R. Miller & N. Heather (Eds.), *Treating addictive behaviors* (2nd ed., pp. 61–73). New York: Plenum Press.

Brown, J. M., & Miller, W. R. (1993). Impact of motivational interviewing on participation and outcome in residential alcoholism treatment. *Psychology of Addictive Behaviors, 7,* 211–218.

Burke, B., Arkowitz, H., & Menchola, M. (2001). *The efficacy of motivational interviewing: A meta-analysis of controlled clinical trials.* Manuscript in preparation.

Butler, C. C., Pill, R., & Stott, N. C. (1998). Qualitative study of patients' perceptions of doctors' advice to quit smoking: implications for opportunistic health promotion. *British Medical Journal, 316,* 1878–1881.

Butler, C. C., Rollnick, S., Cohen, D., Russel, I., Bachmann, M., & Stott, N. (1999). Motivational consulting versus brief advice for smokers in general practice: A randomised trial. *British Journal of General Practice, 49,* 611–616.

Butler, C. C., Rollnick, S., Pill, R., Maggs-Rapport, F., & Stott, N. (1998). Understanding the culture of prescribing: qualitative study of general practitioners' and patients' perceptions of antibiotics for sore throats. *British Medical Journal, 317*(7159), 637–642.

Carbonari, J. P., & DiClemente, C. C. (2000). Using transtheoretical model profiles to differentiate levels of alcohol abstinence success. *Journal of Consulting and Clinical Psychology 68*(5), 810–817.

Carbonari, J. P., DiClemente, C. C., & Sewell, K. B. (1999). Stage transitions and the transtheoretical "stages of change" model of smoking cessation. *Swiss Journal of Psychology, 58*(2), 134–144.

Carey, K. B., Purnine, M. M., Maisto, S. A., & Carey, M. P. (1999). Assessing readiness to change substance abuse: A critical review of instruments. *Clinical Psychology: Science and Practice, 6,* 245–266.

Carey, M. P., Braaten, L. S., Maisto, S. A., Gleason, J. R., Forsyth, A. D., Durant, L. E., &

Jaworski, B. C. (2000). Using information, motivational enhancement, and skills training to reduce the risk of HIV infection for low-income urban women: A second randomized clinical trial. *Health Psychology, 19*(1), 3–11.

Carey, M. P., Kalichman, S. C., Forsyth, A. D., Wright, E. M., & Johnson, B. T. (1997). Enhancing motivation to reduce the risk of HIV infection for economically disadvantaged urban women. *Journal of Consulting and Clinical Psychology, 65*(4), 531–541.

Carey, M. P., Maisto, S. A., Kalichman, S. C., Forsyth, A. D., Wright, E. M., & Johnson, B. T. (1997). Enhancing motivation to reduce the risk of HIV infection for economically disadvantaged urban women. *Journal of Consulting and Clinical Psychology, 65*(4), 531–541.

Carkhuff, R. R. (1969). Helper communication as a function of helper affect and content. *Journal of Counseling Psychology, 16*(2, Pt. 1), 126–131.

Carkhuff, R. R., Anthony, W. A., Cannon, J. R., Pierce, R. M., & Zigon, F. J. (1979). *The skills of helping: An introduction to counseling skills.* Amherst, MA: Human Resource Development Press.

Carney, M. M., & Kivlahan, D. R. (1995). Motivational subtypes among veterans seeking substance abuse treatment: Profiles based on stages of change. *Psychology of Addictive Behaviors, 9*, 1135–1142.

Carr, V. C. (1985). Telephone prompting to reduce missed CMHC appointments. *Hospital and Community Psychiatry, 36*, 1217–1218.

Carroll, K. (1997). Compliance and alcohol treatment: An overview. In K. Carroll (Ed.), *Improving compliance with alcoholism treatment* (Project MATCH Monograph Series, 6, pp. 5–12, NIH: Publication No. 97–4143). Rockville, MD: National Institute on Alcohol Abuse and Alcoholism. National Institutes of Health.

Cashin, J. R., Presley, C. A., & Meilman, P. W. (1998). Alcohol use in the Greek system: Follow the leader? *Journal of Studies on Alcohol, 59*(1), 63–70.

Centers for Disease Control (2000). *CDC fact book 2000/2001.* Washington, DC: Department of Health and Human Services.

Chafetz, M. E. (1961). A procedure for establishing therapeutic contact with the alcoholic. *Quarterly Journal of Studies on Alcohol, 22*, 325–328.

Chafetz, M. E. (1968). Research in the alcohol clinic of an around-the-clock psychiatric service of the Massachusetts General Hospital. *American Journal of Psychiatry, 124*, 1674–1679.

Chafetz, M. E., Blane, H. T., Abram, H. S., Clark, E., Golner, J. H., Hastie, E. L., & McCourt, W. F. (1964). Establishing treatment relations with alcoholics: A supplementary report. *Journal of Nervous and Mental Disease, 138*, 390–393.

Chafetz, M. E., Blane, H. T., Abram, H. S., Golner, J. H., Hastie, E. L., & Meyers, W. (1962). Establishing treatment relations with alcoholics. *Journal of Nervous and Mental Disease, 134*, 395–409.

Chamberlain, P., Patterson, G., Reid, J., Kavanagh, K., & Forgatch, M. (1984). Observation of client resistance. *Behavior Therapy, 15*, 144–155.

Chen, A. (1991). Noncompliance in community psychiatry: A review of clinical interventions. *Hospital and Community Psychiatry, 42*, 282–287.

Chen, K., & Kandel, D. B. (1995). The natural history of drug use from adolescence to the mid-thirties in a general population sample. *American Journal of Public Health, 85*(1), 41–47.

Cherpitel, C. J. (1994). Injury and the role of alcohol: County-wide emergency room data. *Alcoholism: Clinical and Experimental Research, 18*(3), 679–684.

Christensen, A., & Shenk, J. L. (1991). Communication, conflict, and psychological distance in nondistressed, clinic, and divorcing couples. *Journal of Consulting and Clinical Psychology, 59,* 458–463.

Claussen, B., & Aasland, O. G. (1993). The Alcohol Use Disorders Identification Test (AUDIT) in a routine health examination of long-term unemployed. *Addiction, 88,* 363–368.

Cohen, S., Doyle, W., Skoner, D. P., Rabin, B. S., & Gwaltney, J. M. (1997). Social ties and susceptibility to the common cold. *Journal of the American Medical Association, 277,* 1940–1944.

Cohen, S., & Willis, T. A. (1985). Stress, social support, and the buffering hypothesis. *Psychological Bulletin, 98,* 310–357.

Colby, S. M., Monti, P. M., Barnett, N. P., Rohsenow, D. J., Weissman, K., Spirito, A., Woolard, R. H., & Lewander, W. J. (1998). Brief motivational interviewing in a hospital setting for adolescent smoking: A preliminary study. *Journal of Consulting and Clinical Psychology, 66*(3), 574–578.

Connors, G. J., Donovan, D. M., & DiClemente, C. C. (2001). *Substance abuse treatment and the stages of change: Selecting and planning interventions.* New York: Guilford Press.

Connors, G. J., Walitzer, K. S., & Derman, K. H. (2000, November). *Preparation for alcoholism treatment: Effects on treatment attendance and posttreatment drinking.* Paper presented at the annual meeting of the Society for Study of Alcohol and Other Drugs, Leeds, UK.

Conroy, W. J. (1979). Human values, smoking behavior, and public health programs. In M. Rokeach (Ed.), *Understanding human values.* New York: Macmillan.

Cooney, N. L., Zweben, A., & Fleming, M. F. (1995). Screening for alcohol problems and at risk-taking in health care settings. In R. K. Hester & W. R. Miller (Eds.), *Handbook of alcoholism treatment approaches: Effective alternatives* (2nd ed., pp. 45–60), New York: Allyn & Bacon.

Corrao, G., Bagnardi, V., Zambon, A., Arico, S., Dall'Aglio, C., Addolorato, G., Giorgi, I., & the ASSALT Group. (1999). Outcome variables in the evaluation of alcoholics' treatment: Lessons from the Italian Assessment of Alcoholism Treatment (ASSALT) project. *Alcohol and Alcoholism, 34,* 873–881.

Cramer, J., Mattson, R., Prevey, M., Scheyer, R., & Ouellette, U. (1989). How often is medication taken as prescribed? *Journal of the American Medical Association, 261*(22), 3273–3277.

Creer, T., & Levstek, D. (1997). Adherence to asthma regimes. In D. S. Gochman (Ed.), *Handbook of health behavior research II: Provider determinants* (Vol. 2, pp. 269–284). New York: Plenum Press.

Crits-Christoph, P., Siqueland L., Blaine, J., Frank, A., Luborsky, L., Onken, L. S., Muenz, L. R., Thase, M. E., Weiss, R. D., Gastfriend, G. R., Woody, G. E., Barber, J. P., Butler, S. F., Daley, D., Salloum, I., Bishop, S., Najavits, L. M., Lis, J., Mercer, D., Griffin, M. L., Moras, K., & Beck, A. T. (1999). Psychosocial treatments for cocaine dependence: National Institute on Dug Abuse collaborative cocaine treatment study. *Archives of General Psychiatry, 56,* 493–502.

CSAT Treatment Improvement Protocol No. 35. (1999). *Enhancing motivation for change in substance abuse treatment* (DHHS Publication No. (SMA) 99–3354). Washington, DC: U.S. Government Printing Office.

Daley, D. C., & Zuckoff, A. (1998). Improving compliance with the initial outpatient session among discharged inpatient dual diagnosis clients. *Social Work, 43*(5), 470–473.

Daley, D. C., & Zuckoff, A. (1999). *Improving treatment compliance: Counseling and systems strategies for substance abuse and dual disorders.* Center City, MN: Hazelden.

Daley, D. C., Salloum, I. M., Zuckoff, A., Kirisci, L., & Thase, M. E. (1998). Increasing treatment adherence among outpatients with depression and cocaine dependence: A pilot study. *American Journal of Psychiatry, 155,* 1611–1613.

Darley, J. M., & Batson, C. D. (1973). From Jerusalem to Jericho: A study of situational and dispositional variables in helping behavior. *Journal of Personality and Social Psychology, 27,* 100–119.

Darley, J. M., & Latane, B. (1968). Bystander intervention in emergencies: Diffusion of responsibility. *Journal of Personality and Social Psychology, 8,* 377–383.

De Francesco, C. (2001). Reflections on the values card sort. *Motivational Interviewing Newsletter: Updates, Education and Training* [Online]. Edition 8.2. Richmond, VA: Mid-Atlantic Addiction Technology Transfer Center/Center for Substance Abuse Treatment. Available: www.motivationalinterview.org

Deci, E. L., & Ryan, R. M. (1985). *Intrinsic motivation and self-determination in human behavior.* New York: Plenum Press.

Dempsey, R. (1996). Using motivational interviewing techniques in a prison setting and in the community with a partner. In R. E. Mann (Ed.), *Motivational interviewing with sex offenders: A practice manual* (pp. 30–35). Hull, UK: National Organisation for the Treatment of Abusers.

Dench, S., & Bennett, G. (2000). The impact of brief motivational intervention at the start of an outpatient day programme for alcohol dependence. *Behavioural and Cognitive Psychotherapy, 28,* 121–130.

Dennis, M. L. (2000). *The Cannabis Youth Treatment (CYT) experiment: Preliminary findings.* Washington, DC: Center for Substance Abuse Treatment, Substance Abuse and Mental Health Services Administration, Department of Health and Human Services.

Department of Health and Human Services. (2000). *10th special report to the United States Congress on alcohol and health: Highlights from current rearch.* Washington DC: National Institutes of Health.

deShazer, S., Berg, I. K., Lipchik, E., Nunnally, E., Molnar, A., Gingerich, W., & Weiner-Davis, M. (1986). Brief therapy: Focused solution development. *Family Process, 25,* 201–211.

DiClemente, C. C. (1994). If behaviors change, can personality be far behind. In T. Heatherton & J. Weinberger (Eds.), *Can personality change* (pp. 175–198). Washington, DC: American Psychological Association.

DiClemente, C. C. (1999a). Motivation for change: Implications for substance abuse. *Psychological Science, 10*(3), 209–213.

DiClemente, C. C. (1999b). Prevention and harm reduction for chemical dependency: A process perspective. *Clinical Psychology Review* [Special issue: prevention of children's behavioral and mental health problems: New horizons for psychology], *19*(4), 473–486.

DiClemente, C. C. (forthcoming). *Addiction and change: A transtheoretical analysis.* New York: Guilford Press.

DiClemente, C. C., Carbonari, J. P., & Velasquez, M. M. (1992). Alcoholism treatment mismatching from a process of change perspective. In R. R. Watson (Ed.), *Treatment of drug and alcohol abuse* (pp. 115–142). Totowa, NJ: Humana Press.

DiClemente, C. C., Carbonari, J., Zweben, A., Morrel, T., & Lee, R. E. (2001). Motivation hypothesis causal chain analysis. In R. Longabaugh & P. W. Wirtz (Eds.), *Project MATCH: A priori matching hypotheses, results, and mediating mechanisms* (National Institute on Alcohol Abuse and Alcoholism, Project MATCH Monograph Series, Vol. 8). Rockville, MD: National Institute on Alcohol Abuse and Alcoholism.

DiClemente, C. C., & Hughes, S. O. (1990). Stages of change profiles in outpatient alcoholism treatment. *Journal of Substance Abuse, 2,* 217–235.

DiClemente, C. C., Marinilli, A. S., Singh, M., & Bellino, L. E. (2001). The role of feedback in the process of health behavior change. *American Journal of Health Behavior, 25,* 217–227.

DiClemente, C. C., & Prochaska, J. O. (1985). Processes and stages of change: Coping and competence in smoking behavior change. In S. Shiffman & T. A. Wills (Eds.), *Coping and substance abuse* (pp. 319–342). New York: Academic Press.

DiClemente, C. C., & Prochaska, J. O. (1998). Toward a comprehensive, transtheoretical model of change: Stages of change and addictive behaviors. In W. R. Miller & N. Heather (Eds.), *Treating addictive behaviors* (2nd ed., pp. 3–24). New York: Plenum Press.

DiClemente, C. C., & Scott, C. W. (1997). Stages of change: Interaction with treatment compliance and involvement. In L. S. Onken, J. D. Blaine, & J. J. Boren (Eds.), *Beyond the therapeutic alliance: Keeping the drug-dependent individual in treatment* (pp. 131–156). Rockville, MD: National Institute on Drug Abuse.

DiClemente, C. C., Story, M., & Murray, K. (2000). On a roll: The process of initiation and cessation of problem gambling among adolescents, *Journal of Gambling Studies, 16*(2/3), 289–313.

DiIorio, C., Faherty, B., & Manteuffel, B. (1994). Epilepsy self-management: Partial replication and extension. *Research in Nursing and Health, 17,* 167–174.

Dimeff, L. A. (1998). Brief intervention for heavy and hazardous college drinkers in a student primary health care setting. *Dissertation Abstracts International: The Sciences and Engineering, 58*(12–B), 6805.

Dishion, T. J. (in press). *The family checkup: A brief family intervention for adolescent problem behavior.* New York: American Academy of Child and Adolescent Psychiatry.

Dishion, T. J., & Kavanaugh, K. (in press). *Adolescent problem behavior: An intervention and assessment sourcebook.* New York: Guilford Press.

Diwan, S., & Littrell, J. (1996). Impact of small group dynamics on focus group data: Implications for social work research. *Journal of Applied Social Sciences, 20*(2), 95–106.

Dobscha, S. K., Delucchi, K., & Young, M. L. (1999). Adherence with referrals for outpatient follow-up from a VA psychiatric emergency room. *Community Mental Health Journal, 35,* 451–458.

Doherty, Y., Hall, D., James, P., Roberts, S., & Simpson, J. (2000). Change counselling in diabetes: The development of a training programme for the diabetes team. *Patient Education and Counseling, 40,* 263–278.

Donovan, D. M., Rosengren, D. B., Downey, L., Cox, G. B., & Sloan, K. L. (2001). Attrition prevention with individuals awaiting publicly funded drug treatment. *Addiction, 96,* 1149–1160.

Dowden, C., & Andrews, D. A. (2000). Effective correctional treatment and violent reoffending: A meta-analysis. *Canadian Journal of Criminology, 42*(4), 449–467.

Downey, L., Rosengren, D. B., & Donovan, D. M. (2000). To thine own self be true: Self-concept and motivation for abstinence among substance abusers. *Addictive Behaviors, 25,* 743–757.

Drake, R. E., Mercer-McFadden, C., Mueser, K., McHugo, G. J., & Bond, G. R. (1998). Review of integrated mental health and substance abuse treatment for patients with severe mental illness: A review of recent research. *Schizophrenia Bulletin, 24*(4), 589–608.

Dunn, C., DeRoo, L., & Rivara, F. P. (2001). The use of brief interventions adapted from motivational interviewing across behavioral domains: A systematic review. *Addiction, 96*(12), 1725–1742.

Easton, C., Swan, S., & Sinha, R. (2000). Motivation to change substance use among offenders of domestic violence. *Journal of Substance Abuse Treatment, 19,* 1–5.

Edwards, A. L. (1953). *Edwards Personal Preference Schedule.* New York: Psychological Corporation.

Edwards, G., & Orford, J. (1977). A plain treatment for alcoholism. *Proceedings of the Royal Society of Medicine, 70,* 344–348.

Ellickson, P. L., & Bell, R. M. (1990). Drug prevention in junior high: A multi-site longitudinal test. *Science, 247*(4948), 1299–1305.

Emmons, K. M., Hammond, S. K., Fava, J. L., Velicer, W. F., Evans, J. L., & Monroe, A. D. (in press). A randomized trial to reduce passive smoke exposure in low income households with young children. *American Journal of Preventive Medicine.*

Emmons, K. M., & Rollnick, S. (2001). Motivational interviewing in health care settings: Opportunities and limitations. *American Journal of Preventive Medicine, 20*(1), 68–74.

Ershoff, D. H., Quinn, V. P., Boyd, N. R., Stern, J., Gregory, M., & Wirtschafter, D. (1999). The Kaiser Permanente prenatal smoking cessation trial: When more isn't better, what is enough? *American Journal of Preventive Medicine, 17*(3), 161–168.

Farrall, M. (2001). The use of motivational interviewing techniques in offending behaviour group work. *Motivational Interviewing Newsletter: Updates, Education and Training, 8*(1), 8–12.

Fazio, R., & Zanna, M. (1981). Direct experience and attitude behavior consistency. In L. Berkowitz (Ed.), *Advances in experimental social psychology* (Vol. 14, pp. 162–202). New York: Academic Press.

Feather, N. T. (1992). Values, valences, expectations, and actions. *Journal of Social Issues, 48* 109–124.

Ferguson, R. T. (1998). Motivational interviewing with less motivated driving under the influence of alcohol second offenders with an exploration of the processes related to change (Doctoral dissertation, University of Wyoming, 1998). *Dissertation Abstracts International, 59*(1–B), 0415.

Festinger, L. (1957). *A theory of cognitive dissonance.* Stanford, CA: Stanford University Press.

Fiester, A. R., Cooley, M. L., & Bausinger, L. (1979). The effect of phone prompts on nonattendance rates at a CMHC aftercare center. *Hospital and Community Psychiatry, 30,* 312.

Fiorentine, R., & Anglin, M. D.(1996). More is better: Counseling participation and the effectiveness of outpatient drug treatment. *Journal of Substance Abuse Treatment, 13,* 341–348.

Fisch, R., Weakland, J. H., & Segal, L. (1982). *The tactics of change: Doing therapy briefly*. San Francisco: Jossey-Bass.

Fishman, P., Taplin, S., Meyer, D., & Barlow, W. (2000). Cost-effectiveness of strategies to enhance mammography use. *Effective Clinical Practice, 4*, 213–220.

Foote, J., DeLuca, A., Magura, S., Warner, A., Grand, A., Rosenblum, A., & Stahl, S. (1999). A group motivational treatment for chemical dependency. *Journal of Substance Abuse Treatment, 17*, 181–192.

Frank, J. D., & Frank, J. B. (1991). *Persuasion and healing: A comparative study of psychotherapy* (3rd ed.). Baltimore: Johns Hopkins University Press.

Frankl, V. E. (1963). *Man's search for meaning*. Boston: Beacon Press.

Fromm, E. (1956). *The art of loving*. New York: Harper & Row.

Garfield, S. L. (1994). Research on client variables in psychotherapy. In A. E. Bergin & S. L. Garfield (Eds.), *Handbook of psychotherapy and behavior change* (4th ed.). New York: Wiley.

Garland, R. J., & Dougher, M. J. (1991). Motivational intervention in the treatment of sex offenders. In W. R. Miller, & S. Rollnick, *Motivational interviewing: Preparing people to change addictive behavior* (pp. 303–313). New York: Guilford Press.

Gaylin, N. L., Esser, U., Schneider, I., Rombauts, J., & Devriendt, M. (1990). Couple and family therapy. In G. Lietaer & J. Rombauts (Eds.), *Client-centered and experiential psychotherapy in the nineties* (pp. 813–863). Leuven, Belgium: Leuven University Press.

Gendreau, P. (1996). Offender rehabilitation. What we know and what needs to be done. *Criminal Justice and Behavior, 23*(1), 144–161.

Gentilello, L. M., Rivara, F. P., Donovan, D. M., Jurkovich, G. J., Daranciang, E., Dunn, C. W., Villaveces, A., Copass, M., & Ries, R. (1999). Alcohol interventions in a trauma center as a means of reducing the risk of injury recurrence. *Annals of Surgery, 230*(4), 473–483.

George, W. H., & Marlatt, G. A. (1989). Introduction. In D. R. Laws (Ed.), *Relapse prevention with sex offenders* (pp. 1–31). New York: Guilford Press.

Gfroerer, J. C., Greenblatt, J. C., & Wright, D. A. (1997). Substance use in the U. S. college-age population: Differences according to educational status and living arrangement. *American Journal of Public Health, 87*(1), 62–65.

Ginsburg, J. I. D. (2000). *Using motivational interviewing to enhance treatment readiness in offenders with symptoms of alcohol dependence*. Unpublished doctoral dissertation, Carleton University, Ottawa, Ontario, Canada.

Glanz, K. (1979). Strategies for nutritional counseling: Dietitians' attitudes and practice. *Journal of the American Dietetic Association, 74*(4), 431–437.

Glanz, K., Patterson, R. E., Kristal, A. R., DiClemente, C. C., Heimendinger, J., Linnan, L., & Ockene, J. (1994). Stages of change in adopting healthy diets: Fat, fiber and correlates of nutrient intake. *Health Education Quarterly, 21*(4), 499–519.

Glasgow, R. E., & Rosen, G. M. (1978). Behavioral bibliotherapy: A review of self-help behavior therapy manuals. *Psychological Bulletin, 85*, 1–23.

Glasgow, R., Whitlock, E., Eakin, E., & Lichtstein, E. (2000). A brief smoking cessation intervention for women in low-income planned parenthood clinics. *American Journal of Public Health, 90*(5), 786–789.

Goldstein, M., DePue, J., Monroe, A., Willey Lesne, C., Rakowski, W., Prokhorov, A., Niaura, R., & Dube, C. (1998). A population-based survey of physician smoking cessation counseling practices. *Preventive Medicine, 27*, 720–729.

Golombeck, H., Marton, P., Stein, B. A., & Korenblu, M. (1989). Adolescent personality development: Three phases, three courses, and varying turmoil. *Canadian Journal of Psychiatry, 34*(6), 500–504.

Gordon, T. (1970). *Parent effectiveness training*. New York: Wyden.

Gould, R. A., & Clum, G. A. (1993). A meta-analysis of self-help treatment approaches. *Clinical Psychology Review, 13*, 169–186.

Graeber, D. A., Moyers, T. B., Griffith, G., Guajardo, E., & Tonigan, S. (2000, June). *Comparison of motivational interviewing and educational intervention in patients with schizophrenia and alcoholism*. Paper presented at the scientific meeting of the Research Society on Alcoholism, Denver, CO.

Granfield, R., & Cloud, W. (1996). The elephant that no one sees: Natural recovery among middle-class addicts. *Journal of Drug Issues, 26*, 45–61.

Greenberg, L. S., Elliott, R., & Lietaer, G. (1994). Research on experiential psychotherapies. In A. E. Bergin & S. L. Garfield (Eds.), *Handbook of psychotherapy and behavior change* (4th ed., pp. 509–539). New York: Wiley.

Grimley, D. M., Riley, G. E., Bellis, J. M., & Prochaska, J. O. (1993). Assessing the stages of change and decision-making for contraceptive use for the prevention of pregnancy, sexually transmitted diseases, and acquired immunodeficiency syndrome. *Health Education Quarterly, 20*(4), 455–470.

Haley, J. (1963). *Strategies of psychotherapy*. New York: Grune & Stratton.

Handmaker, N. S., Miller, W. R., & Manicke, M. (1999). Findings of a pilot study of motivational interviewing with pregnant drinkers. *Journal of Studies on Alcohol, 60*, 285–287.

Hansen, W. B., & Graham, J. W. (1991). Preventing alcohol, marijuana, and cigarette use among adolescents: Peer pressure resistance training versus establishing conservative norms. *Preventive Medicine, 20*, 414–430.

Hanson, R. K., & Bussière, M. T. (1998). Predicting relapse: A meta-analysis of sexual offender recidivism studies. *Journal of Consulting and Clinical Psychology, 66*(2), 348–362.

Harland, J., White, M., Drinkwater, C., Chinn, D., Farr, L., & Howel, D. (1999). The Newcastle exercise project: A randomized controlled trial of methods to promote physical activity in primary care. *British Medical Journal, 319*, 828–831.

Harper, R., & Hardy, S. (2000). An evaluation of motivational interviewing as a method of intervention with clients in a probation setting. *British Journal of Social Work, 30*, 393–400.

Harris, K. B., & Miller, W. R. (1990). Behavioral self-control training for problem drinkers: Components of efficacy. *Psychology of Addictive Behaviors, 4*, 82–90.

Hayward, P., Chan, N., Kemp, R., & Youle, S. (1995). Medication self-management: A preliminary report on an intervention to improve medication compliance. *Journal of Mental Health, 4*(5), 511–517.

Heather, N., Rollnick, S., & Bell, A. (1993). Predictive validity of the Readiness to Change Questionnaire. *Addiction, 88*, 1667–1677.

Heather, N., Rollnick, S., Bell, A., & Richmond, R. (1996). Effects of brief counselling among male heavy drinkers identified on general hospital wards. *Drug and Alcohol Review, 15*(1), 29–38.

Hermans, H. J. (1987). Self as an organized system of valuations: Toward a dialogue with the person. *Journal of Counseling Psychology, 34*, 10–19.

Hochstadt, N. J., & Trybula, Jr., J. (1980). Reducing missed initial appointments in a community mental health center. *Journal of Community Psychology, 8*, 261–265.

Hogue, T. E., & Mann, R. E. (2000, November). *Working with sexual offenders: Can we predict who makes a good therapist?* Workshop presented at the 19th Annual Research and Treatment Conference of the Association for the Treatment of Sexual Abusers, San Diego, CA.

Horn, J. L., Wanbe. G., K. W., & Foster, F. M. (1990). *Guide to the Alcohol Use Inventory*. Minneapolis: National Computer Systems.

Hser, Y., Maglione, M., Polinsky, M. L., & Anglin, M. D. (1997). Predicting drug treatment entry among treatment-seeking individuals. *Journal of Substance Abuse Treatment, 15*, 213–220.

Hu, T-w, Hunkeler, E. M., Weisner, C., Li, E., Grayson, D. K., Westphal, J., & McClellan, A. T. (1997). Treatment participation and outcome among problem drinkers in a managed care alcohol outpatient treatment program. *Journal of Mental Health Administration, 24*, 23–34.

Hughes, R. (1987). *The fatal shore: The epic of Australia's founding*. New York: Knopf.

Husby, R. (1985). Short-term dynamic psychotherapy: III. A 5–year follow-up of 36 neurotic patients. *Psychotherapy and Psychosomatics, 43*, 17–22.

Ingersoll, K. S., Wagner, C. C., & Gharib, S. (2000). *Motivational groups for community substance abuse programs*. Richmond, VA: Mid-Atlantic Addiction Technology Transfer Center/Center for Substance Abuse Treatment.

Isenhart, C. E. (1994). Motivational subtypes in an inpatient sample of substance abusers. *Addictive Behaviors, 19*, 463–475.

Ito, J. R., Donovan, D. M., & Hall, J. J. (1988). Relapse prevention in alcohol aftercare: Effects on drinking outcome, change process, and aftercare attendance. *British Journal of Addictions, 83*, 171–181.

Jacob, T., & Leonard, K. (1988). Alcoholic-spouse interaction as a function of alcoholism subtype and alcohol consumption interaction. *Journal of Abnormal Psychology, 97*, 231–237.

Jacobson, N. S., & Christensen, A. (1996). *Integrative couple therapy: Promoting acceptance and change*. New York: Norton.

Jacobson, N. S., Roberts, L. J., Berns, S. B., & McGlinchey, J. B. (1999). Methods for defining and determining the clinical significance of treatment effects: Description, application, and alternatives. *Journal of Consulting and Clinical Psychology, 67*(3), 300–307.

Jamieson, Beals, Lalonde, & Associates. (2000). *Motivational enhancement treatment (MET) manual. Theoretical foundation and structured curriculum. Individual and group sessions*. Developed for the State of Maine, Department of Mental Health, Mental Retardation and Substance Abuse Services, Office of Substance Abuse. Ottawa, Ontario, Canada: Author.

Janis, I. L., & Mann, L. (1977). *Decision-making: A psychological analysis of conflict, choice, and commitment*. New York: Free Press.

Jerrell, J. M., & Ridgely, M. S. (1995). Comparative effectiveness of three approaches to serving people with severe mental illness and substance abuse disorders. *Journal of Nervous and Mental Disease, 183*, 566–576.

Jessor, R. (1991). Risk behavior in adolescence: A psychosocial framework for understanding and action. *Journal of Adolescent Health, 12*(4), 374–390.

Johnson, V. E. (1986). *Intervention: How to help those who don't want help*. Minneapolis, MN: Johnson Institute.

Johnston, L. D., O'Malley, P. M., & Bachman, J. G. (2000a). *Monitoring the future national results on adolescent drug use: Overview of key findings*. Bethesda, MD: National Institute on Drug Abuse.

Johnston, L. D., O'Malley, P. M., & Bachman, J. G. (2000b). *Monitoring the future national results on adolescent drug use: 1975–1999. Vol. II: College students and young adults.* Bethesda, MD: National Institute on Drug Abuse.

Jones, R. A. (1977). *Self-fulfilling prophecies: Social, psychological and physiological effects of expectancies.* Hillsdale, NJ: Erlbaum.

Joseph, J., Breslin, C., & Skinner, H. (1999). Critical perspectives on the transtheoretical model and stages of change. In J. A. Tucker, D. M. Donovan, & G. A. Marlatt (Eds.), *Changing addictive behavior: Bridging clinical and public health strategies* (pp. 160–190). New York: Guilford Press.

Joyce, L. T. (1990). The new revolving-door patients: Results from a national cohort of first Admissions. *Acta Psychiatrica Scandinavia, 82,* 130–135.

Juárez, P. (2001). *A randomized trial of motivational interviewing and feedback on heavy drinking college students.* Unpublished master's thesis, University of New Mexico, Albuquerque.

Kadden, R., Carroll, K. M., Donovan, D., Cooney, N., Monti, P., Abrams, D., Litt, M., & Hester, R. (1992). *Cognitive-behavioral coping skills therapy manual: A clinical research guide for therapists treating individuals with alcohol abuse and dependence* (NIAAA Project MATCH Monograph Series, Vol. 3, DHHS Publication No. ADM 92–1895). Washington, DC: U.S. Government Printing Office.

Kanfer, F. H. (1986). Implications of a self-regulation model of therapy for treatment of addictive behaviors. In W. R. Miller & N. Heather (Eds.), *Treating addictive behaviors* (pp. 29–47). New York: Plenum Press.

Kazdin, A. E. (1992). *Research design in clinical psychology* (2nd ed.). Needham Heights, MA: Allyn & Bacon.

Kear-Colwell, J., & Pollock, P. (1997). Motivation or confrontation. Which approach to the child sex offender? *Criminal Justice and Behavior, 24*(1), 20–33.

Kelly, J. A. (1995). *Changing HIV risk behavior: Practical strategies.* New York: Guilford Press.

Kemp, R., David, A., & Hayward, P. (1996). Compliance therapy: An intervention targeting insight and treatment adherence in psychotic patients. *Behavioural and Cognitive Psychotherapy, 24,* 331–350.

Kemp, R., Hayward, P., Applewhaite, G., Everitt, B., & David, A. (1996). Compliance therapy in psychotic patients: Randomised controlled trial. *British Medical Journal, 312,* 345–349.

Kemp, R., Kirov, G., Everitt, B., Hayward, P., & David, A. (1998). Randomised controlled trial of compliance therapy: 18–month follow-up. *British Journal of Psychiatry, 172,* 413–419.

Kennerley, R. J. (2000). The ability of a motivational pre-group session to enhance readiness for change in men who have engaged in domestic violence (Doctoral dissertation, University of South Carolina, 2000). *Dissertation Abstracts International, 60*(7–B), 3569.

Konopasky, R. J., & Konopasky, A. W. B. (2000). Remaking penile plethysmography. In D. R. Laws, S. M. Hudson, & T. Ward (Eds.), *Remaking relapse prevention with sex offenders* (pp. 257–284). Thousand Oaks, CA: Sage.

Koumans, A. J. R., & Muller, J. J. (1965). Use of letters to increase motivation in alcoholics. *Psychological Reports, 16,* 1152.

Koumans, A. J. R., Muller, J. J., & Miller, C. F. (1967). Use of telephone calls to increase motivation for treatment in alcoholics. *Psychological Reports, 21,* 327–328.

Kreuter, M. W., Strecher, V. J., & Glassman, B. (1999). One size does not fit all: The case for tailoring print materials. *Annals of Behavioral Medicine, 21*(4), 276–283.

Kristiansen, C. M. (1985). Value correlates of preventive health behavior. *Journal of Personality and Social Psychology, 49,* 748–758.

Krulee, D. A., & Hales, R. E. (1988). Compliance with psychiatric referrals from a general hospital psychiatry outpatient clinic. *General Hospital Psychiatry, 10,* 339–345.

Kuchipudi, V., Hobein, K., Fleckinger, A., & Iber, F. L. (1990). Failure of a 2–hour motivational intervention to alter recurrent drinking behavior in alcoholics with gastrointestinal disease. *Journal of Studies on Alcohol, 51,* 356–360.

Lambert, M. J. (1976). Spontaneous remission in adult neurotic disorders: A revision and summary. *Psychological Bulletin, 81,* 107119.

Lando, H. A., Valanis, B. G., Lichtenstein, E., Curry, S. J., McBride, C. M., Pirie, P. L., & Grothaus, L. C. (2001). Promoting smoking abstinence in pregnant and postpartum patients: A comparison of two approaches. *American Journal of Managed Care, 7*(7), 685–693.

Larimer, M. E., Turner, A., Anderson, B., Lydum, A., Kilmer, J. R., Palmer, R. S., & Fader, J. (2001). Brief motivational intervention for alcohol abuse prevention in college fraternities. *Journal of Studies on Alcohol, 62*(3), 370–380.

Larivière, M., & Robinson, D. (1996). *Attitudes of federal correctional officers towards offenders* (Research Report No. R-44). Ottawa, Ontario, Canada: Correctional Service of Canada.

Lash, S. J. (1998). Increasing participation in substance abuse aftercare treatment. *American Journal of Drug and Alcohol Abuse, 24,* 31–36.

Lash, S. J., & Blosser, S. L. (1999). Increasing adherence to substance abuse aftercare group therapy. *Journal of Substance Abuse Treatment, 16,* 55–60.

Latane, B., & Darley, J. M. (1968). Group inhibition of bystander intervention in emergencies. *Journal of Personality and Social Psychology, 10,* 215–221.

Laws, D. R. (1989). *Relapse prevention with sex offenders.* New York: Guilford Press.

Leake, G. J., & King, A. S. (1977). Effect of counselor expectations on alcoholic recovery. *Alcohol Health and Research World, 11*(3), 16–22.

Lincourt, P., Kuettel, T. J., & Bombardier, C. H. (in press). Motivational interviewing in a group setting with mandated clients: A pilot study. *Addictive Behaviors.*

Lipsey, M. W., & Wilson, D. B. (1993). The efficacy of psychological, educational, and behavioral treatment. Confirmation from meta-analysis. *American Psychologist, 48*(12), 1181–1209.

Locke, E. A., & Latham, G. P. (1990). Work motivation and satisfaction: Light at the end of the tunnel. *Psychological Science, 1,* 240–246.

Longabaugh, R., & Beattie, M. (1985). Optimizing the cost-effectiveness of alcoholism treatment. In *Future directions in alcohol abuse treatment* (ADAMHA Research Monograph, No. 15, DHHS Publication No. ADM 85–1322, pp. 104–136). Washington, DC: U. S. Government Printing Office.

Longabaugh, R., Beattie, M., Noel, N., Stout, R., & Malloy, P. (1993). The effect of social investment on treatment outcome. *Journal of Studies on Alcohol, 54* (4), 465–478.

Longabaugh, R., Wirtz, P. W., & Clifford, P. R. (1995). *The important people and activities instrument.* Providence, RI: Brown University.

Luborsky, L., Diguer, L., Seligman, D. A., Rosenthal, R., Krause, E. D., Johnson, S., Halperin, G., Bishop, M., Berman, J. S., & Schweizer, E. (1999). The researcher's own therapy allegiances: A "wild card" in comparisons of treatment efficacy. *Clinical Psychology: Science and Practice, 6*(1), 95–106.

Luborsky, L., McLellan, A. T., Woody, G. E., O'Brien, C. P., & Auerbach, A. (1985). Therapist success and its determinants. *Archives of General Psychiatry, 42,* 602–611.

Ludman, E., Curry, S., Meyer, D., & Taplin, S. (1999). Implementation of outreach telephone counseling to promote mammography participation. *Health Education and Behavior, 26*(5), 689–702.

Maio, R. F., Portnoy, J., Blow, F. C., & Hill, E. (1994). Injury type, injury severity, and repeat occurrence of alcohol-related trauma in adolescents. *Alcoholism: Clinical and Experimental Research, 18,* 261–264.

Malan, D. H., Heath, E. S., Bacal, H. A., & Balfour, F. H. (1975). Psychodynamic changes in untreated neurotic patients: II. Apparently genuine improvements. *Archives of General Psychiatry, 32,* 110–126.

Mann, R. E. (Ed.). (1996). *Motivational interviewing with sex offenders: A practice manual.* Hull, UK: National Organisation for the Treatment of Abusers.

Mann, R. E. (2000). Managing resistance and rebellion in relapse prevention intervention. In D. R. Laws, S. M. Hudson, & T. Ward (Eds.), *Remaking relapse prevention with sex offenders* (pp. 187–200). Thousand Oaks, CA: Sage.

Mann, R. E., Ginsburg, J. I. D., & Weekes, J. (2002). Motivational interviewing with offenders. In M. McMurran (Ed.), *Motivating offenders to change: A guide to enhancing engagement in therapy.* Chichester, UK: Wiley.

Mann, R. E., & Rollnick, S. (1996). Motivational interviewing with a sex offender who believed he was innocent. *Behavioural and Cognitive Psychotherapy, 24,* 127–134.

Mann, R. E., & Shingler, J. (2001). *Collaborative risk assessment with sexual offenders.* Unpublished manuscript.

Manohar, V. (1973). Training volunteers as alcoholism treatment counselors. *Quarterly Journal of Studies on Alcohol, 34,* 869–877.

Marcus, B. H., Rossi, J. S., Selby, V. C., Niaura, R. S., & Abrams, D. B. (1992). The stages and processes of exercise adoption and maintenance in a worksite sample. *Health Psychology, 11*(6), 386–395.

Markham, M. R., Miller, W. R., & Archiniega, L. (1993). BACCuS 2. 01: Computer software for quantifying alcohol consumption. *Behavior Research Methods, Instruments, and Computers, 25,* 420–421.

Marlatt, G. A., Baer, J. S., Kivlahan, D. R., Dimeff, L. A., Larimer, M. E., Quigley, L. A., Somers, J. M., & Williams, E. (1998). Screening and brief intervention for high-risk college student drinkers: Results from a two-year follow-up assessment. *Journal of Consulting and Clinical Psychology, 66*(4), 604–615.

Marlatt, G. A., & Gordon, J. R. (Eds.). (1985). *Relapse prevention: Maintenance strategies in the treatment of addictive behaviors.* New York: Guilford Press.

Marques, J. K., Nelson, C., Alarcon, J.-M., & Day, D. M. (2000). Preventing relapse in sex offenders: What we learned from SOTEP's experimental treatment program. In D. R. Laws, S. M. Hudson, & T. Ward (Eds.), *Remaking relapse prevention with sex offenders* (pp. 321–340). Thousand Oaks, CA: Sage.

Marshall, W. L., Anderson, D., & Fernandez, Y. M. (1999). *Cognitive behavioural treatment of sexual offenders.* Chichester, UK: Wiley.

Marshall, W. L., Thornton, D., Marshall, L. E., Fernandez, Y. M., & Mann, R. E. (2001). Treatment of sexual offenders who are in categorical denial: A pilot project. *Sexual Abuse: A Journal of Research and Treatment, 13*(3), 205–216.

Martin, J. E., Calfas, K. J., Patten, C. A., Polarek, M., Hofstetter, R., Noto, J., & Beach, D. (1997). Prospective evaluation of three smoking interventions in 205 recovering alcoholics: One-year results of Project SCRAP-tobacco. *Journal of Consulting and Clinical Psychology, 65,* 190–194.

Martin, J. E., Noto, J. V., & Walters, S. T. (2000, September). *A controlled trial of motivational feedback-based group vs. written intervention in heavy drinking college students: Project AIM-Greek collaboration.* Paper presented at the international conference on Treatment of Addictive Behaviors, Cape Town, South Africa.

Martino, S., Carroll, K. M., O'Malley, S. S., & Rounsaville, B. J. (2000). Motivational interviewing with psychiatrically ill substance abusing patients. *American Journal on Addictions, 9,* 88–91.

Maslow, A. (1967). Neurosis as a failure of personal growth. *Humanitas, 3,* 153–170.

Maslow, A. (1970). *Motivation and personality* (2nd ed.). New York: Harper & Row.

Matas, M., Staley, D., & Griffin, W. (1992). A profile of the noncompliant patient: A thirty-month review of outpatient psychiatry referrals. *General Hospital Psychiatry, 14,* 124–130.

Mattson, M. E. (1998). Finding the right approach. In W. R. Miller & N. Heather (Eds.), *Treating addictive behaviors* (2nd ed., pp. 163–172). New York: Plenum Press.

Mattson, M., DelBoca, F., Cooney, N., DiClemente, C. C., Donovan, D. M., Rice, C. L., & Zweben, A. (1998). Patient compliance in Project MATCH: Session attendance predictors and relationship to outcome. *Alcoholism Clinical and Experimental Research, 11*(6), 1328–1339.

McCaskill, P. A., Toro, P. A., & Wolfe, S. M. (1998). Homeless and matched housed adolescents: A comparative study of psychopathology. *Journal of Clinical Child Psychology, 27*(3), 306–319.

McConnaughy, E. A., DiClemente, C. C., Prochaska, J. O., & Velicer, W. F. (1989). Stages of change in psychotherapy: A follow-up report. *Psychotherapy Practice and Research, 26,* 494–503.

McCrady, B. S., & Epstein, E. E. (1995). Directions for research on alcoholic relationships: Marital- and individual-based models of heterogeneity. *Psychology of Addictive Behaviors, 9,* 157–166.

McCullough, J. P., McCune, K. J., Kaye, A. L., Braith, J. A., Friend, R., Roberts, W. C., Belyea-Caldwell, S., Norris, S. L., & Hampton, C. (1994). One-year prospective replication study of an untreated sample of community dysthymia subjects. *Journal of Nervous and Mental Disease, 182,* 396–401.

McMurran, M., & Hollin, C. R. (1993). *Young offenders and alcohol related crime: A practitioner's guidebook.* Chichester, UK: Wiley.

Mercer-McFadden, C., Drake, R. E., Brown, N. B., & Fox, R. S. (1997). The Community Support Program demonstrations of services for young adults with severe mental illness and substance use disorders. *Psychiatric Rehabilitation Journal, 20*(3), 13–24.

Mhurchu, C. N., Margetts, B. M., & Speller, V. (1998). Randomized clinical trial comparing the effectiveness of two dietary interventions for patients with hyperlipidaemia. *Clinical Science, 95*(4), 479–487.

Milgram, S. (1963). Behavioral study of obedience. *Journal of Abnormal and Social Psychology, 67,* 371–378.

Miller, E. T. (1999). *Preventing alcohol abuse and alcohol-related negative consequences among freshman college students: Using emerging computer technology to deliver and evaluate the effectiveness of brief intervention efforts.* Seattle: University of Washington Press.

Miller, W. R. (1983). Motivational interviewing with problem drinkers. *Behavioural Psychotherapy, 11,* 147–172.

Miller, W. R. (1985). *Living as if: How positive faith can change your life*. Philadelphia: Westminster Press.

Miller, W. R. (1987). Techniques to modify hazardous drinking patterns. In M. Galanter (Ed.), *Recent developments in alcoholism* (Vol. 5, pp. 425–438). New York: Plenum Press.

Miller, W. R. (1991). Emergent treatment concepts and techniques. *Annual Review of Addictions Research and Treatment, 2,* 283–295.

Miller, W. R. (1992). *Stages of Change Readiness and Treatment Eagerness Scale (SOCRATES)*. Albuquerque, NM: Center on Alcoholism, Substance Abuse, and Addictions.

Miller, W. R. (1994). Motivational interviewing: III. On the ethics of motivational intervention. *Behavioural and Cognitive Psychotherapy, 22,* 111–123.

Miller, W. R. (1996a). Manual for Form 90: A structured assessment interview for drinking and related behaviors (NIAAA Project MATCH Monograph Series, Vol. 5, DHHS Publication No. ADM 96–4004). Washington, DC: U.S. Government Printing Office.

Miller, W. R. (1996b). Motivational interviewing: Research, practice, and puzzles. *Addictive Behaviors, 21*(6), 835–842.

Miller, W. R. (1998a). Enhancing motivation for change. In W. R. Miller & N. Heather (Eds.), *Treating addictive behaviors* (2nd ed., pp. 121–132). New York: Plenum Press.

Miller, W. R. (1998b). Toward a motivational definition and understanding of addiction. *Motivational Interviewing Newsletter for Trainers, 5,* 3.

Miller, W. R. (Ed.). (1999a). *Enhancing motivation for change in substance abuse treatment* (Treatment Improvement Protocol [TIP] Series No. 35). Rockville, MD: Center for Substance Abuse Treatment.

Miller, W. R. (1999b). Pros and cons: Reflections on motivational interviewing in correctional settings. *Motivational Interviewing Newsletter for Trainers, 6*(1), 2–3.

Miller, W. R. (2000). Rediscovering fire: Small interventions, large effects. *Psychology of Addictive Behaviors, 14,* 6–18.

Miller, W. R. (Ed.). (in press). *Project COMBINE Combined Behavioral Intervention: Therapist manual*. Rockville, MD: National Institute on Alcohol Abuse and Alcoholism.

Miller, W. R., Andrews, N. R., Wilbourne, P., & Bennett, M. E. (1998). A wealth of alternatives: Effective treatments for alcohol problems. In W. R. Miller & N. Heather (Eds.), *Treating addictive behaviors: Processes of change* (2nd ed., pp. 203–216). New York: Plenum Press.

Miller, W. R., & Baca, L. M. (1983). Two-year follow-up of bibliotherapy and therapist-directed controlled drinking training for problem drinkers. *Behavior Therapy, 14,* 441–448.

Miller, W. R., Benefield, R. G., & Tonigan, J. S. (1993). Enhancing motivation for change in problem drinking: A controlled comparison of two therapist styles. *Journal of Consulting and Clinical Psychology, 61*(3), 455–461.

Miller, W. R., & Brown, J. M. (1991). Self-regulation as a conceptual basis for the prevention and treatment of addictive behaviours. In N. Heather, W. R. Miller, & J. Greeley (Eds.), *Self-control and the addictive behaviours* (pp. 3–79). Sydney: Maxwell Macmillan Publishing Australia.

Miller, W. R., Brown, J. M., Simpson, T. L., Handmaker, N. S., Bien, T. H., Luckie, L. F., Montgomery, H. A., Hester, R. K., & Tonigan, J. S. (1995). What works? A methodological analysis of the alcohol treatment outcome literature. In R. K. Hester &

W. R. Miller (Eds.), *Handbook of alcoholism treatment approaches: Effective alternatives* (2nd ed., pp. 12–44). Boston: Allyn & Bacon.

Miller, W. R., & C'de Baca, J. (1994). Quantum change: Toward a psychology of transformation. In T. Heatherton & J. Weinberger (Eds.), *Can personality change?* (pp. 252–280). Washington, DC: American Psychological Association.

Miller, W. R., & C'de Baca, J. (2001). *Quantum change: When epiphanies and sudden insights transform ordinary lives.* New York: Guilford Press.

Miller, W. R., & Heather, N. (Eds.). (1998). *Treating addictive behaviors: Processes of change* (2nd ed.). New York: Plenum Press.

Miller, W. R., Heather, N., & Hall, W. (1991). Calculating standard drink units: International comparisons. *British Journal of Addiction, 86*, 43–47.

Miller, W. R., Hedrick, K. E., & Taylor, C. A. (1983). Addictive behaviors and life problems before and after behavioral treatment of problem drinkers. *Addictive Behaviors, 8*, 403–412.

Miller, W. R., & Marlatt, G. A. (1984). *The Comprehensive Drinker Profile.* Odessa, FL: Psychological Assessment Resources.

Miller, W. R., & Marlatt, G. A. (1987). *Manual supplement for the Brief Drinker Profile, Follow-up Drinker Profile, and Collateral Interview Form.* Odessa, FL: Psychological Assessment Resources.

Miller, W., & Mount, K. (2001). A small study of training in motivational interviewing: Does one workshop change clinician and client behavior? *Behavioural and Cognitive Psychotherapy, 29*, 457–471.

Miller, W. R., & Rollnick, S. (1991). *Motivational interviewing: Preparing people to change addictive behavior.* New York: Guilford Press.

Miller, W. R., & Sovereign, R. G. (1989). Check-up: A model for early intervention in addictive behaviors. In T. Loberg, W. R. Miller, P. E. Nathan, & G. A. Marlatt (Eds.), *Addictive behaviors: Prevention and early intervention* (pp. 219–231). Amsterdam: Swets and Zeitlinger.

Miller, W. R., Sovereign, R. G., & Krege, B. (1988). Motivational interviewing with problem drinkers: II. The Drinker's Check-Up as a preventive intervention. *Behavioural Psychotherapy, 16*, 251–268.

Miller, W. R., Taylor, C. A., & West, J. C. (1980). Focused versus broad spectrum behavior therapy for problem drinkers. *Journal of Consulting and Clinical Psychology, 48*, 590–601.

Miller, W. R., Toscova, R. T., Miller, J. H., & Sanchez, V. (2000). A theory-based motivational approach for reducing alcohol/drug problems in college. *Health Education Behavior, 27*, 744–759.

Miller, W. R., Zweben, A., DiClemente, C. C., & Rychtarik, R., (1992). *Motivational enhancement therapy manual: A clinical research guide for therapists treating individuals with alcohol abuse and dependence* (Project MATCH Monograph Series, Vol. 2). Rockville, MD: National Institute on Alcohol Abuse and Alcoholism.

Monti, P. M., Colby, S. M., Barnett, N. P., Spirito, A., Rohsenow, D. J., Myers, M., Woolard, R., & Lewander, W. (1999). Brief intervention for harm reduction with alcohol-positive older adolescents in a hospital emergency department. *Journal of Consulting and Clinical Psychology, 67*, 989–994

Moos, R. H., Finney, J. W., & Cronkite, R. C. (1990). *Alcoholism treatment: Context, process, and outcome.* New York: Oxford University Press.

Moskowitz, J. M. (1985). The primary prevention of alcohol problems: A critical review of the research literature. *Journal of Studies on Alcohol, 50*(1), 54–88.

Moss, M. K., & Arend, R. A. (1977). Self-directed contact desensitization. *Journal of Consulting & Clinical Psychology 45*(5), 730–738.

Mowrer, O. (1945). Time as a determinant in integrative learning. *Psychological Review, 52,* 61–90.

Mowrer, O. (1966). Integrity therapy: A self-help approach. *Psychotherapy: Theory, Research and Practice, 3,* 114–119.

Mrazek, P. J., & Haggerty, R. J. (1994). *Reducing risks for mental disorders.* Washington, DC: National Academy Press, Committee on Prevention of Mental Disorders Division of Biobehavioral Sciences and Mental Disorders, Institute of Medicine.

Mueser, K. T., Bennett, M., & Kushner, M. G. (1995). Epidemiology of substance use disorders among persons with chronic mental illnesses. In A. F. Lehman & L. Dixon (Eds.), *Double jeopardy: Chronic mental illness and substance abuse* (pp. 9–25). New York: Harwood Academic.

Mueser, K. T., Drake, R. E., & Noordsy, D. L. (1998). Integrated mental health and substance abuse treatment for severe psychiatric disorders. *Journal of Practical Psychiatry and Behavioral Health, 4*(3), 129–139.

Mueser, K. T., & Noordsy, D. L. (1996). Group treatment for dually diagnosed clients. In R. E. Drake & K. T. Mueser (Eds.), *Dual diagnosis of major mental illness and substance abuse disorder: II. Recent research and clinical implications* (pp. 33–51). San Francisco: Jossey-Bass.

Murphy, C. M., & Baxter, V. A. (1997). Motivating batterers to change in the treatment context. *Journal of Interpersonal Violence, 12*(4), 607–619.

Murphy, J. G., Duchnick, J. J., Vuchinich, R. E., Davison, J. W., Karg, R. S., Olson, A. M., Fry, A., & Coffey, T. T. (2000). *Relative efficacy of a brief motivational intervention for college students.* Unpublished manuscript, Auburn University.

Murphy, R. T., Cameron, R. P., Rosen, C., & Thompson, K. (2000). *Motivation to change PTSD symptoms: A model of treatment.* Manuscript submitted for publication.

Murphy, R. T., Cameron, R. P., Sharp, L., Rosen, C., Drescher, K., & Gusman, D. F. (2000). *Readiness to change PTSD symptoms and related behaviors among veterans participating in a motivational enhancement group.* Manuscript submitted for publication.

National Institute on Alcohol Abuse and Alcoholism, U.S. Department of Health and Human Services. (1995). *Motivational enhancement therapy manual: A clinical research guide for therapists treating individuals with alcohol abuse and dependence* (Project MATCH Monograph Series, NIH Publication No. 94-3723). Rockville, MD: Author.

Newcomb, M. D., & Bentler, P. M. (1988). *Consequences of adolescent drug use: Impact on the lives of young adults.* Newbury Park, CA: Sage.

Nielson, B., Nielson, A. S., & Wraae, O. (2000). Factors associated with compliance of alcoholics in outpatient treatment. *Journal of Nervous and Mental Disease, 188,* 101–107.

NIMH Multisite HIV Prevention Trial. (1998). The NIMH Multisite HIV prevention trial: Reducing HIV sexual risk behavior. *Science, 280,* 1889–1994.

Noonan, W. C. (1995a). *Group motivational enhancement therapy.* Unpublished manuscript.

Noonan, W. C. (1995b). *Group motivational interviewing as an enhancement to outpatient alcohol treatment.* Unpublished doctoral dissertation, University of New Mexico, Albuquerque.

Noonan, W. C., & Moyers, T. B. (1997). Motivational interviewing: A review. *Journal of Substance Misuse, 2,* 8–16.

Nowinski, J., Baker, S., & Carroll, K. (1992). *Twelve step facilitation therapy manual: A clinical research guide for therapists treating individuals with alcohol abuse and dependence* (NIAAA Project MATCH Monograph Series, Vol. 1, DHHS Publication No. ADM 92–1893). Washington, DC: U.S. Government Printing Office.

Nye, E. C., Agostinelli, G., & Smith, J. E. (1999). Enhancing alcohol problem recognition: A self-regulation model for the effects of self-focusing and normative information. *Journal of Studies on Alcohol, 60,* 685–693.

O'Farrell, T. J., & Maisto, S. A. (1987). The utility of self-report and biological measures of alcohol consumption in alcoholism treatment outcome studies. *Advances in Behaviour Research and Therapy* [Special Issue: Two decades of behavioral research in the alcohol field: Change, challenge, and controversy], *9*(2–3), 91–125.

Offer, D., & Schonert-Reichl, K. A. (1992). Debunking the myths of adolescence: findings from recent research. *Journal of the American Academy of Child and Adolescent Psychiatry, 31*(6), 1003–1014.

O'Hanlon, W., & Weiner-Davis, M. (1989). *In search of solutions: A new direction in psychotherapy.* New York: Norton.

Olfson, M., Mechanic, D., Boyer, C. A., & Hansell, S. (1998). Linking inpatients with schizophrenia to outpatient care. *Psychiatric Services, 49,* 911–917.

Onken, L. S., Blaine, J. D., & Boren, J. J. (Eds.). (1997). *Beyond the therapeutic alliance: Keeping the drug-dependent individual in treatment* (NIDA Research Monograph 165, NIH Publication No. 97–4142). Washington, DC: U.S. Government Printing Office.

Owen, C., Rutherford, V., Jones, M., Tennant, C., & Smallman, A. (1997). Noncompliance in psychiatric aftercare. *Community Mental Health Journal, 33,* 25–34.

Owen, R. R., Fischer, E. P., Booth, B. M., & Cuffel, B. J. (1996). Medication noncompliance and substance abuse among patients with schizophrenia. *Psychiatric Services, 47*(8), 853–858.

Parker, M. W., Winstead, D. K., & Willi, F. J. P. (1979). Patient autonomy in alcohol rehabilitation: I. Literature review. *International Journal of the Addictions, 14,* 1015–1022.

Patterson, G. R., & Forgatch, M. S. (1985). Therapist behavior as a determinent for client noncompliance: A paradox for the behavior modifier. *Journal of Consulting and Clinical Psychology, 53,* 846–851.

Peele, S. (1990). Addiction as a cultural concept. *Annals of the New York Academy of Sciences, 602,* 205–220.

Pentz, M. A., Dwyer, J. H., MacKinnon, D. P., Flay, B. R., Hansen, W. B., Wang, Y. U, & Johnson, A. (1989). A multicommunity trial for primary prevention of adolescent drug abuse: Effects of drug use prevalence. *Journal of the American Medical Association, 22,* 3259–3266.

Perz, C. A., DiClemente, C. C., & Carbonari, J. P. (1996). Doing the right thing at the right time? Interaction of stages and processes of change in successful smoking cessation. *Health Psychology, 15,* 462–468.

Peterson, A. C. (1993). Presidential address: Creating adolescents: The role of context and process in developmental trajectories. *Journal of Research on Adolescence, 3,* 1–18.

Peterson, P. L. (1998). *Motivational enhancement to reduce risk of street youth.* Grant proposal funded by National Institute on Alcoholism and Alcohol Abuse (No. 5 R01 112167).

Pill, R., Rees, M. E., Stott, N. C., & Rollnick, S. R. (1999). Can nurses learn to let go? Issues arising from an intervention designed to improve patients' involvement in their own care. *Journal of Advanced Nursing, 29*(6), 1492–1499.

Pillay, A. L., & Wassenaar, D. R. (1995). Psychological intervention, spontaneous remission, hopelessness, and psychiatric disturbance in adolescent parasuicides. *Suicide and Life-Threatening Behavior, 25,* 386–392.

Premack, D. (1970). Mechanisms of self-control. In W. A. Hunt (Ed.), *Learning mechanisms in smoking* (pp. 107–123). Chicago: Aldine.

Prochaska, J. O., & DiClemente, C. C. (1982). Transtheoretical therapy: Toward a more integrative model of change. *Psychotherapy: Theory, Research, and Practice, 19,* 276–288.

Prochaska, J. O., & DiClemente, C. C. (1983). Stages and processes of self-change of smoking: Toward an integrative model of change. *Journal of Consulting and Clinical Psychology, 51,* 390–395.

Prochaska, J. O., & DiClemente, C. C. (1984). *The transtheoretical approach: Crossing the traditional boundaries of therapy.* Malabar, FL: Krieger.

Prochaska, J. O., DiClemente, C. C., & Norcross, J. C. (1992). In search of how people change: Applications to the addictive behaviors. *American Psychologist, 47,* 1102–1114.

Prochaska, J. O., DiClemente, C. C., Velicer, W. F., & Rossi, J. S. (1993). Standardized individualized, interactive and personalized self-help programs for smoking cessation. *Health Psychology, 12,* 399–405.

Prochaska, J. O., Velicer, W. F., DiClemente, C. C. Guadagnoli, J. O., & Rossi, J. S. (1991). Patterns of change: Dynamic typology applied to smoking cessation. *Multivariate Behavioral Research, 26,* 83–107.

Prochaska, J. O., Velicer, W. F., Rossi, J. S., Goldstein, M. G., Marcus, B. H., Rakowski, W., Fiore, C., Harlow, L. L., Redding, C. A., Rosenbloom, D., & Rossi, S. R. (1994). Stages of change and decisional balance for twelve problem behaviors. *Health Psychology, 13*(1), 39–46.

Project MATCH Research Group. (1997a). Matching alcoholism treatments to client heterogeneity: Project MATCH posttreatment drinking outcomes. *Journal of Studies on Alcohol, 58,* 7–29.

Project MATCH Research Group. (1997b). Project MATCH secondary a priori hypotheses. *Addiction, 92,* 1671–1698.

Project MATCH Research Group. (1998a). Matching alcoholism treatments to client heterogeneity: Project MATCH three-year drinking outcomes. *Alcoholism: Clinical and Experimental Research, 23*(60), 1300–1311.

Project MATCH Research Group. (1998b). Matching alcoholism treatments to client heterogeneity: Treatment main effects and matching effects during treatment. *Journal of Studies on Alcohol, 59,* 631–639.

Project MATCH Research Group. (1998c). Therapist effects in three treatments for alcohol problems. *Psychotherapy Research, 8,* 455–474.

Rakowski, W., Dube, C. E., Marcus, B. H., Prochaska, J. O., Velicer, W. F., & Abrams, D. B. (1992). Assessing elements of women's decisions about mammography. *Health Psychology, 11*(2), 111–118.

Rao, S. A. (1999). The short-term impact of the family check-up: A brief motivational intervention for at-risk families. *Dissertation Abstracts International: The Sciences and Engineering, 59*(7–B), 3710.

Regier, D. A., Farmer, M. E., Rae, D. S., Locke, B. Z., Keith, S. J., Judd, L. L., &

Goodwin, F. K. (1990). Comorbidity of mental disorders with alcohol and other drug abuse. *Journal of the American Medical Association, 264,* 2511–2518.

Resnicow, K., Coleman-Wallace, D., Jackson, A., DiGirolamo, A., Odom, E., Wang, T., Dudley, W., Davis, M., & Baranowski, T. (2000). Dietary change through black churches: Baseline results and program description of the Eat for Life trial. *Journal of Cancer Education, 15,* 156–163.

Resnicow, K., DiIorio, C., Soet, J., Borrelli, B., Ernst, D., & Hecht, J. (2001). *Motivational interviewing in health promotion: It sounds like something is changing.* Manuscript under review.

Resnicow, K., Jackson, A., Braithwaite, R., DiIorio, C., Blisset, D., Perisamy, S., & Rahotep, S. (in press). Healthy Body/Healthy Spirit: Design and evaluation of a church-based nutrition and physical activity intervention using motivational interviewing. *Health Education Research.*

Resnicow, K., Jackson, A., Wang, T., Dudley, W., & Baranowski, T. (2001). A motivational interviewing intervention to increase fruit and vegetable intake through black churches: Results of the Eat for Life trial. *American Journal of Public Health, 91,* 1686–1693.

Resnicow, K., Odom, E., Wang, T., Dudley, W., Mitchell, D., Vaughan, R., Jackson, A., & Baranowski, T. (2000). Validation of three food frequency questionnaires and twenty-four hour recalls with serum carotenoids in a sample of African American adults. *American Journal of Epidemiology, 152,* 1072–1080.

Richmond, R. L., Bell, A. P., Rollnick, S., & Heather, B. B. (1996). Screening for smokers in four Sydney teaching hospitals. *Journal of Cardiovascular Risk, 3,* 199–203.

Roberts, L. J., Neal, D. J., Kivlahan, D. R., Baer, J. S., & Marlatt, G. A. (2000). Individual drinking changes following a brief intervention among college students: Clinical significance in an indicated preventive context. *Journal of Consulting and Clinical Psychology, 68*(3), 500–505.

Roberts, M. (1997). *The man who listens to horses.* New York: Random House.

Roffman, R. (2000). *The Teen Marijuana Check-up.* Grant proposal submitted to the National Institute on Drug Abuse.

Rogers, C. R. (1951). *Client-centered therapy.* Boston: Houghton-Mifflin.

Rogers, C. R. (1959). A theory of therapy, personality, and interpersonal relationships as developed in the client-centered framework. In S. Koch (Ed.), *Psychology: The study of a science*: Vol. 3. *Formulations of the person and the social contexts* (pp. 184–256). New York: McGraw-Hill.

Rogers, C. R. (1961). *On becoming a person.* Boston: Houghlin Mifflin.

Rogers, C. R. (1964). Toward a modern approach to values: The valuing process in the mature person. *Journal of Abnormal and Social Psychology, 68*(2), 160–167.

Rogers, E. M. (1995). *Diffusion of innovations* (4th ed.). New York: Free Press.

Rokeach, M. (1973). *The nature of human values.* New York: Free Press.

Rokeach, M. (Ed.). (1979). *Understanding human values.* New York: Macmillan.

Rollnick, S. (1996). Behaviour change in practice: Targeting individuals. *International Journal of Obesity and Related Metabolic, 20*(Suppl. 1), S22–S26.

Rollnick, S. (1998). Readiness, importance, and confidence: Critical conditions of change in treatment. In W. R. Miller & N. Heather (Eds.), *Treating addictive behaviors* (2nd ed., pp. 49–60). New York: Plenum Press.

Rollnick, S., & Bell, A. (1991). Brief motivational interviewing for use by the nonspecialist. In W. R. Miller, & S. Rollnick, *Motivational interviewing: Preparing people to change addictive behavior* (pp. 203–213). New York: Guilford Press.

Rollnick, S., Butler, C. C., & Stott, N. (1997). Helping smokers make decisions: The enhancement of brief intervention for general medical practice. *Patient Education and Counseling, 31*(3), 191–203.

Rollnick, S., Heather, N., & Bell, A. (1992). Negotiating behaviour change in medical settings: The development of brief motivational interviewing. *Journal of Mental Health, 1,* 25–39.

Rollnick, S., Kinnersley, P., & Butler, C. C. (2002). Context-bound communication skills training: Development of a new method. *Medical Education, 36,* 377–383.

Rollnick, S. Mason, P., & Butler, C. (1999). *Health behavior change: A guide for practitioners.* London: Churchill Livingstone.

Rollnick, S., & Miller, W. R. (1995). What is motivational interviewing? *Behavioural and Cognitive Psychotherapy, 23*(4), 325–334.

Rollnick, S., & Morgan, M. (1995). Motivational interviewing: Increasing readiness for change. In A. M. Washton (Ed.), *Psychotherapy and substance abuse: A practitioner's handbook* (pp. 179–191). New York: Guilford Press.

Ross, R. R., & Lightfoot, L. O. (1985). Developing alcohol abuse programs for offenders. In R. R. Ross & L. O. Lightfoot (Eds.), *Treatment of the alcohol-abusing offender* (pp. 86–144). Springfield, IL: Charles C. Thomas.

Rubino, G., Barker, C., Roth, T., & Fearon, P. (2000). Therapist empathy and depth of interpretation in response to potential alliance ruptures: The role of therapist and patient attachment styles. *Psychotherapy Research, 10,* 408–420.

Rusk, T. N., & Ervin, H. N. (1996). Guiding self-change: A new model for brief psychotherapy. *Journal of Contemporary Psychotherapy, 26,* 327–336.

Ryan, R., Fisher, D., Krutch, B., & Downey, L. (2001, August). *Using assessment and motivational feedback to reduce HIV transmission rates among HIV+ MSM.* Paper presented at the National HIV Prevention Conference, Atlanta.

Ryan, R .M., & Deci, E. L. (2000). Self-determination theory and the facilitation of intrinsic motivation, social development, and well-being. *American Psychologist, 55*(1), 68–78.

Ryan, R. M., Plant, R. W., & O'Malley, S. (1995). Initial motivations for alcohol treatment: Relations with patient characteristics, treatment involvement, and dropout. *Addictive Behaviors, 20*(3), 279–297.

Sanchez, F. (2000). *A values-based intervention for alcohol problems.* Doctoral dissertation, University of New Mexico, Albuquerque.

Saunders, B., Wilkinson, C., & Allsop, S. (1991). Motivational intervention with heroin users attending a methadone clinic. In W. R. Miller & S. Rollnick, *Motivational interviewing: Preparing people to change addictive behavior* (pp. 279–292). New York: Guilford Press.

Saunders, B., Wilkinson, C., & Phillips, M. (1995). The impact of a brief motivational intervention with opiate users attending a methadone programme. *Addiction, 90,* 415–424.

Schmidt, M. M., & Miller, W. R. (1983). Amount of therapist contact and outcome in a multidimensional depression treatment program. *Acta Psychiatrica Scandinavica, 67,* 319–332.

Schneider, R. J., Casey, J., & Kohn, R. (2000). Motivational versus confrontational interviewing: A comparison of substance abuse assessment practices at employee assistance programs. *Journal of Behavioral Health Services and Research, 27*(1), 60–74.

Schuman, H., & Johnson, M. (1976). Attitudes and behavior. *Annual Review of Sociology, 2,* 161–207.

Schwartz, S. H. (1974). Awareness of interpersonal consequences, responsibility denial, and volunteering. *Journal of Personality and Social Psychology, 30,* 57–63.

Schwartz, S. H., & Ames, R. E. (1977). Positive and negative referent others as sources of influence: A case of helping. *Sociometry, 40,* 12–21.

Schwartz, S. H., & Bilsky, W. (1987). Toward a universal psychological structure of human values. *Journal of Personality and Social Psychology, 53,* 550–562.

Schwartz, S. H., & Howard, J. A. (1980). Explanations of the moderating effect of responsibility denial on the personal norm behavior relationship. *Social Psychology Quarterly, 43,* 441–446.

Schwartz, S. H., & Inbar-Saban, N. (1988). Value self-confrontation as a method to aid in weight loss. *Journal of Personality and Social Psychology, 54,* 396–404.

Sefarbi, R. (1990). Admitters and deniers among adolescent sex offenders and their families: A preliminary study. *American Journal of Orthopsychiatry, 60*(3), 460–465.

Selzer, M. (1971). The Michigan Alcoholism Screening Test: The quest for a new diagnostic instrument. *American Journal of Psychiatry, 127,* 1653–1658.

Selzer, M., Vinokur, A., & Van Rooijen, L. (1975). A self-administered Short Michigan Alcoholism Screening Test (SMAST). *Journal of Studies on Alcohol, 36,* 117–126.

Shaffer, H. J. (1992). The psychology of stage change: The transition from addiction to recovery. In J. H. Lowison, P. Ruiz, R. B. Millman, & J. G. Langrod (Eds.), *Substance abuse: A comprehensive textbook* (2nd ed., pp. 100–105). Baltimore: Williams & Wilkins.

Shapiro, A. K. (1971). Placebo effects in medicine, psychotherapy, and psychoanalysis. In A. E. Bergin & S. L. Garfield (Eds.), *Handbook of psychotherapy and behavior change: An empirical analysis* (pp. 439–473). New York: Wiley.

Shiffman, S. (1982). Relapse following smoking cessation: A situational analysis. *Journal of Consulting and Clinical Psychology, 50,* 71–86.

Shoham, V., & Rohrbaugh, M. (1995). Aptitude x treatment interaction research: Sharpening the focus, widening the lens. In M. Aveline & D. Shapiro (Eds.), *Research foundations for psychotherapy research* (pp. 73–95). Sussex, England: Wiley.

Shoham, V., Rohrbaugh, M. J., Stickle, T. R., & Jacob, T. (1998). Demand-withdraw couple interaction moderates retention in cognitive-behavioral versus family-systems treatments for alcoholism. *Journal of Family Psychology, 12*(4), 1–21.

Shope, J. T. (1988). Compliance in children and adults: Review of studies. In D. S. I. E. Leppik (Ed.), *Compliance in epilepsy* (pp. 23–47). Amsterdam: Elsevier.

Simon, S., Howe, L., & Kirschenbaum, H. (1995). *Values clarification: A practical, action-directed workbook.* New York: Warner Books.

Simpson, D. D., Brown, B. S., & Joe, G. W. (1997). Treatment retention and follow-up outcomes in the drug abuse treatment outcome study (DATOS). *Psychology of Addictive Behaviors, 11,* 294–307.

Simpson, D. D., & Joe, G. W. (1993). Motivation as a predictor of early dropout from drug abuse treatment. *Psychotherapy, 30,* 357–368.

Simpson, T. L., Arroyo, J. A., Miller, W. R., & Little, L. M. (1999). [Desired Effects of Drinking Questionnaire]. Unpublished raw data.

Sims, J., Smith, J., Duffy, A., & Hilton, S. (1998). Can practice nurses increase physical activity in the over 65's? Methodologic considerations from a pilot study. *British Journal of General Practice, 48,* 1249–1250.

Singh, N., Squier, C., Sivek, C., & Wagener, M. (1996). Determinants of compliance with antiretroviral therapy in patients with human immunodeficiency virus: Prospective assessment with implications for enhancing compliance. *AIDS Care, 8*(3), 261–269.

Skinner, H. A., & Allen, B. A. (1983). Differential assessment of alcoholism: Evaluation of the Alcohol Use Inventory. *Journal of Studies on Alcohol, 44*(5), 852–862.

Slesnick, N., Meyers, R. J., Meade, M., & Segelken, D. H. (1999). Bleak and hopeless no more: Engagement of reluctant substance-abusing runaway youth and their families. *Journal of Substance Abuse Treatment, 19*, 215–222.

Smart, R. G. (1974). Employed alcoholics treated voluntarily and under constructive coercion: A follow-up study. *Quarterly Journal of Studies on Alcohol, 35*, 196–209.

Smith, D. E., Heckemeyer, C. M., Kratt, P. P., & Mason, D. A. (1997). Motivational interviewing to improve adherence to a behavioral weight-control program for older obese women with NIDDM: A pilot study. *Diabetes Care, 20*(1), 53–54.

Sobell, L. C., & Sobell, M. B. (1992). Timeline follow-back: A technique for assessing self-reported alcohol consumption. In R. Litten & J. P. Allen (Eds.), *Measuring alcohol consumption: Psychological and biochemical methods* (pp. 41–42). Totowa, NJ: Humana Press.

Sobell, L. C., Sobell, M. B., Brown, J. C., Cleland, P. A., & Buchan, G. (1995, November). *A randomized trial comparing group versus individual guided self-change treatment for alcohol and drug abusers.* Paper presented at the annual meeting of the Association for the Advancement of Behavior Therapy, Washington, DC.

Sobell, L. C., Sobell, M. B., & Leo, G. I. (1993). *Spousal support: A motivational intervention for alcohol abusers.* Poster session presented at the annual meeting of the Association for the Advancement of Behavior Therapy, Atlanta, GA.

Sobell, L. C., Sobell, M. B., & Toneatto, T. (1992). Recovery from alcohol problems without treatment. In N. Heather, W. R. Miller, & J. Greely (Eds.), *Self-control and the addictive behaviors.* New York: Maxwell Macmillan.

Sobell, L. C., Sobell, M. B., Toneatto, T., & Leo, G. I. (1993). What triggers the resolution of alcohol problems without treatment? *Alcoholism: Clinical, Experimental, and Research, 17*, 217–224.

Sobell, M. B., & Sobell, L. C. (1993). *Problem drinkers.* New York: Guilford Press.

Sobell, M. B., & Sobell, L. C. (1998). Guiding self change. In W. R. Miller & N. Heather (Eds.), *Treating addictive behaviors* (2nd ed., pp. 189–202). New York: Plenum Press.

Soet, J. E., & Basch, C. E. (1997). The telephone as a communication medium for health education. *Health Education and Behavior, 24*(6), 759–772.

Solomon, P., & Gordon, B. (1988). Outpatient compliance with psychiatric emergency room Patients by presenting problems. *Psychiatric Quarterly, 59*, 271–283.

Spielberger, C. D. (1988). *Manual for the State-Trait Anger Expression Scale (STAX).* Odessa, FL: Psychological Assessment Resources.

Stall, R., & Biernacki, P. (1986). Spontaneous remission from the problematic use of substances: An inductive model derived from a comparative analysis of the alcohol, opiate, tobacco, and food/obesity literatures. *International Journal of the Addictions, 21*, 1–23.

Stanton, M. D., Todd, T. C., & Associates (1982). *The family therapy of drug abuse and addiction.* New York: Guilford Press.

Stark, M. J. (1992). Dropping out of substance abuse treatment: A clinically oriented review. *Clinical Psychology Review, 12*, 93–116.

Stephens, R. S., Roffman, R. A., & Curtin, L. (2000). Comparison of extended versus brief treatments for marijuana use. *Journal of Consulting and Clinical Psychology, 68*(5), 898–908.

Stephens, R. S., Roffman, R. A., & Simpson, E. E. (1994). Treating adult marijuana dependence: A test of the relapse prevention model. *Journal of Consulting and Clinical Psychology, 62,* 92–99.

Stewart, L., & Millson, W. A. (1995). Offender motivation for treatment as a responsivity factor. *Forum on Corrections Research, 7*(3), 5–7.

Stewart, L., & Montplaisir, G. (1999). *Reasons for drop- outs among participants in the Cognitive Skills and Anger and Other Emotions Management programs.* Unpublished manuscript.

Stewart, M., Brown, J. B., Weston, W. W., McWhinney, I. R,, McWilliam, C. L., & Freeman, T. R. (Eds.). (1995). *Patient-centered medicine: Transforming the clinical method.* Thousand Oaks, CA: Sage.

Stott, N. C. H., Rollnick, S., & Pill, R. M. (1995). Innovation in clinical method: Diabetes care and negotiating skills. *Family Practice, 12*(4), 413–418.

Suris, A. M., Trapp, M. C., DiClemente, C. C., & Cousins, J. (1998). Application of the transtheoretical model of behavior change for obesity in Mexican American women. *Addictive Behaviors, 23*(4), 655–668.

Swanson, A. J., Pantalon, M. V., & Cohen, K. R. (1999). Motivational interviewing and treatment adherence among psychiatric and dually diagnosed patients. *Journal of Nervous and Mental Disease, 187,* 630–635.

Taplin, S., Barlow, W., Ludman, E., MacLehose, R., Meyer, D., Seger, D., Herta, D., Chin, R., & Curry, S. (2000). Testing reminder and motivational telephone calls to increase screening mammography: A randomized study. *Journal of the National Cancer Institute, 92*(3), 233–242.

Thase, M. E., Weiss, R. D., Gastfriend, G. R., Woody, G. E., Barber, J. P., Butler, S. F., Daley, D., Salloum, I., Bishop, S., Najavits, L. M., Lis, J., Mercer, D., Griffin, M. L., Moras, K., & Beck, A. T. (1999). Psychosocial treatments for cocaine dependence: National Institute on Drug Abuse collaborative cocaine treatment study. *Archives of General Psychiatry, 56,* 493–502.

Thevos, A. K., Kaona, F. A. D., Siajunza, M. T., & Quick, R. E. (2000). Adoption of safe water behaviors in Zambia: Comparing educational and motivational approaches. *Education for Health, 13*(3), 366–376.

Thevos, A. K., Olsen, S. J., Rangel, J., Kaona, F. A. D., Tembo, M., & Quick, R. E. (2001). *Social marketing and motivational interviewing as community interventions for safe water behaviors: Follow-up surveys in Zambia.* Unpublished manuscript.

Thevos, A. K., Quick, R. E., & Yanduli, V. (2000). Application of motivational interviewing to the adoption of water disinfection practices in Zambia. *Health Promotion International, 15*(3), 207–214.

Thornton, D. (in press). Constructing and testing a framework for dynamic risk assessment. *Sexual Abuse: A Journal of Research and Treatment.*

Tonigan, J. S., Miller, W. R., & Brown, J. M. (1997). The reliability of Form 90: An instrument for assessing alcohol treatment outcome. *Journal of Studies on Alcohol, 58*(4), 358–364.

Treasure, J. L., Katzman, M., Schmidt, U., Troop, N., Todd, G., & de Silva, P. (1999). Engagement and outcome in the treatment of bulimia nervosa: First phase of a sequential design comparing motivation enhancement therapy and cognitive behavioural therapy. *Behaviour Research and Therapy, 37,* 405–418.

Trice, H. M., & Beyer, J. M. (1983). Social control in worksettings: Using the constructive confrontation strategy with problem-drinking employees. In D. A. Ward (Ed.),

Alcoholism: Introduction to theory and treatment (Rev. ed., pp. 314–339). Dubuque, IA: Kendall/Hunt.

Trigwell, P., Grant, P. J., & House, A. (1997). Motivation and glycemic control in diabetes mellitus. *Journal of Psychosomatic Research, 43,* 307–315.

Trostle, J. (1988). Doctors' orders and patients' self-interest: Two views of medication usage? In D. S. I. E. Leppik (Ed.), *Compliance in epilepsy* (pp. 57–69). Amsterdam: Elsevier.

Truax, C. B., & Carkhuff, R. R. (1967). *Toward effective counseling and psychotherapy.* Chicago: Aldine.

Truax, C. B., & Mitchell, K. M. (1971). Research on certain therapist interpersonal skills in relation to process and outcome. In A. E. Bergin & S. L. Garfield (Eds.), *Handbook of psychotherapy and behavior change: An empirical analysis* (pp. 299–344). New York: Wiley.

Turner, A. J., & Vernon, J. C. (1976). Prompts to increase attendance in community mental health center. *Journal of Applied Behavioral Analysis, 9,* 141–145.

Turner, J. G., Nokes, K. M., Corless, I. B., Holzemer, W. L., Inouye, J., Brown, M. A., & Powell-Cope, G. M. (1998). *History of drug use and adherence in HIV+ persons.* Paper presented at the 12th International Conference on AIDS, Geneva.

U.S. Department of Health and Human Services. (2000). *Treating tobacco and dependence: Clinical practice guideline.* Rockville, MD: U.S. Department of Health and Human Services, Public Health Service.

Vaillant, G. E. (1995). *The natural history of alcoholism revisited.* Cambridge, MA: Harvard University Press.

Valle, S. K. (1981). Interpersonal functioning of alcoholism counselors and treatment outcome. *Journal of Studies on Alcohol, 42,* 783–790.

Velasquez, M. M., Carbonari, J. P., & DiClemente, C. C. (1999). Psychiatric severity and behavior change in alcoholism: The relation of transtheoretical model variables to psychiatric distress in dually diagnosed patients. *Addictive Behaviors, 24*(4), 481–496.

Velasquez, M. M., Hecht, J., Quinn, V. P., Emmons, K. M., DiClemente, C. C., & Dolan-Mullen, P. (2000). Application of motivational interviewing to prenatal smoking cessation: Training and implementation issues. *Tobacco Control, 9*(Suppl. 3), 36–40.

Velasquez, M. M., Maurer, G. G., Crouch, C., & DiClemente, C. C. (2001). *Group treatment for substance abuse: A stages-of-change therapy manual.* New York: Guilford Press.

Velicer, W. F., & DiClemente, C. (1993). Understanding and intervening with the total population of smokers. *Tobacco Control, 2,* 95–96.

Velicer, W. F., Prochaska, J. O., Bellis, J. M., DiClemente, C. C., Rossi, J. S., Fava, J. L., & Steiger, J. H. (1993). An expert system intervention for smoking cessation. *Addictive Behaviors, 18,* 269–290.

Volpicelli, J. R., Alterman, A. I., Hayasguda, M., & O'Brien, C. P. (1997). Naltrexone and alcohol dependence: Role of subject compliance. *Archives of General Psychiatry, 54,* 737–74.

Waldorf, D., Reinarman, C., & Murphy, S. (1991). *Cocaine changes: The experience of using and quitting.* Philadelphia: Temple University Press.

Walizter, K. S., Dermen, K. H., & Connors, G. J. (1999). Strategies for preparing clients for treatment—A review. *Behavior Modification, 23,* 129–151.

Walker, R., Minor-Schork, D., Bloch, R., & Esinhart, J. (1996). High-risk factors for rehospitalization within six months. *Psychiatric Quarterly, 67,* 235–242.

Walker Daniels, J. (1998). *Coping with the health threat of smoking: An analysis of the precontemplation stage of smoking cessation.* Doctoral dissertation, Psychology Department, University of Maryland, Baltimore County.

Walker Daniels, J., & Murphy, C. M. (1997). Stages and processes of change in batterers' treatment. *Cognitive and Behavioral Practice, 4,* 123–145.

Walters, S. T. (1998). *Manual for the SDSU Alcohol Information and Motivation (AIM) program.* Unpublished manuscript.

Walters, S. T. (2000). In praise of feedback: An effective intervention for college students who are heavy drinkers. *Journal of American College Health, 48,* 235–238.

Walters, S. T., & Bennett, M. E. (2000). Addressing drinking among college students: A review of the empirical literature. *Alcoholism Treatment Quarterly, 18*(1), 61–77.

Walters, S. T., Bennett, M. E., & Miller. J. E. (2000). Reducing alcohol use in college students: A controlled trial of two brief interventions. *Journal of Drug Education, 30*(3), 361–372.

Walters, S. T., Gruenewald, D. A., Miller, J. H., & Bennett, M. E. (2001). Early findings from a disciplinary program to reduce problem drinking by college students. *Journal of Substance Abuse Treatment, 20*(1), 89–91.

Weakland, J. H., & Fisch, R. (1992). Brief therapy—MRI style. In S. H. Budman, M. F. Hoyt, and S. Friedman (Eds.), *The first session in brief therapy* (pp. 306–323). New York: Guilford Press.

Weinstein, N. D., Rothman, A. J., & Sutton, S. R. (1998). Stage theories in health behavior: Conceptual and methodological issues. *Health Psychology, 17*(3), 290–299.

Werch, C. E., & DiClemente, C. C. (1994). A multi-component stage model for matching drug prevention strategies and messages to youth stage of use. *Health Education Research: Theory and Practice, 9*(1), 37–46.

Westerberg, V. S. (1998). What predicts success? In W. R. Miller & N. Heather (Eds.), *Treating addictive behaviors* (2nd ed., pp. 301–315). New York: Plenum Press.

Willoughby, R. W., & Edens, J. F. (1996). Construct validity and predictive utility of the stages of change scale for alcoholics. *Journal of Substance Abuse, 8*(3), 275–291.

Winters, K. C., Latimer, W. L., & Stinchfield, R. D. (1999). Adolescent Treatment. In P. J. Ott, R. E. Tarter, & R. T. Ammerman (Eds.), *Sourcebook on substance abuse: Etiology, epidemiology, assessment, and treatment* (pp. 350–361). Boston: Allyn & Bacon.

Wojciszke, B. (1987). Ideal-self, self-focus and value-behavior consistency. *European Journal of Social Psychology, 17,* 187–198.

Wolpe, P. R., Gorton, G., Serota, R., & Sanford, B. (1993). Predicting compliance of dual diagnosis inpatients with aftercare treatment. *Hospital and Community Psychiatry, 44,* 45–49.

Woollard, J., Beilin, L., Lord, T., Puddey, I., MacAdam, D., & Rouse, I. (1995). A controlled trial of nurse counselling on lifestyle change for hypertensives treated in general practice: Preliminary results. *Clinical and Experimental Pharmacology and Physiology, 22*(6–7), 466–468.

Wright, E. C. (1993). Non-compliance—or how many Aunts has Matilda? *The Lancet, 342,* 909–913.

Yahne, C. E., & Miller, W. R. (1999). Evoking hope. In W. R. Miller (Ed.), *Integrating spirituality into treatment: Resources for practitioners* (pp. 217–233). Washington, DC: American Psychological Association.

Yalom, I. (1995). *The theory and practice of group psychotherapy* (4th ed.). New York: Basic Books.

Yates, F. (1984). Does treatment work? Yes, but not the way we plan it. In N. Heather, I. Robertson, & P. Davies (Eds.), *Alcohol misuse: Three crucial questions* (pp. 148–157). London: Methuen.

Zuckoff, A., & Daley, D. C. (1999, March/April). Dropout prevention and dual diagnosis clients. *The Counselor*, pp. 23–27.

Zuckoff, A., & Daley, D. C. (2001). Engagement and adherence in treating persons with non-psychosis dual disorders. *Psychiatric Rehabilitation Skills, 5*, 131–162.

Zuckoff, A., Ryan, C. M., & Thoma, F. (2000). *HIV risk reduction in gay men: Use of motivational interviewing to facilitate attendance in interventions.* Paper presented at the 23rd annual meeting of the Research Society on Alcoholism, Denver, CO.

Zweben, A. (1991). Motivational Counseling with Alcoholic Couples. In W. R. Miller & S. Rollnick, *Motivational interviewing: Preparing people to change addictive behavior* (pp. 225–235). New York: Guilford Press.

Zweben, A., & Barrett, D. (1993). Brief couples treatment for alcohol problems. In T. R. O'Farrell (Ed.), *Treating alcohol problems: Marital and family interventions* (pp. 353–380). New York: Guilford Press.

Zweben, A., Bonner, M., Chaim, G., & Santon, P. (1988). Facilitative strategies for retaining the alcohol-dependent client in outpatient treatment. *Alcoholism Treatment Quarterly, 5*, 3–24.

Zweben, A., & Li, S. (1981). The efficacy of role induction in preventing early drop-out from outpatient treatment of drug dependency. *American Journal of Drug and Alcohol Abuse, 8*(2), 71–83.

Zweben, A., & Pearlman, S. (1983). Evaluating the effectiveness of conjoint treatment of alcohol complicated marriages: Clinical and methodological issues. *Journal of Marital and Family Therapy, 9*, 61–72.

Index

Page numbers followed by "b" indicate box, "f" indicate figure, and "t" indicate table.